PERMANENTE IN THE NORTHWEST

IAN C. MACMILLAN, MD

WITH CONTRIBUTIONS FROM
KITTY EVERS, MD & ALLAN J. WEILAND, MD

EDITED BY JUDY HAYWARD

The Permanente Press

Oakland, California • Portland, Oregon

About the Author: Ian C. MacMillan, MD has never authored *anything* before. He was born and raised in Regina, Saskatchewan where he was influenced by his physician father to become a doctor. He received his MDCM from Queen's University, Kingston, Ontario and interned at University of Alberta Hospital where he met his future wife Shirley on the pediatric ward. A Fellowship in Internal Medicine at the Mayo Clinic convinced him of the desirability of group practice and, after a pathology residency in Victoria B.C. where he was impressed with the beauty of the Pacific Northwest, he joined The Permanente Clinic in 1961.

© 2010 by The Permanente Press

Published 2010 by The Permanente Press
Oakland, California • Portland, Oregon

The Permanente Press is owned by The Permanente Federation, LLC
Oakland, California

PERMANENTE IN THE NORTHWEST

14 13 12 11 10   1 2 3 4 5

ISBN: 0-9770463-3-8
Library of Congress Control Number: 2009937531

Book design by Lynette Leisure
Printed in the United States of America

PERMANENTE
IN THE
NORTHWEST

TO THE PHYSICIANS, NURSES,
AND OTHER PERSONNEL
WHO MET AND STILL MEET
THE CHALLENGE OF PROVIDING
HEALTH CARE CONSISTENT WITH
THE CONCEPTS SET FORTH
BY SIDNEY R. GARFIELD
MANY YEARS AGO.

TABLE OF CONTENTS

—ᶆ—

FOREWORD

What would later become Kaiser Permanente (KP) began as something of an afterthought for Henry Kaiser and as a job opportunity for young surgeon Sidney Garfield; Kaiser, the industrialist who drove himself and others to "Think Big," couldn't afford to let illness and injury among workers drain productivity on his big projects. Medical care had to be readily available in remote sites and capable of keeping workers healthy and on the job. For his part, the recently trained Garfield imagined a job that offered key features he'd enjoyed in his training: predictable pay, camaraderie with fellow physicians, and reliable cross-coverage during off hours.

By 1933, Garfield had already opened a practice to serve workers constructing the Los Angeles aqueduct in the Mojave Dessert. When Kaiser needed medical care for workers building the Grand Coulee Dam in Eastern Washington in 1938, he negotiated with Garfield to pay pennies per month per worker to provide this care. Prepaying for medical service to a defined population thus became the practical arrangement by which Kaiser and Garfield accomplished their objectives.

Kaiser's emphasis on productivity became even more critical in World War II, when he was assigned important projects in the Pacific Northwest. At his shipyards in Portland, Oregon and Vancouver, Washington, Kaiser sought to replicate his previous arrangement with Garfield to assure medical service to workers. The collaboration between the two led to the hiring, in 1945, of internist Ernest Saward, who became Chief of Medicine.

The KP Northwest (KPNW) organization did not come into being at that moment. It wasn't until after war's end that Saward and others realized that the plan for shipyard workers also suited a civilian population: not only the salaried physicians, but also workers and their families whose costs for medical care would be predictable and shared among many others. A novel model for prepaid medical care emerged, linking physicians to groups of peace-time civilians. The history of this Northwest physician group parallels that of Garfield's physicians in California; two groups with separate beginnings shared a template and later became affiliated as geographic Regions in a national Kaiser Permanente.

The author of this account, Ian MacMillan, for many years confined his writing to notes in medical charts as an internist and rheumatologist with KP. For 14 of those years he was the well-regarded Chief of the Department of Medicine at Kaiser Sunnyside Medical Center. He occupied the position when I joined the department until I succeeded him in 1989. He was a proper and humane physician, born and reared in Saskatchewan, trained at Mayo Clinic, and proud of his Scottish antecedents—a red-head who invariably dressed in a trademark suit of muted color. He was unfailingly warm and encouraging to his younger peers and relished sharing stories that footnoted the humor and small surprises in our daily lives.

In his narrative covering six decades of KPNW history, MacMillan exploits the opportunity to tell the stories of physicians and others in both major and minor roles. Testament to his broad curiosity, he enriches his archive with historical detail and context. The early concepts and arrangements by KP founders are tested by dramatic changes in public attitudes and expectations about health care and its costs and benefits.

Prepayment was a cardinal feature of the arrangements Kaiser made with Garfield and Saward and, as described by MacMillan, the issue that inspired hostility from the medical establishment of the day. Two other key features of the model were putting physicians on salary in an era of fee-for-service and assigning them shared responsibility for the ostensibly healthy in addition to the sick and injured. The implications of these have only gradually come to influence how physicians practice in KP.

The use of collective resources for collective benefit turns physicians into trustees of members' prepaid contributions or "resource stewards" in KP vernacular. The arrangement ought to encourage efficiency and health promotion—putting more emphasis on preventing disease or treating it early, refraining from unnecessary testing and procedures, finding the simplest remedies, cutting out redundancy, and sharing important patient information among treating physicians.

Permanente in the Northwest relates through small stories how a change in financing medical care, implemented 60 years ago, created a rationale, and drove physicians to collaborate to deliver care to a population that included both the sick and the well. In telling this story, MacMillan has made the book relevant not only to past and present physicians who will find their names in the text, but also to the current national discussion of health care reform.

Arthur D. Hayward, MD
Medical Director, Continuing Care Services
Kaiser Permanente Northwest

PREFACE

"No book can be fully understood
unless the writer discloses the motivation
that led him to embark on his onerous task"
— *The Trials of Socrates*, I.F. Stone.

In 1982, I met Jack Smillie at a meeting of Permanente Medical Directors in Colorado. At the time, Smillie was writing the history of The Permanente Medical Group of Northern California. He shared with me audiotapes from his 1982 interview with Ernest Saward about The Permanente Clinic in the Northwest. Fascinated by Smillie's project, I returned to Portland where I tried, without success, to organize a Northwest Permanente history project. Twenty-seven years later, with encouragement and support of many, the history has at last been written.

This work brings together the myriad stories of the past to provide a definitive history of Northwest Permanente and its physicians. It describes both conflicts within the Medical Group and hostility to Permanente by the medical establishment. It tells Permanente's steady advancement, despite these challenges, toward Sidney Garfield's vision, articulated in his 1945 address to the Multnomah County Medical Society. In that address he described Permanente's guiding principles: prevention, prepayment, and group practice. My hope is that the book accurately depicts Northwest Permanente physicians' extraordinary range of talents, their achievements, their innovations, and even their occasional missteps. I hope, too, that the book captures the complexities of a large group practice like ours, as well as the limitless opportunities within such a practice for professional development.

Ernest Saward looms as the dominant figure in the history of the Northwest Region. It was he who almost single-handedly held a small group of discouraged physicians together in 1945, when the future looked most bleak. It was his strong hand that guided Northwest Permanente's growth from uncertain beginnings to the robust position it had achieved by the time Saward departed in 1970.

ACKNOWLEDGMENTS

I would like to thank Al Weiland, who as Medical Director of Northwest Permanente (NWP) enabled this project, and Tom Janisse who enthusiastically saw it through. The encouragement at the beginning by Jon Stewart and the support of Harvey Klevit, Kitty Evers, Ek Ursin, Al Martin, and Seth Garber was vital to set the process in motion, as was the help of Vivian Terral and Jean Bradley. Of great benefit has been the friendship and collegiality I was able to develop with historian Steve Gilford who inspired in me the passion that sustains historians. It was such a pleasure to share with him historical discoveries along the way. The support of Tom Debley and his staff at Kaiser Permanente Heritage Resources was invaluable. The enthusiasm of Lady Elizabeth Saward was infectious. Thanks to Tom Saward for providing family photos. The assistance of NWP administrative staff was immeasurable: Lori Byers arranged meetings; Linda Battaglini oversaw the early logistics of the project and provided transcription services; Ann Swindler faithfully transcribed endless interviews; Darlene Hartley researched files, managed to find a corner for the archives, and later was the sole transcriptionist; Sue Christianson was always a smiling face at the reception desk and was a source to locate interviewees; Helena Purcell and Deborah Hedges provided advocacy and leads for historical sources. Credit goes to Al Martin for his major contribution to Chapter 8: The ER and the OR, and to Ek Ursin for the use of his *Tribute To A Beloved Physician: Norbert Fell*. Thanks to Margaret Zeps for serving as a research librarian.

Lunch with Morris Collen and Cecil Cutting, who provided perspective, was a memorable experience. Thanks to Jim Gersbach and the staff at Media Relations for providing access to their archives and special thanks to Jim DeLong whose long service to Kaiser Permanente provided unique insight into our history. Charles Grossman provided numerous documents, which were able to fill out previously blank pages in our history and I am thankful for his friendship. Thanks to Permanente Press editor Max McMillen for her extensive manuscript preparation and copyediting. I cannot thank my editor Judy Hayward enough for all the hours she devoted to the project, the patience she had dealing with an amateur author who sometimes strayed. If you find the book readable, it is because of her talent, and if there are parts difficult to read it is because I went against her advice. Finally, I am indebted to my wife Shirley who for six years learned to live with the focus and preoccupation of an author.

INTRODUCTION

On the evening of March 2, 1989, Ernest Saward, the first Medical Director for the Kaiser Permanente Northwest Region, spoke about the social mission of medicine in the first Ernest W. Saward Lecture. He decried the inequities and high cost of health care in America. He described to his audience a plague of the "high and ever-rising health care costs" afflicting Portlanders and compared their dilemma to that of the citizens of Rochester, New York. In Rochester, said Saward, people had joined to share costs more equitably and to extend health insurance to more of their fellow citizens. Weak from inoperable cancer and sitting in a chair rather than standing at a podium, Saward compared the prevailing American model of health care to a California gold rush and pictured an elephant dancing among mice shouting "Every man for himself!"

Saward was uniquely qualified to talk about financing health care and to speak with authority about Portland and Rochester. It was Saward who organized a group of physicians in 1945 and served as their Medical Director for 25 years. He then returned to the medical school where he had graduated and served as Associate Dean and Professor of Social Medicine for 18 years. Saward had based the Permanente Medical Care Program on practices that were novel at the time—sharing prepaid costs and health care benefits and paying physicians by salary. The mission was to make health care available and affordable for members. Starting with seven physicians, the group Saward saved from dissolution by a parliamentary maneuver has grown to 750 physicians serving 475,000 members.

Twenty years after Saward's inaugural lecture, Atul Gawande, an endocrine surgeon, health policy expert, and frequent contributor to the *New Yorker* and other publications, delivered the 2009 Saward Lecture. Gawande echoed Saward's warning and spoke of an explosive, unsustainable rise in health care costs. Gawande cited Portland, Oregon, as a city where costs of care had been relatively contained. In contrast, Gawande cited a town in Texas; the town where costs, among the highest in the country, did not result in any better health outcomes for its local population.

Both physicians were curious about elements that have contributed to shortcomings and excessive costs of the modern American health care system. *The History of Permanente in the Northwest* spans the life of Northwest Permanente's unique health care model and tells the stories of those physicians who, like Saward, believed that prepayment, salaries, and group practice could result in affordable health care for their members and satisfying careers for themselves.

NORTHWEST PERMANENTE CHRONOLOGY

1933 – Sidney Garfield provides medical care to Los Angeles aqueduct workers in the Mojave Desert, which becomes a prepaid group practice plan.

1938 – Edgar Kaiser engages Garfield to provide a prepaid medical plan to care for Grand Coulee construction workers in central Washington State.

1942 – Henry Kaiser arranges Garfield's discharge from the Army Medical Corp. so he can organize medical care for shipyard workers in San Francisco Bay area and in Portland/Vancouver.
– The Permanente Foundation and the Northern Permanente Foundation are created.
– The Northern Permanente Foundation Hospital is constructed in Vancouver.
– "Vanport City"—housing for shipyard workers construction begins; there will be an eventual population of 50,000.

1945 – Ernest Saward leaves Hanford to join the Vancouver Medical Group as Chief of Medicine.
– WW II ends.
– Seven physicians remain to provide a public Permanente Health Plan with Wallace Neighbor as Medical Director.
– Northwest Health Plan membership: 2,500.

1947 – Neighbor leaves for California and Saward becomes Medical Director.
– The Broadway Clinic opens in Portland.

1948 – Memorial Day flood destroys Vanport including the Permanente Vanport hospital.
– The first partnership is formed: The Permanente Medical Association.

1950 – Second partnership is formed with Saward as Medical Director: The Permanente Clinic.

1955 – Tahoe Agreement.

1959 – Bess Kaiser Hospital opens.
– Northwest Health Plan membership: 25,000.

1961 – Saward helps reorganize Kaiser Hawaii medical plan.
– Northwest Health Plan membership: 50,000.

1963 – Multnomah County Medical Association accepts Permanente physicians.

1966 – Medicare begins.

1967 – Northwest Health Plan membership: 100,000.

1970 – Saward takes leave of absence and Lewis Hughes is appointed Medical Director.

1973 – Anderson quintuplets delivered at Bess Kaiser Hospital.

1975 – Kaiser Sunnyside Medical Center construction completed.

1976 – Marvin Goldberg replaces Hughes as Medical Director, reorganizes Medical Group, improves morale and encourages involvement in the medical community.

1977 – Northwest Health Plan membership: 200,000.

1978 – Medical Group incorporates: Northwest Permanente, P.C.

1980 – Medical office opens in Salem.

1981 – AIDS epidemic begins.
 – David Lawrence hired as Bess Kaiser Hospital Area Medical Director.
 – NWP physicians total 245.

1984 – Longview medical office opens.

1985 – David Lawrence leaves to become Regional Manager for Colorado.
 – Northwest Health Plan membership: 300,000.

1986 – Fred Nomura replaces Goldberg as Medical Director.

1988 – Nurses and SEIU strike.

1991 – David Lawrence becomes CEO of Kaiser Permanente Medical Care Program.
 – NWP physicians total 501.

1992 – Allan J. Weiland elected Regional Medical Director.

1993 – Clinton health plan is introduced and, though it fails, it stimulates growth of managed care and increased competition for Kaiser Permanente.

1995 – Institution of EPICARE electronic records begins, directed by Homer Chin.
 – Northwest Health Plan membership: 384,000.

1996 – Bess Kaiser Hospital closes.
 – 250 Permanente physicians obtain privileges at Providence St. Vincent Hospital.
 – Other Permanente physicians obtain privileges at Southwest Washington Medical Center in Vancouver.

 – KPNW attempts affiliation with Group Health Cooperative of Puget Sound. Group Health Medical Group became Group Health Permanente.

1997 – January 6: The Permanente Federation formed.

1998 – Health Plan Central Office freezes capital expenditure for facilities in response to financial crisis.

1999 – Dale Crandall becomes Health Plan President.

2002 – David Lawrence replaced by George Halvorson as CEO of Kaiser Foundation Hospitals and Health Plan.
 – Cynthia Fintner replaces Barbara West as KPNW Regional President.

2003 – The partnership of the Health Plan and Medical Group is once again tested by large restructure in operations.

2005 – Andrew Lum, from the Colorado Permanente Medical Group, elected Regional Medical Director.
 – Personal Health Link allows members to communicate with physician by Internet.

2006 – Fintner replaced by Andrew McCullouch as President of Kaiser Foundation Hospitals and Health Plan of the Northwest.

2007 – Sharon Higgins, long-standing ENT surgeon with NWP, elected Executive Medical Director, becoming the first woman to lead the Medical Group.

2008 – Brookside Center for residential care of mental health patients opens on Sunnyside campus.
 – Northwest Health Plan membership: 472,555.

2009 – Center for Heart and Vascular Surgery opens on Sunnyside campus.
 – Construction for Westside Medical Center in Hillsboro begins.
 – NWP physicians total 865.

PART I:
A LENGTHY
PROLOGUE

CHAPTER 1:
THE ROOTS

—ᗰᐯ—

EARLY PREPAID MEDICINE IN THE NORTHWEST

Although Kaiser Permanente (KP) was thought to be a radical departure from the established model of fee-for-service, its emphasis on prepayment, salaried physicians and preventive health care was certainly not the first time these elements had been incorporated into a plan for delivering health care. Various other historical precedents can be found for an alternative health care model.

In 1883 St. Joseph's Hospital in Victoria, British Columbia offered a health plan that included doctors' visits, hospitalization, and medicine for one dollar a year. Even earlier, at the beginning of the 19th century, the men who built the railroads established systems to cover their workers' medical expenses, employing company surgeons to treat injuries. By the early 1900s mining and lumber industries, too, were hiring staff physicians, attracting them to isolated areas with guaranteed salaries. At first, facilities in the camps were primitive; physicians used homes or rustic offices as infirmaries. Later, companies built their own hospitals and clinics. Although contract medicine was recognized as a necessity in these isolated areas, medical societies viewed it with hostility. Contract medicine, they said, interfered with the patient-physician relationship and with fee-based remuneration. In addition, the medical community argued that contract physicians offered poor-quality care.

Indeed, the medical community's concerns about the general quality in medicine were justified. At the time, the profession of medicine was rife with unscientific practitioners and quacks promising unsound and unproven cures. Others, self-taught, with some knowledge of anatomy and pharmacy, passed themselves off as physicians. Unregulated medical schools proliferated. Until the late 1800s even regulated medical schools awarded an MD after just one year of post-graduate study.

At the same time that industries were contracting for physician care for their workers, fraternal organizations and lodges were becoming popular in American life—especially among immigrants. Fraternal groups offered their own version of contract or "lodge" medicine. With dues collected from members, they placed physicians under contract to provide medical care and the prerequisite physical exams for life insurance benefits available to members.[1] Physicians willing to work in this way bid among themselves for lodge contracts, sometimes charging annual fees as low as one or two dollars per member per year.

One organization, the Workers Party of American Finns, later affiliated with the American Socialist Party, built Finnish Hall in 1909 at a cost of $11,000 in Portland on the corner of North Fremont and Montana streets. The barnlike, two-story structure with meeting rooms, living quarters, a kitchen, and a grand ballroom, was a social and political center for its members. In 1917, the United Finnish Kaleva Brothers and Sisters Lodge #23 formed and began to schedule activities at Finn Hall. However, whereas the Finnish Workers Association and the Industrial Workers of the World[2] agitated for social change, the United Finns was a benevolent organization, its focus on members' health. To that end, it regularly sponsored lectures on preventive medicine and "nature's remedies." Dentist Toivo Johnson lectured on dental care.

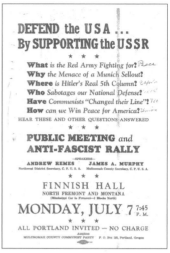

DEFEND the USA ...
By SUPPORTING the USSR

* * *

What is the Red Army Fighting for?
Why the Menace of a Munich Sellout?
Where is Hitler's Real 5th Column?
Who Sabotages our National Defense?
Have Communists "Changed their Line"?
How can we Win Peace for America?

HEAR THESE AND OTHER QUESTIONS ANSWERED

* * *

PUBLIC MEETING *and*
ANTI-FASCIST RALLY

SPEAKERS
ANDREW REMES   JAMES A. MURPHY
Northwest District Secretary, C. P. U. S. A.   Multnomah County Secretary, C. P. U. S. A.

* * *

FINNISH HALL
NORTH FREMONT AND MONTANA
(Mississippi Car is Fremont—4 Blocks North)

MONDAY, JULY 7 7:45 P. M.

* * *

ALL PORTLAND INVITED — NO CHARGE

Auspices
MULTNOMAH COUNTY COMMUNIST PARTY   P. O. Box 183, Portland, Oregon

Communist Party meeting notice at Finn Hall (now Town Hall) circa 1942. *Courtesy of Merle Reinkka.*

Inevitably, political differences caused a divide between the two groups. Beginning in 1955, the Hall went through a series of owners and, in 1968, was renamed Town Hall. Purchased by KP in 1976, the 300-ton building underwent restoration and relocation to KP's North Portland campus in 1990, where it is still regularly used as a site for KP health education programs, meetings, and events. The United Finnish Kaleva Brothers and Sisters Lodge #23 still provides members a prescription drug benefit of $50 and a death benefit of $25. It still holds its regular meetings at Town Hall.

The American Medical Association (AMA) condemned lodge practice, and many medical societies would not accept physicians who contracted with fraternal organizations. Attitudes toward lodge physicians were disdainful; their skills were reputed to be substandard: the care they provided suitable for only the working classes—"the lower orders," as some referred to them. In general, the medical profession viewed contract and socialized medicine as one and the same—both anathema.

FOR-PROFIT HEALTH CARE CORPORATIONS

Still another variation on prepaid medical care was the emergence of for-profit corporations. Although the public generally looked on corporate medicine with disdain and many states prohibited the practice, Oregon passed a Hospital Association Act in 1917 allowing corporations to provide medical care. Initially started by physicians, the corporations eventually came under the control of lay groups that established restrictions unpopular with the doctors. Forerunners of today's for-profit Health Maintenance Organizations (HMOs), these corporations challenged fees that they deemed excessive, required second opinions for major surgeries and reviewed hospital lengths of stay. To compete with the numerous hospital associations, the Multnomah County Medical Society established its own health plan in 1932. Unsuccessful in this effort, the society vigorously criticized the corporations and barred participating physicians from its membership. Then, citing AMA policy, it declared that physicians employed by profit-making associations were unethical. Finally, it organized a statewide prepaid program, Oregon Physicians Service, which, it claimed, "did not interfere with the doctor-patient relationship." Determined in their efforts to quash the for-profit associations, Medical Society members started to bill patients directly, requiring patients to obtain reimbursement from the associations. Unable to enforce its controls, the beleaguered associations brought a restraint-of-trade suit to court, only to see it defeated. Eventually, the corporations succumbed to takeovers by insurance companies.

A PREPAID MEDICAL PLAN IN CLACKAMAS COUNTY

In the 1930s, physicians in Clackamas County, like most others in the nation, believed in the importance of direct fee-for-service between physician and patient and opposed any government intervention in medical care, believing it would lead to socialized medicine. They were active in their local medical society and in the conservative AMA. They would have scoffed at the idea that by 1938 they would become medical pioneers and form a physician-owned, nonprofit, prepaid medical plan. Physicians Association of Clackamas County (PACC) was, in the words of its sponsors, "the first prepaid medical plan in the nation to have the cooperation of all the doctors in the county."

PACC proved extremely successful, amassing sizable contingency fees and other reserve funds. So great was its success, in fact, that in 1949 the U.S. Justice Department (sponsored by the hospital associations) sued Clackamas County Medical Society in U.S. District Court, alleging that the Society and PACC had violated the Sherman Antitrust Act. The trial ended with acquittal of all 14 charges.

Nearly a half century later, PACC adopted a more corporate model; this departure from its original model and its eventual demise is described in Chapter 18, "The Eighties: New Directions."

GROUP HEALTH COOPERATIVE OF PUGET SOUND

Although the modern cooperative movement dates from nineteenth-century England, a small farming community in the U.S. was the setting for the first medical cooperative. The cooperative health plan established in 1929 at Elk City, Oklahoma was the creation of socialist physician Michael Shadid, author of *A Doctor for the People*. Shadid wanted to reorganize medical care on a prepaid, comprehensive basis. Medical cooperatives, he explained, emphasized four principles: group practice, prepayment, preventive medicine, and consumer participation. As in so many instances where non-traditional approaches to providing medical care were attempted, the local medical profession began a long campaign of sabotage.

In August 1945 Shadid lectured in Seattle. His message resonated with his audience, and soon thereafter, leaders of farm granges, the Aeromechanics Union, and local supply and food co-ops met in a Seattle union hall and formed the Seattle Hospital Committee—the genesis of the first meeting of Group Health Cooperative (Group Health). Each of the 400 charter members contributed $100 to provide capital. One year later an opportunity arose to purchase Medical Security Clinic—a 15-physician proprietary prepaid group practice, together with a 60-bed hospital. After a stormy 1946 meeting, Group Health won approval to purchase the clinic. In the interim between approval and actual ownership on January 1, 1947, Medical Security Clinic began to provide care for the 400 co-op members as well as 8,000 non-co-op member enrollees from industrial contracts.

What evolved was a coalition among medical staff, administrators, and consumers, whose active voting membership elected trustees to run the organization but whose physicians and medical professionals were self-governing. A unionized nursing group and a core of professional business administrators and support staff came later.

Annual meetings of Group Health were anything but dull. Members hotly debated social issues and voted on various resolutions, including coverage for contraception, access to medical records, whether to provide abortion services (a motion to withhold abortion services was always defeated), nuclear disarmament, bans on handguns, labeling of irradiated food, and more.

Opposition to Group Health from the King County Medical Society and the medical community at large was immediate, fierce, and predictable. The Society refused membership to Group Health physicians, and most Seattle-area hospitals refused staff privileges. Virginia Mason Clinic was the exception, having itself been shunned as an

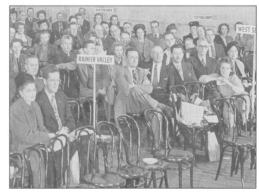

Group Health Cooperative meeting, circa 1950.
Courtesy of Group Health Cooperative.

outcast for engaging in group practice. In 1948, King County Medical Society tried unsuccessfully to block Group Health's hospital accreditation. In November 1949, Group Health took legal action against the local medical society for conspiring to monopolize contracts. Losing the suit in 1950, it won on appeal the following year. King County Medical Society was ordered to cease monopolistic action. One year later, in July 1952, it finally opened membership to qualified Group Health physicians.[3]

In 1952 various actions by the Group Health Board of Trustees precipitated a crisis in its relationship with its Medical Group, whose members objected to the Board's non-medical expenditures on political campaigns and on various activities of the cooperative. One affront followed another; against the Medical Group's advice, the Board enrolled dependents of longshoremen enrollees. Then it forced the resignation of a manager popular among the physicians. The last straw occurred when the Board reversed the medical staff's dismissal of an unpopular chief of surgery—a clear trespass into the Medical Group's area of control. The impasse was broken only when three physicians acquired seats on the Board with the understanding that physicians were to have a substantive voice in Board decisions.

Group Health prospered; in 1960 it completed, at a cost of $2.5 million, a 173-bed central hospital. Stagnant growth in 1961 was worrisome to administrators, but physicians were even more concerned about too much growth. Consequently, the cooperative reached a decision to limit membership to co-op enrollees, rather than to recruit new groups. Ernest Saward, Medical Director for the Permanente Clinic, based in Portland-Vancouver, saw an opportunity. A visit by a delegation

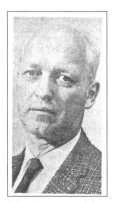

led by Saward gave Group Health second thoughts about this strategy. Saward announced that KP would be only too pleased to enter the Seattle market if Group Health intended to restrict new membership to its co-op enrollees. He went so far as to propose that Group Health collaborate with— even become part of—the KP organization. Group Health's rejection of this offer was swift, and it quickly reevaluated its plans for growth. In no way did the Seattle cooperative want to lose its identity or lose its consumer-directed policies. The two groups did, however, agree to treat each other's patients for emergencies. More will be said about Group Health developments in later chapters.

Prime promoter of the Clackamas Plan, Walter Noehren, MD, 1962. *Courtesy of* The Oregonian.

THE CLACKAMAS PLAN

Largely through the dream of Permanente physician Walter Noehren, an idea for a national health care delivery system called the Clackamas Plan gained support in the early

1960s. Here is its genesis: In the December 1947 issue of the *Journal of Pediatrics*, Noehren promoted a national prepaid medical insurance. His plan required that everyone with sufficient income enroll in a local prepaid medical program. Those unable to pay would apply to the federal government for help. Always an idealist, Noehren left Permanente in 1948 after an unsuccessful attempt to achieve an open-physician panel system. In Troutdale, Oregon, he tried to establish a comprehensive community health center, converting a house to a small medical facility that offered limited inpatient services, calling it the Troutdale Hospital Project. Though his project failed to prosper, he nevertheless drew favorable attention for his ideas from such luminaries as editor of the *Journal of the American Medical Association* (*JAMA*) Morris Fishbein, architect Frank Lloyd Wright, and publisher of *The Oregonian* Philip Parrish. Thus encouraged, he tried but failed to gain further support, and he moved to the small community of Sandy, Oregon, where he opened a private practice. In the idealism of the early Kennedy years, he dreamed again and promoted his plan for those 65 and older. The resulting Clackamas County Oregon Proposal (Medical Care for Every Man) won the support of the Clackamas County Medical Society, the Oregon Medical Association (OMA), and the AMA in November 1961. The passage of the Medicare bill of 1965 eclipsed the local Clackamas Plan.

SIDNEY GARFIELD AND DESERT CENTER 1933-1938

The story of Sidney Garfield and his venture in the Mojave Desert to provide medical care for the workers of the Los Angeles aqueduct has been told many times—most recently in *The Story of Dr. Sidney R. Garfield: The Visionary Who Turned Sick Care into Health Care* by Tom Debley. In 1933 five years before Garfield would meet and partner with industrialist Henry J. Kaiser and his son Edgar, he launched his first medical practice in the Mojave Desert in Southern California. Introduced as a fee-for-service plan, it struggled and proved financially unsustainable until Garfield replaced fee-for-service with prepayment—only then did the new plan flourish. The 12-bed Contractors General Hospital near Desert Center, 50 miles east of Indio, California, had the latest x-ray equipment, Venetian blinds, and air conditioning—an innovation at the time.

The agreed-on premium was set at five cents per day per worker for job-related medical problems and ten cents per day for non-job related illnesses. Garfield was now able to provide medical care in the way he wanted, free from the dictates of the insurance companies. Prepayment triggered the realization that, if fewer workers suffered injuries, a focus on prevention would improve both finances and the workers' lives. Thus, prevention and prepayment became two of the basic principles for what would later become Kaiser Permanente.

Today Desert Center is again the quiet place it was before thousands of workers and an innovative health care system transformed it for a few years in the 1930s. Except for two cafes, a market, a post office, and a gas station, little remains. A plaque on a solitary boulder, California Historical Site 992, commemorates the opening of that long-ago hospital and the medical care that briefly flourished there. In 1991, Steve Gilford, whose historical studies focus significantly on KP, guided by local residents, located the former hospital site. Aside from a crumbling foundation, all that remains are some syringes and instruments lying forlornly in the sand. The syringes, Gilford noted, were premium quality—BD Luer-Lok.

HENRY KAISER AND SIDNEY GARFIELD AT GRAND COULEE 1938-1941

In 1934 Six Companies, a consortium of contractors that included the Henry J. Kaiser Company, lost the bid to construct the foundation for Grand Coulee Dam to Mason, Walsh, Atkenson-Kier (MWAK). Preliminary construction began that year, and three communities sprang from the desert west of Spokane, Washington, to accommodate the influx of workers. Engineers Town for employees of the Bureau of Reclamation was on the western side of the Columbia. Grand Coulee, to the south and high above the river, quickly garnered a reputation for its saloons, gambling joints, nightclubs, dance halls and B-street brothels. Journalist Richard Neuberger,[4] in the first of several *Oregonian* articles about dam construction, called Grand Coulee "the toughest town in North America." Unlike the other two communities, Mason City on the other side of the river was a company town—built and managed by MWAK—with 360 houses, numerous dormitories, a cookhouse, a mess hall,

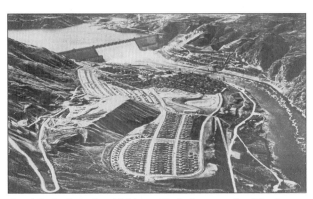

and a 35-bed hospital. To provide health care for its workers, MWAK adopted its own prepaid system, providing medical services for non-job-related illness or injury, including hospitalization, for forty-five cents per week. On-the-job illness and accidents were covered by state-sponsored workers insurance.

In 1935 Congress authorized construction of

Grand Coulee Dam site with Mason City in foreground and Engineer Town on the other side of the Columbia River.
Courtesy of Kaiser Permanente Heritage Resources.

the "high dam," and a call went out for bids. This time, Kaiser was determined not to miss out. He coordinated a merger to include Six Companies and MWAK, and the newly formed Consolidated Builders Incorporated won the bid. Kaiser's son Edgar was named general manager of the project and Clay Bedford, a Kaiser Industries employee since 1925, its general superintendent. Bedford had worked with Edgar on the construction of the Bonneville Dam, completed in 1938.

The following July, having heard how Garfield had organized a health care system for workers in the desert, Kaiser sent word through A.B. Ordway,[5] his right-hand man, to young Garfield, asking him to set up a similar program for workers at Grand Coulee. Garfield was preparing to open his long-delayed private practice in the Los Angeles area and received the word from Kaiser with something less than enthusiasm, but, despite his misgivings, he agreed to visit the Grand Coulee site.

Garfield flew to Portland to meet Edgar Kaiser; with Edgar's wife, they drove the 200 miles to Grand Coulee. They arrived late in the day at construction headquarters at Mason City, a community of 15,000. Garfield observed a dilapidated 35-bed hospital where salaried physicians received additional income by providing fee-for-service care. Patients capable of paying were given the red-carpet treatment; construction workers stood in line, literally at the rear of the hospital. The two-tier system was cause for considerable dissatisfaction among the workers. It didn't take Garfield

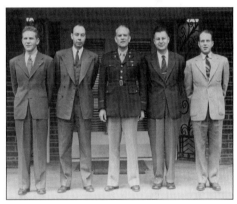

Grand Coulee Physicians: (left to right) Garfield, Cutting, Neighbor, Gillette, Wiley.
Courtesy of Kaiser Permanente Heritage Resources.

long to see another opportunity, and he agreed to take on the project. Thus began the long collaboration between Henry Kaiser, Edgar Kaiser, and Sidney Garfield that was to become Kaiser Permanente—the prototype of the modern health maintenance organization.

Garfield started by refurbishing the hospital, installing air conditioning, and making other improvements. Next, he persuaded his friend Wallace Neighbor to become Medical Director. Garfield still retained responsibilities for supervising surgical residents at Los Angeles County General Hospital. Neighbor, who had practiced at the luxurious Arrowhead Springs Resort in California for five years, was ready to leave behind the care of those he termed the "worried well" for a clinical challenge with a big industrial project.

Recruitment of other physicians was a struggle. Medical residents in both Seattle and Portland were unwilling to join an experimental program. Undaunted, Garfield looked to California. There he recruited Stanford University surgical resident Cecil Cutting. (Cutting, a brilliant surgeon, later became Executive Director of The Permanente Medical Group [TPMG]). Next he recruited Raymond Gillette, Chief of Ob/Gyn residents at San Francisco General Hospital and a friend and classmate of Cutting. Still another recruit was a classmate of Garfield from Iowa, Gene Wiley, a general practitioner and surgeon who, like Gillette, would later practice at Northern Permanente Foundation Hospital during the war years.

· ·

And on up the river is Grand Coulee Dam
The mightiest thing ever built by man
To run the great factories and water the land
It's roll on, Columbia, Roll on
      — Woodie Guthrie *(Permission: Ludlow Music, Inc)*

· ·

Those physicians who practiced at Grand Coulee later recalled the fundamental satisfaction of practicing within a prepaid, hospital-based group practice. A close-knit group, they were pioneers of sorts, even forming their own Grant County Medical Society.

By 1941 the huge project was nearing completion. Construction activities slowed and workers began to disperse. Physicians sought opportunities elsewhere. Cutting accepted an orthopedic position at the multispecialty Virginia Mason Clinic in Seattle, Washington. Neighbor joined the Army Medical Corps. Garfield returned to Los Angeles County to a teaching assignment at the University of Southern California (USC) and joined a University of Southern California Army Reserve medical unit.

PREPAID HEALTH PLANS AT MANHATTAN PROJECT SITES

As German aggression mounted in the late 1930s amid growing reports of German experiments with nuclear fission with uranium, Albert Einstein, in his now-famous 1939 letter, urged President Roosevelt to fund research to develop an atomic bomb.[6] Six weeks after Hitler's army invaded Poland the Advisory Council on Uranium met for the first time, setting in motion plans to develop an atomic bomb. With the attack on Pearl Harbor in 1941 and the U.S. entry in World War II, President Roosevelt approved the plan and appointed Army Corps of Engineers General Leslie R. Groves to head the Manhattan Project. Groves wasted no time. In August, he appropriated 54,000 acres of Appalachian land 20 miles west of Knoxville, Tennessee (to be known as Oak Ridge) for the production of uranium. In November, he acquired Los Alamos, New Mexico for the laboratory to design the bomb. Within another three months, the government acquired land at Hanford, a remote site in the dusty flats of eastern Washington state. With its isolation, its abundant water supply, and its nearby hydroelectric power from Grand Coulee, the Hanford location was an ideal site for plutonium production.

And so began the massive undertaking known as the Manhattan Project. To build the first atomic weapons the U.S. would invest more than $2 billion and construct an industrial complex that spread from Tennessee to New Mexico to Washington state. By 1945 it would rival the American automobile industry in scale. With the government's acquisition of the Hanford, Washington site, construction began on massive production reactors and plutonium extraction structures. Scientists threw themselves into producing the first nuclear reactor to manufacture large quantities of plutonium. At Oak Ridge, a vast tract of land known as "Site X," workers were engaged in a deadly business, separating U235 from natural uranium.[7] Depression-era workers came from every part of the country to work at the Manhattan Project sites, attracted as much by the government wages as by patriotic fervor. Populations at both Hanford and Oak Ridge exploded. The original population of less than 1,000 at Hanford-Richland swelled within months to 45,000. The need for a medical care program for workers and their families in these otherwise isolated areas was obvious and urgent. Two prepaid community health care programs emerged at both new communities.

ERNEST SAWARD AT HANFORD ENGINEERING WORKS 1943-1945

Ernest Saward, who figures so prominently in the history of Northwest Permanente, was a seemingly improbable choice for participating in a prepaid health care program at Hanford. Born in Brooklyn in 1914, Saward, like Sidney Garfield, was the son of European immigrants determined to succeed in their adopted country. They had even greater expectations for their children. Saward's great grandfather had emigrated from England to New York, where he established a coal brokerage business. Saward's father had made a successful career as an engineer for the city of New York. Saward was a frail child; he suffered from ear infections—for which he eventually underwent a mastoidectomy—and from rheumatic fever with a residual heart murmur. At age 15, his worried parents sent him to Franklin, a rural village in upstate New York, to board and to complete his high school education. One of his teachers, recognizing the boy's intellectual gifts, encouraged him to pursue his education and probably helped him obtain a scholarship to Colgate College.

John Chaffee, Saward's roommate at Colgate was very different from Saward. He was a member of the Beta Theta Pi fraternity, was a playboy, a dapper dresser, and owned an automobile. Saward, recently schooled in a farming community, was unfashionable and studious, but Chaffee liked him and recognized his abilities. The fraternity, about to lose its accreditation because of low grade-point averages, recruited Saward to boost their overall grade-point average. Thus he was introduced to a different lifestyle. Despite the chaos at the fraternity house, he was able to teach Chaffee how to study properly, which he attributed to his acceptance at medical school. At Colgate, a professor of zoology suggested Saward apply to the University of Rochester School of Medicine, even before he had completed his undergraduate course work. He interviewed at Rochester with George Whipple who the previous year, together with George Minot and William Murphy, had received the 1934 Nobel Prize in medicine. (In 1920 Whipple had discovered that a high-liver diet could prevent pernicious anemia in dogs. Six years later, Minot and Murphy found that the high-liver diet could control the disease in humans.) At one point in the interview, Whipple asked the young Saward what he did best, to which Saward replied that he had some skill in hunting woodchucks. Whipple himself loved to hunt woodchucks and the interview ended with a discussion on the subject. Saward later credited his acceptance to the medical school, at least in part, to this common interest.

Receiving his MD in 1939—simultaneously with his Artium Baccalauretus from Colgate University—Saward interned at Barnes Hospital in St. Louis, Missouri, and completed his residency at Peter Bent Brigham Hospital in Boston. On the basis of a brief summer experience as a medical student at a tuberculosis sanitarium, he was recruited as a pulmonary expert and chief resident at a tuberculosis center in Waltham, Massachusetts. This clinical experience would later become valuable in the struggle for the survival of the Northwest Permanente Clinic.

Now married[8] and with a family, Saward accepted a staff assignment at the Mary Imogene Basset Hospital, in Cooperstown, New York. George McKenzie, the Director of the hospital, was a Fabian socialist. As early as 1929, McKenzie had written, "Is it visionary to think of the hospital of the future, and perhaps the not very distant future, as a socially progressive health center?" McKenzie envisioned a rural hospital pursuing patient care, education, and research with full-time, salaried physicians. By 1930, he had already developed a revolutionary prepaid self-insurance plan, an early version of today's health maintenance organizations (HMOs). Subscribers paid in advance an annual premium of $25 for singles and $100 for families that covered physician fees, hospitalization, including surgery, and preventive care. The experimental plan, though successful, was terminated in 1940 by the New York State Department of Social Welfare because of pressure from the competing Blue Cross insurance plan.

Early in 1943 Stafford Warren was named chief of the medical section of the Manhattan Project. In March a handful of cases of meningococcal meningitis broke out in the barracks at the Project's Hanford site, which housed 6,000 workers. At the time, there were no known effective drugs to combat the bacteria with the possible exception of sulfa. Warren visited the camp and initiated isolation procedures, but the increasing number of cases called for additional medical help. Warren contacted Saward, one of his former students at University of Rochester Medical School, and requested a meeting. He described a secret project that he hoped Saward would join. Saward, now happy with his present position and proximity to Harvard, demurred. After a second call two weeks later, the still-reluctant Saward agreed to a meeting at the DuPont corporate headquarters in Wilmington, Delaware, to hear more about the project. Before the meeting, he was required to undergo an extensive FBI security clearance after which he was briefed about the Manhattan Project, the Hanford site, and the need for someone to help provide medical care for thousands of Hanford workers. Despite his earlier disinclination, he found himself intrigued with the prospect. He agreed to accept the position.

And so it was that in the spring of 1943 the 29-year-old Saward, product of an elite East Coast medical education and training, traveled to Hanford, a dusty, uncivilized eastern Washington town, to organize health care for DuPont workers and their families. A stopover in Chicago on his long train journey allowed him to visit the Chicago Public Library on Michigan Avenue. Anticipating the primitive conditions at Hanford, he asked for information on hospital design. Given a stack of books on the subject, he read through them for an entire day. Later, as he resumed his journey west, he got out a pencil and drew his own plans for a hospital.

At the time of Saward's arrival, a temporary camp for construction workers had already been built at the Hanford site. Another more permanent "government city" was built around the small town of Richland, population 250, located 20 miles south of Hanford. But the hurried construction of 3 plutonium production piles or reactors and 4 chemical separation plants required thousands of workers. By August 1943 the hastily erected construction camp already housed 12,500 workers and by June 1944 the number would swell to 45,000, with 131 barracks for men, 64 barracks for women, 880 Quonset huts, and 3,600 house trailers. Additional facilities included an infirmary, a clinic, a recreational hall, a theatre, 8 mess halls, and 8 schools. One of the barracks buildings doubled as a hospital.

General Groves ordered that Richland Village be built as inexpensively as possible, but DuPont corporate leaders insisted that housing for managers and professionals be constructed for permanence and comfort. No barracks or dormitories. Employees were assigned to 1 of 8 models according to status. An "A" house was a 3-bedroom, 2-story duplex with electric heat. Prefabricated Engineering Company of Portland provided 2,300 housing units. Community services at Richland included 3 schools, a hospital, a movie theatre and a combined police and fire station. Commercial development included retail stores for groceries and drugs, barber and beauty shops, and restaurants.[9]

Saward's arrival at Hanford must have given him pause. Assigned to live in one of the barracks, he would later recall that weeds and asparagus grew between the floorboards of his new home. The landscape in every direction was desert and scrubland; choking dust storms aggravated by construction made daily life almost intolerable. Brawls and fights were commonplace. Disconcerting signs of the volatile atmosphere were all too evident. Saloon windows, for example, were specially designed so that tear gas canisters could easily be thrown into the saloons to quell fights. The women's barracks, Saward noted uneasily, were surrounded by barbed wire, and a resolute guard stood around the clock at the gate. Husbands and wives were required to live in separate barracks—only those married couples living in the trailer camp were exceptions to this rule. Still, such was the urgency of the mission at Hanford that, despite the lawlessness in the workforce, police were instructed to keep offenders in jail for a minimum time so as to hasten their return to work. Saward sent for his family when he obtained an "A" house in Richland.

His to-do list was daunting. It was obvious that a community certain to grow by many thousands required a proper hospital and with the help of DuPont ad-

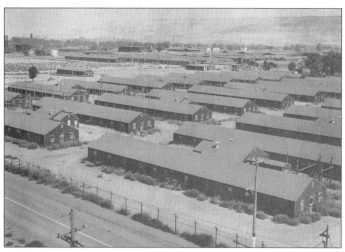

Workers barracks at Hanford construction site.
Courtesy of the Museum of History and Industry.

ministrator Gilbert Church, the Army engineers quickly constructed one. Physicians at Hanford were a mixed group. Although some were reasonably competent practitioners, others were marginal at best. Still others, he suspected, were primarily interested in avoiding the draft. One physician operated a syphilis clinic 3 nights a week. His treatment was

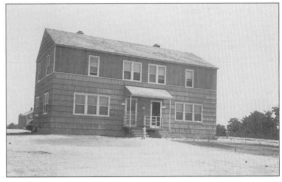

Saward House in Richland. *Courtesy of Tom Saward.*

arsphenamine (arsenic) injections, commonly used before the availability of penicillin, for which he shamelessly charged $10. Worse, he did no serological tests but merely collected his fees from those who thought they might have contracted syphilis. Saward, who had worked in a syphilis control program at Barnes Hospital, was dismayed. But it was the containment of the meningitis epidemic that was his first priority, and by isolating cases in separate tents, he and his staff were able to contain the epidemic at 67 deaths and avoid panic within the labor force. Richland residents then and later were, for the most part, unaware of the meningitis epidemic that, gone untreated, would almost certainly have taken a heavier toll on the work force and on the project itself.

DuPont had hired William "Dag" Norwood in February 1943 to be Medical Director at both Hanford and Richland. Norwood's arrival at Hanford was delayed until March the following year so that he could receive additional training at Manhattan Project sites at Chicago and Oakridge. Meanwhile, Saward, already on site and Chief of Medicine, had some autonomy to help organize the new health care program. As he did, he began to shape his ideas for a prepaid, community health care program. The medical system had two divisions: one, the Village Medical Division, was to provide for the needs of the Richland residents. The other, the Industrial Medicine Division, was to see to the safety and health care needs of the workers.

The Hanford program, though slow to do so, eventually organized a psychiatric service. Severe cases were hospitalized at first in a barracks building formerly used to isolate infectious diseases. Later, a well-designed hospital included a 25-bed psychiatric ward. Still, psychiatric clinicians at Hanford were limited to one half-time physician, a nurse, and a social worker. Regular inpatient nursing staff filled the gaps. A sample month of psychiatric admissions indicates that staffing for mental health diagnoses was thin. Hanford psychiatric admissions for May 1944 included alcoholism (60), epilepsy (19), psychopathic personality (7), schizophrenia (6), other psychoses (5), and luetic G.P.I (1).

Saward persuaded the reluctant physicians that cooperation with the prepaid program was preferable to being drafted into the Pacific war arena. Coverage was extended to families of workers. Saward assigned work according to skills and established a triage system. Eventually, according to Saward, physicians' initial resentment toward prepayment and group practice dissipated. In time, they began to view the prepaid group practice as a sensible—even superior—alternative to fee-for-service. (Interestingly, Garfield's last proprietary medical venture took him, too, to Hanford—but nearly a decade after Saward's departure—when Kaiser engineers were building nuclear reactors: KW in 1954 and KE in 1955.)

PART II:
THE EARLY
DECADES

CHAPTER 2:
WARTIMES 1941-1945

In 1936, Congress passed the Merchant Marine Act to encourage America's shipbuilders to enlarge the peacetime Merchant Marines, authorizing the building of 500 additional Merchant Marine ships over a ten-year period. They were to be "owned and operated by citizens of the United States" and, eerily prescient, capable of "serving as a naval and military auxiliary in time of war." Recognizing the Merchant Marine Act as a lucrative opportunity, in 1937 Henry Kaiser and two other contractors in the Six Companies consortium decided to turn from the building of dams to shipbuilding. It was a bold venture, for Kaiser knew virtually nothing about the building of ships.

By 1940 Adolph Hitler had conquered Europe and turned his attention to England. The German Luftwaffe with its superior air power was inflicting heavy damage to British shipyards, and Nazi U-boats were sinking British ships three times faster than they could be built. Representatives of the British Ministry of War Transport arrived in the U.S. with the urgent request for 60 ships. Two companies formed by Todd Shipbuilding Corporation and Six Companies bid the job and won the contract. Thirty ships were to be built at a Todd-based shipyard in Portland, Maine and another 30 at a yet-to-be constructed shipyard in Richmond, California. With the awarding of the contract in 1940, furious construction began on the Richmond shipyard on the eastern shore of San Francisco Bay. A mere four months later in April 1941, the keel of the Ocean Vanguard, the first British Liberty Ship, was laid.

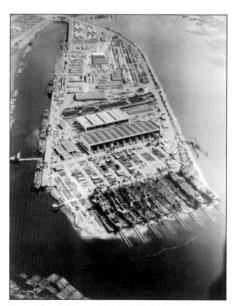

Swan Island Shipyard during World War II.
Courtesy of the Oregon Historical Society, OrHi 49686.

NORTHWEST SHIPYARDS

With the January 1941 official announcement of the Liberty ship program, Kaiser lost no time. He acquired an 87-acre site on the Willamette River in the St. Johns area of North Portland,[1] and yard construction began there almost immediately. With its completion, Oregon Shipbuilding Corporation began building Liberty ships for Great Britain. After the December 7th bombing of Pearl Harbor, Kaiser opened two more shipyards—one on 186 acres of waterfront farmland one mile east of Vancouver, Washington,[2] and another on Swan Island, site of the

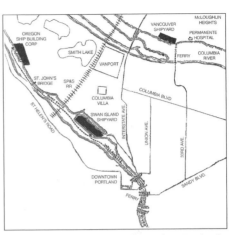

Location of the three Kaiser shipyards in Portland and Vancouver.

former Portland Municipal Airport. Having bought out Todd's interest in the company, Kaiser placed his son Edgar in charge of the three Portland-Vancouver shipyards. Clay Bedford, Edgar's friend and colleague from the Bonneville and Grand Coulee projects, was already on site at the Richmond yard. The two now entered a period of intense competition for speed in building ships. In 1942 Portland set a shipbuilding record when the Joseph Teal, built in just 10 days, was launched during a secret visit by President Roosevelt. But that record did not stand; Bedford's Richmond workers then built a ship in just 4 days, 15 hours, and 26 minutes.

Kaiser shipyards in Oregon, Washington, and California produced nearly 1,500 ships during the war—27% of those commissioned by the U.S. Maritime Commission. Of these, 743—nearly half—were built in the Portland-Vancouver shipyards between 1941 and 1945. What's more, Kaiser's shipyards built them at 25% less than the average cost of all other American shipyards and in two-thirds the time. Oregon Shipbuilding launched 332 Merchant Marine Liberty ships—hard-working vessels that carried crucial supplies throughout the war.

SHIPYARD WORKERS

World War II spawned the biggest on-the-job training project in history. Railroads carried workers by the thousands to West Coast plane factories, military bases, and shipyards. A quarter of the shipyard workers were women, and only 2% of them had previously worked in a shipyard. Kaiser created special trains called "Magic Carpet Specials" to haul new workers from the East and the South. New arrivals came every corner of the country in response to advertisements like this one in the September 20, 1942 edition of the *Oregon Journal*: "10,000 Shipyard

Workers wanted at Swan Island, Vancouver, Oregon Shipyards … Previous experience is not necessary. Training will be given on the job. Willingness to work and a desire to do that work where it will do the maximum good—those are the things that count." And so they came: bartenders from Montana, taxi drivers from Boston, African Americans from the South, struggling families from the Dakotas, housewives from Michigan, farmers from Arkansas. They came for better wages, for a fresh start, for a change of scenery. They came, too, because of a sense of duty to the war effort.

SHIPYARD HOUSING

At their peak, the Portland-Vancouver shipyards employed nearly 100,000 workers, 28,000 of them women. Shifts ran around the clock. The influx of so many people—more than 200,000 counting spouses and children—created a massive housing crisis.

From its 1940 prewar population of 18,000, Vancouver more than quadrupled in size to 90,000 by 1944, and Portland grew by 54,000 people—at least 40,000 of them shipyard workers and their families. As workers streamed by the thousands from the East, Midwest and South, Kaiser rushed to fill the demand for housing and infrastructure. In Vancouver, dormitory buildings—barracks-like row houses and single-family houses—proliferated. McLoughlin Heights, developed from 1,000 acres of farmland and brushland east of Vancouver, was a step up from the other complexes with 5,000 single-family dwellings and views of Mt. Hood. Its temporary prefabricated houses became the largest such development east of New York. Unique was the Boulevard Shopping Center with 33 merchants, one of the first multistore shopping centers in the nation designed by soon-to-be famous Pietro Belluschi. It received recognition from the New York Museum of Modern Art as an example of things to come. Edgar Kaiser's home on nearby Wauna Vista Drive overlooked the Columbia River.

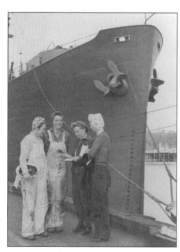

Women workers at Kaiser Shipyards.
Courtesy of The Oregonian.

Portland's Columbia Villa was an 82-acre housing complex with 462 homes and duplexes. Built by the federal government expressly for shipyard workers, its plywood barracks-style structures were meant to last only 10 years. A signature feature of the Villa was its looping streets, connecting to the surrounding grid in only 4 places and producing a pastoral, if isolating, effect. Later the Villa became Oregon's largest public housing project.

The city of Vanport—the name a hybridization of Vancouver and Portland—was the world's largest housing project at the time, a planned community for shipyard workers. Built on a flood plain north of Portland city limits, Vanport was protected from the Willamette and Columbia rivers by dikes. For a time, Vanport was Oregon's second largest city, with a shipyard population that swelled to 50,000. Housing designs were limited to 3 configurations: 2-story buildings with 8 or 14 units, as well as small 1-story multi-unit dwellings. Vanport had its own police force, fire department, post office, and hospital. It also had 5 elementary schools, 6 preschools, 5 recreational centers, an 800-seat movie theatre, and a 10-acre park. The initial publicity for Vanport called it "a masterpiece of urban planning," but adults who lived there remember it as far from idyllic. Because of wartime shortages of manpower and material, construction was shabby. In addition, commercial services were inadequate to serve the population's needs. Two washing machines served 56 families. The units were built so close together that residents found the noise a continual nuisance. Insects and rodents were constant, if unwelcome, companions. Still, those who remember a childhood at Vanport recall it with a wistful nostalgia. Gary Sowles, a child in the largest Vanport family, spent happy hours playing on homemade rafts on the numerous waterways and sloughs. Jack Dick, later a Lake Oswego barber, climbed the water tower to catch pigeons and played in freight cars that stood on the railroad dike. Siblings Hal Freitag and Barbara Sims played baseball on a diamond adjacent to the hospital; they remember an errant ball that once flew onto the roof of the operating room during a surgery. Former Portland Metro counselor Ed Washington thought of Vanport as a magical place for kids; he made pocket money by fetching ice for his neighbors.

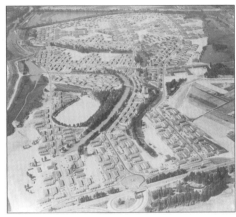

Vanport during World War II.
Courtesy of the Oregon Historical Society, OrHi 49686.

SHIPYARD LIFE

Despite the fact that the country was at war, the atmosphere in the shipyards could be surprisingly festive, with entertainment and ceremonial activities interrupting the daily work routine. Dignitaries came regularly to perform the time-honored ritual of breaking a bottle of champagne to launch a ship. President Roosevelt himself arrived in his ten-car presidential train on a day in September 1942 as part of a two-week inspection of factories, military bases, and shipyards. His presence was intended to be

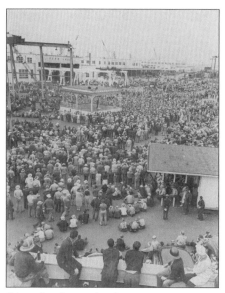

Shipyard workers gather for announcements and entertainment.
Courtesy of the Oregon Historical Society.

secret, but word spread quickly and thousands of workers lined the route, cheering as he rode in an open car with Henry and Edgar Kaiser. On a later occasion Eleanor Roosevelt, escorted by Edgar Kaiser, visited the Vancouver yards and toured a first-aid station and the Northern Permanente Foundation Hospital.

War bond drives brought celebrities to the shipyard, including comedian Jack Benny's wife Mary Livingston; actors Walter Pigeon, Ethel Barrymore, Joan Leslie, Adolf Monjou; and ecdysiast Gypsy Rose Lee. Eleven-year-old Jane Powell, a local girl destined for later Hollywood fame, sang with four shipyard security guards, The Singing Sentinels, who entertained for visiting notables at ship launchings. Among them were Lord Halifax, Winston Churchill's cabinet minister; opera singer Lily Pons; and General Jonathan Wainwright.

Eighteen-year-old James DeLong, in his summer job as shipyards chauffeur, announced coming entertainment acts for shipyard workers from a sound truck. Sidney Garfield and Wallace Neighbor were frequent speakers at ceremonies. Sometimes children participated in the activities, as when obstetrician Ray Gillette's 11-year-old daughter attended as flower girl for the launching of the first A-P 5 attack transport U.S.S. Oconto.

ARTISTS IN THE SHIPYARDS

Portland enjoyed a rich, diverse, and distinctive art scene before the war, thanks in part to its well-established Museum Art School. In addition, the Depression-era Works Progress Administration (WPA) provided work for serious artists. Those employed by federal programs were required to limit their work to portrayals of American scenes from daily life. Among WPA artists were studious painters of Oregon life. During the war years, Martina Gangle (1906-1994), a deeply committed social activist and communist, and brothers Arthur Runquist (1891-1971) and Albert Runquist (1894-1971) worked in the Vancouver yards; Gangle as a welder, the elder Runquist as a foreman. During breaks from work, the three painted and drew, leaving a vivid and often poignant record of shipyard life. Gangle's favorite subjects, working-class people and social realism, characterizes much of her art. Albert Runquist's art reveals a strong interest in landscape; his brother Arthur was drawn more to the figure.[3] The book *Waging War on the Home Front* by Arsdol and Mack includes some of Gangle's and the Runquist brothers' art.

DAY CARE FOR WORKERS' CHILDREN

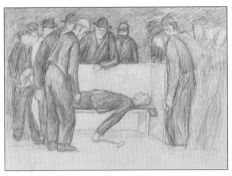

Sketch of a shipyard injury by Arthur Runquist. *From the author's collection.*

When Eleanor Roosevelt visited Vancouver in April 1943 for the launching of the U.S.S. Alazon Bay, she had a more serious purpose in mind. Earlier in the year she had visited the Portland, Maine, shipyards during the graveyard shift, ascending a gangplank to talk to women welders working on platforms four feet above ground. She listened as they described their problems as working mothers. The difficulty of their dual role strengthened her conviction that day nurseries and play schools should be located at factories and shipyards where mothers worked.

But public opinion was not on Eleanor Roosevelt's side. Fierce objection arose over the idea of working mothers. New York Mayor Fiorella LaGuardia opined, "The worst mother is better than the best institution." Even the lone woman member of President Roosevelt's cabinet objected to the development of day care centers. With so much opposition, only six government-sponsored day care centers were built.

Undeterred by the strident critics of childcare centers, during her visit to the Vancouver shipyards Mrs. Roosevelt talked at length with Edgar and Henry Kaiser about the problems of working mothers and urged them to develop a model childcare center. Within weeks, Edgar began planning to build centers at the entrance to Swan Island and Oregon shipyards. Architect George Wolff's unique, octagonal building design was praised by *Architectural Record* and *Parents Magazine*. Its 15 playrooms surrounded a central outside playground. Children's bathrooms were equipped with child-size toilets and washbasins. Forrest Rieke, MD, and one or more nurses staffed an infirmary.[4] Again at Mrs. Roosevelt's urging, Edgar implemented another innovation: pre-cooked meals for mothers to take home at the end of their shifts. Still, these humanitarian measures, unremarkable by today's standards, met with fierce resistance and often from surprising quarters. Protest arose, for example, from Multnomah County, the U.S. Children's Bureau, and from the Oregon State Medical Society (later to become the Oregon Medical Association) on the grounds that childcare centers would encourage mothers to work outside the home—an idea at odds with the idealized notion of motherhood at the time.

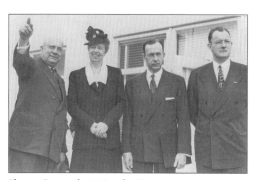

Eleanor Roosevelt visiting the Kaiser Vancouver Shipyard, April 1943; (left to right) Henry J. Kaiser, Eleanor Roosevelt, Edgar Kaiser, and Henry J. Kaiser, Jr. *Courtesy of the Oregon Historical Society, OrHi 49686.*

GARFIELD'S HEALTH CARE PROGRAM FOR SHIPYARD WORKERS

With the anticipated influx of 100,000 workers, the need for a health care program quickly became a matter of urgency. In January 1941 Henry Kaiser once again contacted Garfield to help provide medical care for his rapidly growing labor force. Garfield arranged contracts with insurance companies to cover medical and hospital care for on-the-job illness and injury. The first group sickness and accidental insurance plan went into effect December 7, 1941. The cost was fifty cents per worker per day.

By January 1942 the senior Kaiser and Edgar could see that medical care for the legions of men and women at the yards was still woefully inadequate. Again, Kaiser turned to Garfield for help. Making preparations for a tour of duty in India with the U.S. Army Reserve Medical Corps in Southern California, Garfield nevertheless responded to his former partner's call. This time he developed a far more comprehensive plan, using as his blueprint the basic health care concepts he had implemented for the huge construction projects at Desert Center and at Grand Coulee.

By now influential in Washington DC, Kaiser was able to secure Garfield's release from the army so that he might continue to organize health care for shipyard workers in California, Oregon, and Washington. Garfield believed that health care funding could be provided through a nonprofit medical foundation. Henry Kaiser must have concurred; in July 1942, they established The Permanente Foundation in California with Kaiser named Chairman of the Board of Trustees and his wife Bess a trustee.

Within months Garfield established a similar Northern Permanente Foundation for the care of Portland-Vancouver shipyard workers, already numbering 10,000 and expected to grow to over 50,000. At first, both physicians and other health care workers were employed by the foundation. But because of American Medical Association objections to physicians employed by a lay organization, the physicians became employees of Garfield himself.

Next Garfield arranged a separate prepaid health plan for shipyard workers at Swan Island and at St. Helens with Oregon Physicians Service, an organization of the Oregon State Medical Society. Its agreement with Oregon Ship Corporation stipulated that Oregon Physician Service would provide care for more than

25,000 employees—the biggest single contract ever written by a physicians' mutual service bureau for prepaid medical care. On-the-job care was to be compensated by the Oregon State Industrial Commission. Workers themselves paid for non-job-related care through monthly deductions from their wages. Worker influx soon created a strain on area hospitals. One well-publicized incident graphically portrayed the problem: a 14-year-old boy died from critical burns sustained in a house fire after the six local hospitals, all at capacity, denied his admission.

The boy's death acted as a catalyst to create additional hospital beds. In 1943 the Housing Authority of Portland commissioned architect George Wolff to design a hospital in Vanport, to be administered and controlled by Oregon Physician Service and open to all licensed physicians. A well-designed facility, it was modeled after the Northern Permanente Foundation Hospital, built the previous year in Vancouver, Washington. The Vanport Hospital provided medical and maternity care, with a nursery, operating rooms, a pharmacy, and outpatient facilities. The Multnomah County Health Department clinic even had a designated space. Unfortunately, the hospital could not escape the taint of socialized medicine; few doctors—even those in Vanport—were willing to admit patients there, choosing instead to admit to the overcrowded Portland-area hospitals. When few Vanporters signed up for the prepaid plan, Oregon Physician Service adopted a fee-for-service plan. Still, paying patients were infrequent, and the occupancy rate averaged only 60%. Hospital staffing worsened during the winter of 1944-1945, with continual staff turnover. Just one physician—usually a moonlighting military doctor—provided weekend coverage.

WARTIME PHYSICIAN RECRUITMENT

At Richmond, Garfield had been able to recruit a core group of physicians who had experience with, or were committed to, group practice. But physicians in the Portland-Vancouver program were unfamiliar with, or lacked enthusiasm for, group practice. To exacerbate Garfield's troubles, a 1942-1943 flu epidemic stretched resources sufficiently that the new Northern Permanente Foundation Health Plan was forced to refer members to other community hospitals and doctors. This caused confusion among members who had assumed they would continue to be cared for by non-plan physicians.

Finally, Garfield called upon his old friend Wallace Neighbor, who had worked with him at Los Angeles County General Hospital and at Grand Coulee. Neighbor had joined the U.S. Army Medical Corps, where he had been based at Fort MacArthur in San Pedro, California. There he enjoyed an administrative position, with housing services and regular afternoon tennis. Somehow, Garfield and Edgar Kaiser influenced the Surgeon General to release Neighbor, and he became CEO and Medical Director of the Northern Permanente Foundation

Health Plan. His challenge was to administer and organize a diverse group of physicians, some of questionable competence and others with little motivation. Nevertheless, despite these formidable challenges, Neighbor eventually assembled a core of dependable physicians, some of whom were Grand Coulee veterans. Gradually, a functional organization emerged.

MEDICAL SOCIETIES AND DISCRIMINATION

By November 1942, 35% of America's 120,000 physicians had been inducted into the armed forces. With the expectation that many more would be called to military duty, the Federal War Manpower Commission initiated the Procurement and Assignment Service (PAS) to determine those physicians essential to the war effort and those deemed ineligible. Medical societies were influential with local branches of the PAS. The King County Medical Society exerted significant control over physician allocation in Washington State. Garfield decried what he saw as medical society and PAS discrimination toward Permanente, claiming that PAS assigned to him only the most poorly trained physicians. (At the time, physicians assigned by PAS could obtain temporary licenses by mail before they had taken their state board examinations.)

Kaiser and Garfield had had enough. In November 1943 Senator Claude Pepper, Chair of a Subcommittee on Education and Labor, held hearings on war manpower resources. Both Garfield and Henry Kaiser testified about the opposition they faced from medical societies as well as from the AMA, which influenced the PAS. Garfield pointed out that the chairman of the PAS was also president of the King County Medical Society—a clear conflict of interest. He went on to testify that the Washington State Medical Association officials had threatened Permanente physicians with induction into the army if Kaiser extended its prepaid medical program to families of workers. Morris Fishbein, editor of the *Journal of the American Medical Association* asked derisively for proof of alleged threats. Had the officials placed these threats in writing? Kaiser shot back, "They wouldn't dare!" Later that month an editorial in *JAMA*, in a not-so-subtle reference to Kaiser, railed against "the desire of some industrial leaders and staff of physicians to maintain their individual empires without regard to the war effort." In turn, Kaiser challenged Fishbein in subsequent U.S. Senate hearings. Their continuing rancorous debate was reported by *The New York Times, Time Magazine,* and *The New Republic.* In the end, the Senate hearings damaged Fishbein. One AMA physician employee accused him of unethical behavior by using his position to intimidate opponents. Increasingly seen as autocratic and dictatorial, Fishbein eventually became a sufficient liability that in 1949 he was replaced as *JAMA* editor. Ultimately, because of the acute shortage of civilian physicians, the Vancouver medical community grudgingly accepted Permanente physicians and allowed them membership in the Clark County Medical Society, where they served on various committees and presented clinical findings at meetings.

NORTHERN PERMANENTE FOUNDATION HOSPITAL

Garfield wanted to locate a new hospital in Portland where most of the shipyard workers lived. But the Portland medical community, led by Mayo-trained surgeon Thomas Joyce, fought against the intrusion of a prepaid group practice for non-job-related care. Luckily for Garfield, personal relationships intervened. Joyce was Edgar Kaiser's friend, as well as his personal physician. He agreed to a prepaid program limited to industrial care in Oregon. But the medical community remained adamant that a new hospital be located in out-of-the-way Vancouver, rather than in Portland. Reluctantly, Edgar Kaiser agreed, though Garfield was disappointed in the decision: after all, the population in Vancouver at the time was just 18,000. In addition, he recognized the disadvantages inherent in a disjointed program that limited health care in one state to industrial care but allowed for voluntary non-industrial care across the river in another.

Nevertheless, in 1942 a hospital site was purchased on a beautiful 15-acre bluff overlooking the Columbia River. Architect George Wolff won the commission to design the new hospital. Wolff had come to the attention of Henry Kaiser through his friendship with Edgar. Wolff's firm had already won commissions for the layout of the Oregon, Vancouver, and Swan Island shipyards. Later he won the design commission for Vanport City and its

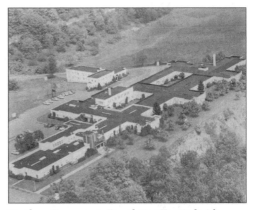

Northern Permanente Foundation Hospital with nurses' residence at top.
Courtesy of Kaiser Permanente Heritage Resources.

50,000 inhabitants. In the ensuing years, Wolff and successors Zimmer, Gunsul, and Frasca would design and build two additional Kaiser Permanente hospitals and numerous medical centers for KP Northwest. In its first phase the new hospital had 70 beds. An attached outpatient facility included physicians' offices, x-ray and physical therapy rooms, and a pharmacy. With wartime limitations on available building materials, including restrictions on nails, contractors resorted to plywood and brick veneer for exterior construction and galvanized steel fixtures, rather than chrome. The assumption was that the building would be temporary—intended to last about eight years. The plan called for an eventual expansion to 300 beds.

Innovative for its time, the new hospital featured six air-conditioned operating rooms centered in a circular pattern ringed by an outside corridor. Each operating room had two entrances, one to the perimeter corridor and another to the inner central supply area. Glass brick provided enhanced lighting. Patient rooms, a combination of private and two and three-bed units, all had bathrooms. Patients had, in addition to call lights, a bedside intercom system to alert nurses. The hospital opened with a medical staff of 20, representing internists and specialties in surgery, orthopedics, obstetrics and gynecology, EENT, and anesthesiology. In time the medical staff would include interns and residents and expand to 45. In 1943 under the auspices of the Northern Permanente Hospital, a convalescent ward, a precursor to what we now refer to as a skilled nursing facility, opened in the lounge of Hudson House Dormitory G with round-the-clock nursing staff. A three-story nurses' residence also housed lab technicians; nurse anesthetists; business office workers; and, in separate quarters, medical residents. The lower level included a spacious lobby, a beauty shop, a gift shop, and a large hall for social events. The group was close-knit. Leora Baldwin Roche worked at the hospital switchboard and admitted patients; she paid $19 a month in rent for her room, for which she received a weekly change of linen. Rabbits ran freely throughout the bucolic rural setting, and tree frogs, unseen, struck up a muted chorus at dusk. An annual visit by the Rose Festival court brought curious cows from the neighboring dairy farm to the fence, where they appeared to watch the proceedings with mild interest.

In this wartime era of food rationing, the hospital cafeteria maintained a reputation for inexpensive meals and good food. A French chef directed the kitchen staff, which included both salad and pastry chefs. Staff members were allowed to bring an occasional guest, a treat for civilian visitors who lacked access to scarce meat. Thursday—hamburger day—was said to be a favorite.

Hospital administrator Rex Hamby, small in stature and soft-spoken, was popular among employees for his enlightened concerns for their welfare. Garfield, universally admired and treated with the deference accorded a dignitary, visited the hospital frequently. With his red hair and somewhat diffident manner, he was known among the staff as "the red fox"; as the years went by and his hair color changed, he became "the gray fox."

THE PHYSICIANS

Ernest Saward later recalled the wartime physicians at Permanente as a mixed group, including some whose main purpose he suspected was to avoid military service. Saward's assessment notwithstanding, Neighbor recruited a number of outstanding doctors. Obstetrician Gillette and surgeon Eugene Wiley, together with

Wiley's brother Dudley, another obstetrician, brought their group-practice experi-ence from Grand Coulee. Walter Noehren, Saward's brilliant classmate at the Uni-versity of Rochester, came from Hanford. Internist Charles Grossman, having just completed his medical residency at Yale where he took part in the first U.S. clinical trial with penicillin, joined the pioneering group in October 1944, induced he said, by the annual salary of $8,400—considerably more than Yale had offered. Radi-ologist Morris Malbin, a graduate of the University of Chicago Medical School, arrived a mere week before Grossman. Rejected for medical reasons by the mili-tary, he determined instead to attend to wartime workers. Frederick Bookhotz, a talented surgeon with a flair for humor, once admitted into the emergency room "a male with chest abscess" for a drainage procedure. The patient was Grossman's dog, an adoptee from the local animal shelter. Its vigorous protests prompted another patient awaiting treatment to remark with alarm that the suffering patient in the adjoining cubicle had begun to bark like a dog.

Endocrinologist Karl Heller was Chief of Medicine during the late war years, be-fore joining the faculty of the Oregon Medical School (later to be renamed Oregon Health and Science University [OHSU]). Internist Joseph Kriss, still a Yale medical student during Grossman's residency, joined the Medical Group before war's end, later accepting a position at Stanford University. Norbert Fell, later to play an impor-tant role in the post-war Pediatric Department, took an externship at Coffey Hospital, (later Portland Physicians and Surgeons Hospital) before coming to the Northern Permanente Foundation Hospital (and to a better paying job as night doctor) in June 1943. Katherine Van Leeuwen, a staff pediatrician during the late war years, later re-called her Permanente experience in the October 1946 issue of *Pediatrics*.

CLINICAL ACHIEVEMENTS

In the early 1940s, Permanente physicians contributed to understanding the cause of pneumonia and pioneering its treatment with sulfa drugs. Seen frequently among shipyard workers, pneumonia was thought to be an occupational hazard until Morris Collen disproved the assumption. In a one-year study at Permanente facilities in Oakland and Richmond, he showed that the incidence and type of pneumonia was no different among shipyard workers than in the general popula-tion. His research was published in the January 1944 issue of the *Journal of Indus-trial Hygiene and Toxicology*.

Existing protocols for treating pneumonia relied on pneumococal type specific anti-serums, which were often ineffective. In a pneumonia study, Collen treated 550 patients aggressively with sulphadiazine. He reported his results in a 1943 is-sue of the *Permanente Foundation Medical Bulletin* and in *The New England Journal of Medicine (NEJM)*.

As late as 1943 no information about penicillin had yet been released to the public. The new antibiotic was a scarce commodity, and 90% of the supply was dedicated to the military. Then, on October 17, 1943, seven-year-old Betty Hall, whose father was a chipper[5] at the Vancouver shipyard, was transported by ambulance from her prefabricated McLoughlin Heights home to the Northern Permanente Foundation Hospital after a mysterious one-day illness. Feverish, her knee swollen, the child lapsed into a coma and convulsed repeatedly. She received high doses of sulfathiazole until her doctors diagnosed osteomyelitis and staphylococcal septicemia. Drainage of the subperiosteal abscess, together with a window cut into the cortex of the femur and holes drilled into the medulla brought little improvement. Her survival appeared doubtful.

Chester Keefer at Boston's Evans Memorial Hospital controlled all penicillin for civilian use. One week after Betty fell ill, he released a supply to Permanente doctors. Twenty-four hours after intramuscular administration of 10,000 units of penicillin at three-hour intervals, the child's condition improved, and her convulsions ceased. After three months, she was discharged from the hospital. This case marked the first civilian use of penicillin on the West Coast, as reported in the 1944 issue of the *Permanente Foundation Medical Bulletin*.

In 1944 Collen garnered another West Coast first with penicillin when he cured a case of type-7 pneumococcal pneumonia with 16,000 units. One year later Grossman, following Collen's guidelines for monitoring blood sulfa levels to avoid renal toxicity, studied the management of lobar pneumonia. His one-year review of 440 cases was published in the October 1945 issue of The *Permanente Foundation Medical Bulletin*.

THE PERMANENTE MEDICAL JOURNALS

Garfield, believing that the Medical Group should promote and participate in research and education, asked Collen to create a publication that would demonstrate to physicians in the community the quality of Permanente medical practice and the achievements within Permanente. The first edition of the *Permanente Foundation Medical Bulletin* was published in July 1943, with Collen as Editor-In-Chief. The third edition included Garfield's first annual report of The Permanente Foundation. The August 24, 1944 issue of the *NEJM* included an endorsement—surprisingly strong, given the general attitude toward prepaid group practice at the time—of the Permanente program. Evidently impressed with Garfield's annual report, its editor called Permanente economic results "amazing" and recommended that the medical profession adopt "some of the methods and principles to obtain the most effective and efficient medical service to large numbers of people at low cost—and at the same time maintain the high standards and dignity of the medical profession." The editorial ended with the question, "Can established practitioners and specialists adapt themselves to this type of medical care?"

Two Permanente physicians, Saward and pediatrician Charles Varga, also joined the editorial staff. Others—surgeons Norman Frink and Gilbert Rogers and orthopedist F.J. Roemer—were *Bulletin* contributors. In 1951 another Permanente publication—*The Educational Proceedings of the Permanente Hospitals*—appeared. It had a 2-year life before combining with the *Bulletin*, to become *The Kaiser Foundation Medical Journal.*[6] *The Journal*, after 4 years, ceased publication in 1958, leaving a void of 36 years. In the absence of a regional or national Permanente publication, several clinical departments in the Northwest Region published monthly clinical newsletters. Then in 1994, Permanente physicians Tom Janisse[7] and Continuing Medical Education (CME) Director Phillip Brenes, in collaboration with Merry Parker, Clinical Publications Editor, consolidated these disparate publications into a new quarterly journal, with each department allotted space for newsletter content. *The Northwest Permanente Journal of Clinical Practice* enjoyed a 3-year run.

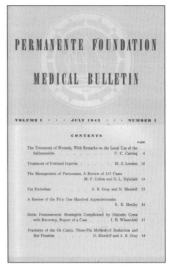

First issue of Permanente Bulletin featuring papers by TPMG pioneer Cecil Cutting on treating wounds of shipyard workers with Sulfonamides and Morris Collen on the treatment of pneumonia. The successes described in the pneumonia paper would draw national medical attention to the new Health Plan.

Permanente Foundation Medical Bulletin courtesy of TPMG Archives.

Then, with support from Regional Medical Director Allan J. Weiland, Janisse, by now Interim CME Director, and his CME Manager counterpart Chris Overton proposed to the Medical Directors of all Regions a national organizational medical journal to focus on physician practice, experience, and innovation. *The Permanente Journal (TPJ)* debuted in the summer of 1997. Published quarterly, *TPJ* enjoys a print circulation of 25,000, with distribution to 16,000 physicians (active and retired), 5,000 clinicians, and 4,000 leaders, managers, and researchers within KP. What Garfield could never have imagined is this: today, 66 years after the 1943 first publication of *The Permanente Foundation Medical Bulletin*, 600,000 people in 164 countries throughout the world access a Permanente Medical Group journal through the Internet.

CHAPTER 3:
HARD TIMES 1945-1950

—ɯ—

In December 1944, with the launching of the last attack transports for the invasion of Japan, workers left the Vancouver shipyards, anticipating the end of wartime ship production. A new contract called for building C-4 transport ships "to bring the boys home." This work sustained the shipyards until Victory in Europe (VE) Day on May 8, 1945, after which a further exodus of workers took place.

Ernest Saward, preparing to end his assignment at Richland and contemplating his future, visited several innovative medical centers in the Northwest, including Roosevelt Hospital in Bremerton, Washington, which served civilian employees of the Navy. He also visited the program at the Kaiser shipyards in Vancouver where his friend and classmate Walter Noehren worked. Like Saward, Noehren had been at Mary Imogene Basset Hospital in Cooperstown, New York. And like Saward, Noehren had been at Hanford. In June 1945 Saward accepted the position of Chief of Medicine for the Northern Permanente program in Vancouver and said goodbye to Richland. At the time, the Medical Group comprised 43 doctors, some of whom, (like Noehren) Saward had known at Hanford. One, whom he had fired at Hanford because of his drug addiction, encountered Saward one day in a corridor; that physician quietly departed the program shortly thereafter.

With the bombing of Hiroshima, World War II came to an end, and with the exodus of workers from Portland and Vancouver shipyards the Northern Permanente Foundation Health Plan appeared to be unsustainable. At a staff meeting called by Wallace Neighbor and attended by 35 to 40 physicians, a motion was made to dissolve the Medical Group. Saward, perhaps the only meeting participant familiar with *Robert's Rules of Order*, moved to table the motion. Seconded by Charles Grossman, the motion to table passed. Just 7 physicians attended the next staff meeting, but all of them wanted to preserve the Medical Group. Neighbor, with something less than enthusiasm, agreed to act as Garfield's surrogate. In late September, 5 of the remaining physicians met with Edgar Kaiser around a beach fire on the north shore of the Columbia River. They wanted to continue the program. Henry Kaiser gave his approval but told them he could not provide financial backing; he was shortly to take charge of the Kaiser-Frazer Automobile Company at Willow Run, Michigan. The core physician group included Norbert Fell, Grossman, Morris Malbin,

Neighbor, Noehren, and Saward. Soon thereafter, they erected a sign on Evergreen Boulevard at the entrance to the Vancouver hospital, announcing a "Community Health Plan: Northern Permanente Hospital."

ASSAULT BY THE WASHINGTON STATE MEDICAL ASSOCIATION AND THE AMERICAN MEDICAL ASSOCIATION

At the time, advertising by the medical profession was viewed as unethical, promotion of a community health plan unthinkable. Within a week, Saward, a member of the Washington State Medical Association, received a letter of disapproval charging him and his small Medical Group with unethical practice. Summoned before the Society's board of censors in Seattle, he argued his position. No conclusive action ensued.

In December 1945 Saward was summoned to a meeting of the Judicial Council of the American Medical Association in Chicago. To prepare his brief, he enlisted the help of Grossman, authorizing a temporary leave for him to conduct research, and that of genial medical librarian Bertha Hallam,[1] who threw her support into the project.

The AMA took the position that "enrolling a membership" was one and the same as soliciting. Further, it opposed the idea of salaried physicians and group practice. Having carefully researched the historical precedents, Saward cited examples of current group practices, including the Mayo Clinic and several other health care programs in industry. He also cited historical legal precedents in England and in the U.S., including an unsuccessful 1939 challenge by the AMA against Group Health Cooperative (Washington, DC) on the basis of restraint of trade. The judicial council engaged him for two and a half hours, the six aging council members contrasting sharply with the 31-year-old Saward. Despite their patronizing manner, occasionally addressing him as "Sonny," Saward held his own. When the council cited his salaried position as unethical, Louis A. Buie, a distinguished Mayo Clinic surgeon and salaried physician, reacted heatedly. During the ensuing arguments—this time among council

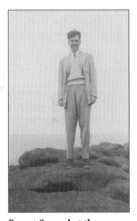

Ernest Saward at the Oregon Coast, circa 1948. *Courtesy of Tom Saward.*

members themselves—the focus shifted from Saward. Council lawyer Joseph Stenton finally advised adjournment. The council dismissed Saward and asked him to return in June 1946 for final disposition of the case. Two weeks later he received a letter from the Washington State Medical Association. All charges against the Permanente physicians had been dropped. Still, this challenge was merely the opening salvo in a 22-year battle between Permanente and the Portland-Vancouver medical community.

CARRYING ON

Neighbor continued as Medical Director, allowing Saward to concentrate on recruiting physicians. Grossman took a temporary leave to help fill a temporary vacancy at the Fontana office of the Southern California Permanente Medical Group (SCPMG) but returned to Permanente in the Northwest the following year. Norman Frink, a graduate of Northwestern Medical School and of residency training at Detroit Receiving Hospital, joined the group as Chief of Surgery. He preceded Roger George by a day. George, a graduate of University of Rochester and a four-year veteran of the Air Force, joined as Chief of Obstetrics and Gynecology. Viennese-trained ophthalmologist Egon Ullman, something of an eccentric according to his contemporaries, was admired for his prodigious work output. Internist Barney Malbin, brother of Morris and a veteran of the Spanish Civil War[2] and of World War II, gave up a private practice in Chicago (where one of his patients was writer-journalist Studs Terkel) to join the group in 1948. The Malbins' arrival was inauspicious; the Memorial Day Flood had devastated the city of Vanport the previous day.

Accredited by the AMA for internships and residencies, the Northern Permanente Foundation Hospital provided training for numbers of doctors. Harold and Charlotte Cohen began their internships in September 1945, temporarily residing in the nurses' residence. Harold then trained with Roger George in obstetrics. Frank Mossman, after an internship in Omaha, intended to train with Frink in chest surgery. Instead, on his arrival in Vancouver in 1946 he trained with Ullman in ENT. David Seligson took his internal medicine residency in the Northern Permanente Foundation Hospital after laboratory and hematological training in Utah. In collaboration with Grossman, he conducted research on amino acid metabolism in tuberculosis patients. At the completion of his residency, he accepted a position at Yale as professor of clinical pathology and internal medicine.

Rex Hamby, who had run the hospital at the Boulder Dam construction site for Six Companies, as well as the Desert Hospital for Garfield at Yuma, Arizona and the Mason City Hospital at Grand Coulee, continued in his role as hospital administrator. Sam Hufford, whose family owned a hotel in Stevenson, Washington and who had become acquainted with the Kaisers during construction of Bonneville Dam, was hired as Health Plan salesman under Manager Bud Bradley. Hufford later became the business manager for Health Plan and, later still, Vice President and Regional Manager of the Northwest Kaiser Foundation Medical Care Program. Bernice Oswald, formerly an IRS auditor, hired as chief accountant in 1945, was later elevated to regional controller. At the time, a woman in such a position was a rarity. (According to one oral history account, she and Lucille Ball were the only women allowed in the Kaiser Executive Dining Room in Oakland.) James DeLong, a student first hired in the shipyards as a chauffeur, served in the Air Force and went on to obtain a degree from the University of Portland. Hired as Permanente credit manager in 1948, he rose to administrator at Bess Kaiser Hospital (BK), a position he held from 1959 to 1977. In 1973, he served as President of the Oregon Association of Hospitals.

HANGING ON

The winter of 1945-1946 was a bleak one for the six doctors providing care for a Health Plan that had dipped to just 2,600 members. These were the beginning of hard times, and they were to continue through the 1950s. The Permanente physicians received no financial support from the Foundation or from Henry Kaiser; they were dependent on Health Plan dues—and on what they could earn through private practice fees—for their salaries. Morris Malbin regularly drove to McMinnville, where he maintained a part-time radiology practice; he contributed this income to the group. Saward and Grossman traveled to Pendleton and Umatilla, thinking they might open a clinic twice a week for the 2,000 workers building McNary Dam. Health Plan, too, struggled financially; when a portion of the roof blew off the hospital, Edgar Kaiser paid $6,000 from his personal funds for the repairs.

Saward and Frink devised another way to keep their small Health Plan afloat. Saward had experience in treating tuberculosis, Frink as a thoracic surgeon. Knowing that local Veterans' Administration (VA) hospitals were overcrowded, the two won a VA contract to care for World War II veterans, including returning prisoners of war who had contracted tuberculosis. The contract specified that the daily charge for care, including room and board, was $13. This fee covered hospital costs and gave the group some small additional earnings. These highly contagious patients—about 100—were confined to an isolated wing at the east end of the hospital. They were not an easy group to care for. No longer under military control, the men sometimes made unauthorized forays from the hospital. Some had to be released from jail and returned to the hospital. Then Saward would assume the role of adjutant general and hold a "court martial," employing young DeLong as "court reporter." Some of those who made unauthorized departures from the hospital simply disappeared.

In its treatment of tuberculosis, Northern Permanente Foundation Hospital was one of the first civilian hospitals to use streptomycin. Until 1947 standard treatment had been pneumothorax, phrenic nerve paralysis, and thoracoplasty. In time, as the medical community learned more about treating tuberculosis with a combination of drugs, patients no longer required hospitalization.

WRONG SIDE OF THE RIVER AND FAILURE TO THRIVE

Just as Garfield had feared, the location of the Northern Permanente Foundation Hospital in small-town Vancouver, rather than in Portland, significantly hampered membership growth. Portland residents were understandably reluctant to travel across the Columbia River to Washington for hospital care. Maternity patients who were Oregon residents objected to a Washington state birth certificate for their children. Whereas membership growth in California rose dramatically, membership in the Northern Permanente Health Plan remained dismally low for over a decade. So serious were the problems of membership that there was discussion about moving the Northwest organization to San Jose, California. Table 1 shows the marked contrast in membership growth between the robust California Regions and their anemic Northwest counterpart from 1945 to 1960.

Table 1. Membership growth in three Kaiser Permanente Regions: 1945-1960			
Year	Northern California	Southern California	Northwest
1945	12,000	3,000	10,000
1950	120,000	20,000	14,000
1555	302,000	199,000	23,000
1960	399,000	321,000	49,000

The Northwest Region suffered because of its isolation from Oakland, the center of influence for the growing Permanente Medical Care Program. Edgar Kaiser, previously helpful to them, was now in Michigan, his attentions turned to managing the Kaiser-Frazer automobile company at Willow Run. Saward recalled that among Kaiser's executives, only Ordway showed any interest in the struggling Northwest program. As part of his itinerary when he traveled to Hanford, where Kaiser engineers were now building nuclear reactors, he would stop in Portland to lunch with Saward. The 1949 balance sheet for The Doctors Clinic[3] showed that private and industrial patient care provided 30% of their income. Contracts with the VA and with Health Plan provided the remainder of the earnings. Expenses included wages, an automobile allowance, and medical society dues. Hope grew for a time when faculties at Reed College and Vanport College (later to become Portland State University) joined the Permanente program in 1945 and when the Bonneville Power Administration signed in 1947. Still, membership remained stubbornly stagnant.

Then, in 1950 the International Longshoremen Workers Union (ILWU) joined Health Plan. And although this was a boon to flagging membership, the agreement was not wholeheartedly embraced. Union President Harry Bridges was a tough negotiator and he insisted that his conditions be met: first, all union members, regardless of their health status, were to be accepted by the plan; second, there was to be no dual choice in health plans, a condition at odds with a sacred dual-choice feature of Permanente. In addition, Bridges demanded that the plan provide medical coverage for members along the entire West Coast—from Seattle to San Diego.

Despite their concerns about lackluster membership—especially now that the loss of the VA contract was imminent, many in the Medical Group approached the ILWU agreement warily. Bridges and his followers had a reputation for violent tactics to achieve their ends. Even more objectionable was his insistence that Permanente Health Plan be the sole provider of care for ILWU members. Saward was lukewarm about taking on the longshoremen, figuring (rightly, as it turned out) that they would tax the resources of the small Medical Group. Despite misgivings, the lure of the substantial infusion of new members proved, in the end, irresistible.

Permanente agreed to Bridge's terms. To ensure care for longshoremen throughout the Northwest, Garfield had to scramble; in doing so, he forged some innovative partnerships. He arranged for Group Health to provide medical care for 2,000 ILWU workers in Seattle. He contracted with Gray's Harbor Community Hospital to provide care for the 360 union members in Aberdeen, Washington. And he got Coos Bay Hospital Association to care for the 1,330 workers in and around Coos Bay. By 1952 unions would make up 25% of the Permanente Health Plan membership in Portland and Vancouver.

THE VANPORT FLOOD

Additional hardships were in store for the doctors. Vanport Hospital continued to struggle to provide services. Profitable for only three months of its four-year history, the hospital had been kept afloat primarily through provisions of the Lanham Act, which provided federal funds to build public housing for defense workers, and to build hospitals and day care centers. When, in 1946, the 1940 Lanham Act was suspended, a crisis loomed. The Housing Authority of Portland and medical staff searched for solutions. The Multnomah County Medical Society doubted the hospital's ability to become self-supporting; Oregon Physician Service had already abandoned the facility. At its lowest point, the hospital was offered to Vanport physicians for a mere $1 per year. There were no takers. Finally, the Northern Permanente Foundation reached an agreement with the Housing Authority, offering to keep the hospital open and agreeing to pay $1 per year and the additional utility costs. But even with these generous terms, the program was unable to break

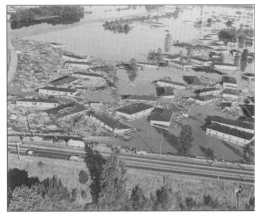

Aftermath of the Vanport Memorial Day Flood, May 30, 1948. *Courtesy of the Oregon Historical Society, OrHi 52427.*

even. Occupancy rates hovered at just 50%. To make financial matters worse, the hospital, rather than turning away non-paying patients, accepted all who came to its doors—a departure from the previous administration's policy. With few remaining options, Permanente received permission from the Housing Authority of Portland to limit its services at Vanport to outpatient and emergency services and to transfer all inpatients to its Vancouver hospital. On May 6 the transfer of patients took place—mere days before the calamitous flooding of Vanport.

Throughout the spring months of 1948, snow continued to fall in the Cascades. Even at the 2,000-foot level, the snow pack was unusually heavy. Then the weather turned suddenly warm, and the snow melted rapidly. This, together with heavy rains, caused a sudden rise in the Columbia River. By May 23, the swollen river was at flood stage, and officials called for evacuation of those most at risk from flooding. On May 27, flood conditions worsened, and calls went out to evacuate areas along the Willamette River in Southwest Portland. Two days later the river was six and a half feet above flood stage. Reports of looting in Camas and Washougal brought out the National Guard. Curiously, the city of Vanport was not thought to be in danger. Officials were lulled into a false sense of security by those who regularly patrolled the dikes and declared them to be sound. Then, on May 30, Memorial Day, at 4:17 p.m., a dike supporting the railroad that separated Smith Lake from Vanport gave way and water tore through the breech. The roiling torrent swept away houses and inundated buildings. Within ten minutes the water level in Vanport rose six feet. Residents fled for their lives.

Meanwhile, Harold Cohen and his wife were marking a pleasant Memorial Day at their Vancouver home, oblivious to the disaster unfolding across the river. Their holiday guests—a medical colleague and his family—had made the short drive from their Vanport home. It was only as they sat down to dinner that they learned from a radio broadcast of the flooding and realized that their home and its contents, including an original Norman Rockwell painting, were being swept away.

The following day, Cohen was forced to detour 100 miles to reach his Portland office from his Vancouver home. With the closure of the Interstate Bridge, his route required that he travel east to the Bridge of the Gods, then west along the Columbia River Highway to Portland. In the days that followed, Cohen sometimes stayed with colleague Frank Mossman who lived beside the Permanente Broadway Clinic. Grossman solved the problem of crossing the river by commuting by sea plane from Vancouver to Swan Island where he kept a car to drive to his Portland clinic. Bernice Oswald, chief accountant, was vacationing at the Oregon coast during the weekend of the flood. A Northern Permanente Foundation purchasing agent owned a plane and told Oswald to get to the Troutdale airport; he would fly her from there to Vancouver.

In the following weeks, DeLong and Oswald worked at the hospital, trying to make sense of sodden paper billing statements. DeLong later conceded that not all of the information they pieced together was accurate, but that they managed to collect on most, if not all, outstanding bills.

Flood conditions remained for nearly a month. By June 23 the Columbia River finally receded to safe levels and the salvage of what remained of the city began. Vanport was never rebuilt. Instead, the land gradually was converted to other uses: the Portland International Raceway, the Multnomah County Exposition Center, and Heron Lakes Golf Course.

. . . .

"… Homeless and scattered
Survivors left that dismal place
Where days after not even a rainbow would dare show its face
Portland opened its homes, its churches
The Y served daily meals
To the thousands of families who ran toward the hills
Red Cross was there too, helping a nation to see
A once hostile community
Responding with love
To this sad tragedy…"

— excerpts from *Vanport Voices*, copyright S. Renee Mitchell

. . . .

FIRST PARTNERSHIP

The reason for Neighbor's decision to leave the Medical Group in 1947 is not entirely clear. It is true that he was disillusioned with membership growth and had talked of returning to California. But Saward may have encouraged his departure. Saward was uncharitable in his assessment of Neighbor and characterized his leadership as ineffective. Other physicians contradicted Saward's view and defended Neighbor as an outstanding leader.

In any case, to encourage membership, a house was purchased on N.E. Weidler Street in Portland to be used as a temporary outpatient office. In 1947 a five-doctor clinic at 2606 N.E. Broadway was built, equipped with x-ray, lab, and pharmacy. Neither Garfield nor Neighbor had an Oregon medical license, a requirement for physicians employed in Oregon. Saward likely used this issue to leverage Neighbor's departure and the Medical Group's eventual break with Garfield, though Saward later cited Neighbor's stress-related pseudo angina and his frustration with conflicts among the physicians as reasons for his leaving. With Neighbor gone, Saward became Medical Director of the physician group and the Northern Permanente Foundation. Preparations then began to form an independent partnership.

In April 1948 the Board of Trustees of Northern Permanente Medical Foundation, meeting for the first time since its 1942 founding, gathered at the Oakland corporate headquarters around a large mahogany table in a meeting room overlooking the city and the San Francisco Bay. There Saward presented his case for partnership. Garfield did not support Saward's request. Nevertheless, The Permanente Medical Association Partnership became official on July 1, 1948. The partnership agreed to pay the Foundation a $5,800 monthly fee for office space and clerical support at the Northern Permanente Hospital and an additional $900 monthly rent for the Broadway Clinic.

No sooner had the partnership formed than the physicians had to confront serious disagreements about its mission and its elemental make up. Some advocated a private-practice model; others, like Noehren, envisioned a socially progressive practice. Other issues that aroused strong views were the optimal number of patients for each physician, the amount of time that should be allotted to each patient visit, and remuneration.

In February 1949 Saward was an overnight guest at Grossman's Berkeley home,[4] in preparation for another meeting with the Board of Trustees. The following morning both men appeared before the Board around the impressive mahogany table in the room with its expansive views. This time, however, Garfield was not present. As part of a reorganized agreement, those assembled agreed to rename the partnership The Permanente Clinic.

Grossman saw nothing unusual in the $1,500 check he received in the mail one month after this meeting. The accompanying explanation that the money was a return of his capital investment in the Permanente Medical Association seemed reasonable, a mere bookkeeping procedure, he thought. Then he received a warning from his friends Morris and Barney Malbin. They claimed that Saward appeared to be threatening Grossman's interest in the partnership. Only later did Grossman learn that his name had been omitted from the new partnership agreement. Looking back, Grossman said that these signals should have aroused his suspicions. As it was, on his return to Vancouver in September, he enjoyed a pleasant evening with Saward and several medical residents who

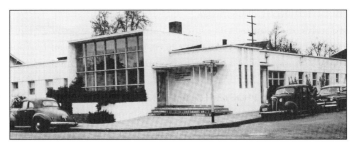

The Broadway Clinic offices, opened in 1947 as the first Kaiser Permanente facility in Portland, Oregon. *Courtesy of Kaiser Permanente Heritage Resources.*

were, he was told, interested in his research. The very next day the unsuspecting Grossman was caught by surprise when Saward, emboldened by advice from legal counsel, announced that Grossman was to be excluded from the partnership.

To this day, the reasons for Grossman's attempted expulsion remain unclear. Did Saward view Grossman as a threat to his leadership? Were Grossman's progressive, left-leaning politics too much

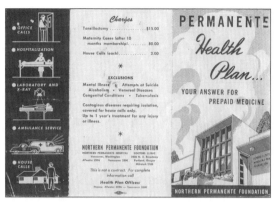

Permanente Health Plan brochure with illustration of the Broadway Clinic.

a liability to the image of the Medical Group? Was his leave of absence during a family illness seen as an abdication of his responsibility to the group? Whatever the reason, his supporters at the partnership meeting objected to his ouster. Morris Malbin asked that the group reaffirm Grossman as a member in good standing. Lucius Button and Frank Mossman also spoke up for Grossman. Saward's response was to call for a vote based on Capital Participation, a tactic that was skewed in favor of Saward's intent. A chorus of dissenters challenged this method of voting as unfair. Grossman, stunned by Saward's betrayal, was by no means prepared to accept dismissal. He announced his intention to mount a legal challenge, and on September 22, the Medical Group received a ten-page brief from Grossman's attorney Chester McCarty stating, in part, "He [Grossman] may seek either to enforce his partnership rights, or, if those are denied him, he may bring suit for an appropriate accounting and for damages against those who seek to exclude him. In my opinion such damages in this instance would be very substantial." Apparently not prepared to risk an expensive legal battle, Saward and his supporters retreated, and the partnership amended its agreement on October 17, 1948, to reinstate Grossman.

This divisive episode was by no means the end of conflict within the Medical Group. Grossman and the Malbins represented a progressive faction, perceived by their more conservative colleagues as too left leaning in their views. Saward, Frink, George, and Frederick Waknitz represented the core of the conservative pro-Saward faction. Votes on major issues were often seven to four, with Saward, George, Frink, and Waknitz in the minority. Looking back 40 years, Frink, in a 1985 memo to the author, characterized these years in the group's history as "years of severe turmoil. ... Ernie Saward's peculiar form of leadership was both a glue and a catalyst. ... Staff meetings often lasted until after midnight and all too often failed to solve controversial issues. When you read the word 'discussion' in the minutes, just think of the final minutes of a tied hockey game."

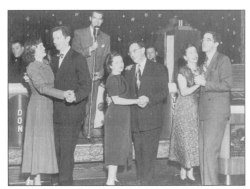

Three of the original Medical Group partners and their wives, 1948: (left to right) Mrs. and Charles Grossman; Mrs. and Barney Malbin; Mrs. and Morris Malbin.
Courtesy of Charles Grossman.

At the December 19, 1949 partnership meeting, Cohen nominated Button for the position of Medical Director. Predictably, Frink nominated Saward. The group elected Button by a vote of seven to three. Next came a motion to replace Saward as Medical Director of the Northern Permanente Foundation. This motion was narrowly carried by a six to five vote, but the tenacious Saward refused to submit his resignation. Hoping to force his removal, the group sent a telegram to Garfield requesting his help to replace Saward as foundation Medical Director. Garfield's reply was carefully worded: "Your wire received advising partnership vote recommending new Medical Director for Northern Permanente Foundation. This probably will require a trip to Vancouver to ascertain merits of such a recommendation. We will plan on doing so sometime in … January or February." True to his word, Garfield attended a special partnership meeting on February 27, 1950. After hearing both criticism of, and support for, Saward, Garfield told Saward's disappointed critics that, although he sympathized with the group's problems, these problems were not his business and must be handled internally. He likened the partnership to a marriage. He hoped that the partners could resolve their differences; failing that, they might find divorce a necessity.

With Garfield's reluctance to involve himself in the group's struggles, the partners again reviewed their options. They could dissolve the partnership and replace it with an organization that would give more authority to one or more leaders. (Saward himself suggested that Garfield take over leadership of such an organizational structure.) Or they could continue with the current partnership structure and remove Saward as Foundation Medical Director.

A March 3, 1950 letter from Garfield stated, in part, "I have discussed the problems that have recently developed at Northern Permanente with the Trustees [and have explained to them] that the medical partners had suggested a dissolution of partnership and a return to the former status where the partners would be employed by the Foundation or somebody suitable to the partners. It was the Trustees' decision that if this was the desire of the partnership that it should be tried as a solution for the impasse that has developed. It should be clearly understood by the physicians that *they* have requested this change from the Trustees."

Eleven attended a May 15 partnership meeting: Button, Cohen, Fell, Frink, Grossman, the two Malbins: Barney and Morris, Mossman, Saward, Ullman, and Waknitz. Cohen and others raised objections to Saward's awarding himself pay for administrative duties—pay that was intended for providing direct patient care. In substituting administrative time for patient care, he was violating partnership orders. The discussion grew heated. The impasse seemed impenetrable. Ullman moved to dissolve the partnership. Grossman moved to table the motion, and the vote to table was carried. Fell then moved to schedule more meetings to work through their differences. Saward and George were to represent one faction, Morris Malbin and Fell, the other. These attempts at reconciliation failed. A letter from one physician who left the group illustrates the rancor that permeated the partnership at the time. His bitterness is palpable. He refers to the controlling faction as "bastards" with "brutal personalities." He accuses them of not carrying their fraction of the burden, creating additional burden for "the socialistic, group-conscious members—the altruistic guys."

Finally, in a May 27 telegram to the group, Edgar Kaiser terminated the agreement with the Foundation, and the Medical Group reverted to a structure under the direction of Garfield. The following month, Garfield negotiated separate contracts with those physicians who wished to stay. Grossman, after an amicable meeting with Garfield, left the group for private practice and research at University of Oregon Medical School. Saward resumed his role as Medical Director. Eventually a new partnership formed, this time with a strong management structure: three permanent members of the executive committee—Saward, Frink, and George—and one elected member. Ultimately the Saward faction, outnumbered at first in the struggle for power, outlasted its adversaries. Saward, Frink, and George were among those who completed their medical careers with the Medical Group. The Malbin brothers, Button, and Mossman eventually left the group.

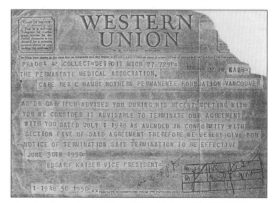

Termination telegram from Edgar Kaiser, May 27, 1950.
From the author's collection.

CHAPTER 4: THE FIFTIES: FIRM FOUNDATION

—~m~—

CONFLICT, CRISIS, COMPROMISE: THE PERMANENTE MEDICAL GROUP

At the same time that the Permanente physicians in Vancouver were forming a partnership plan, the Permanente Foundation Health Plan program in Northern California was undergoing a major reorganization. Sidney Garfield, who had easily managed the medical care programs in the Mojave Desert and at Grand Coulee, was finding it far more difficult to coordinate the growing Permanente program in Northern California. The Alameda County Medical Society continually opposed his efforts, bringing him before its ethics committee several times and going so far as to try to revoke his medical license.

As sole proprietor of Sidney Garfield and Associates, Garfield was an easy target for medical society attacks, so the Medical Group decided to restructure as a partnership. Unlike the Portland-Vancouver partnership whose formation had been protracted and painful, the new California partnership coalesced with relative ease. Cecil Cutting, Garfield, and others had only briefly discussed restructuring; Morris Collen remembered taking a phone call in the hospital dining room from a colleague who told him of the plan to form a partnership—the first Collen had heard of the idea—and asked if he'd like to join. A small nucleus of prospective partners scheduled several meetings and prepared the necessary documents. One day after Permanente Foundation Hospitals incorporated, the new partnership—henceforth to be known as The Permanente Medical Group—replaced Sidney Garfield and Associates. Each of the seven partners contributed $10,000 dollars. The 1948 reorganization of the Northern California Region now comprised three entities: Permanente Health Plan, Permanente Foundation Hospitals, and the newly formed TPMG. Hospitals were foundation-owned but hospital operated. (Garfield, in relinquishing his sole proprietorship of the Medical Group, received no remuneration. He did, however, retain a vested interest in the hospitals.)

Garfield's role was suddenly a problem. His dual responsibilities as executive officer in a nonprofit Health Plan and in a for-profit Medical Group appeared to some to represent a conflict of interest. To eliminate the problem, he resigned as a partner in TPMG but retained his position as medical director of both the Health Plan and Hospitals, a fine distinction that nevertheless remedied the perceived conflict of interest.

WHAT'S IN A NAME? KAISER AND PERMANENTE

Eighteenth century Spanish colonists called the creek in the hills south of San Francisco "Rio Permanente" because it flowed year round—unlike most streams in that dry country. In 1939 Henry Kaiser purchased the land adjacent to the creek for its rich limestone deposits—a necessary ingredient for the cement he produced in his Santa Clara plant. Both Henry Kaiser and Bess liked the Permanente name for its evocative metaphor. They began to incorporate the name in their companies: Permanente Cement Company, Permanente Metals Corporation, and the Permanente Steamship Company, where one of the ships was named the SS Permanente.

Throughout the war years, Kaiser-owned companies continued to use the Permanente name. Then, after the war, Kaiser's companies began to replace the name "Permanente" with "Kaiser." When the Portland-Vancouver Health Plan opened to the public in 1945, its principals wanted to call it the Kaiser Health Plan. But company executives had little faith in the Health Plan's future and feared that using the Kaiser name would associate the industrialist with a failed venture. It wasn't until 1952 that Southern California's Permanente Health Plan and Permanente Foundation Hospitals added the name "Kaiser" and not until 1960 that the less successful Northwest program was permitted to use the revered Kaiser name.

INTERNAL CONFLICTS

TPMG rejected the famous Kaiser name. For one thing, physicians in the partnership were unwilling to be perceived as employees of Henry Kaiser. For another, company administrators—most notably Henry Kaiser himself—had begun to make decisions that intruded on the autonomy of physicians in their medical practice. No longer merely a purchaser of health care, Henry Kaiser was beginning to insist on more direct involvement. Physicians reacted against this intrusion and a loss of autonomy they had enjoyed under Garfield.

When Kaiser's wife Bess fell ill, Garfield suggested that his wife's sister Alyce Chester become Bess's live-in, private-duty nurse. Chester cared for Bess during the last days of her illness; after her death in 1951, Kaiser married Chester, despite the 35-year difference in their ages. Then, a surprise to the physician group, Kaiser announced his intention to build a new hospital—one he intended as a showcase—in Walnut Creek, California. More surprising still, he appointed his new spouse de facto administrator. This decision, coming at a time when Garfield had already begun construction of hospitals in San Francisco and Los Angeles, deflected funds away from these projects. Physician reaction ranged from concern to outrage over these developments. Moreover, Kaiser's decision to build a hospital in rural Walnut Creek seemed to many physicians an irresponsible folly. Equally disturbing, it added to the physicians' growing perception that they were being marginalized from the decision-making process. Additionally, Kaiser began to recruit physicians from within their own ranks for a separate partnership and these newly recruited physicians were rumored to be at a higher pay schedule.

Collen met with Kaiser at his home and in the strongest terms told him that the Medical Group would not tolerate a separate partnership at Walnut Creek. Kaiser held firm, arguing with typical forcefulness that his executives had sufficient expertise to manage any enterprise, including a physician group, in which they had an interest. Collen countered that managing a health care system was a far different matter from overseeing the industrial businesses of ships, steel, and cement. Despite the strong position taken by the two adversaries, both knew that the physicians were vulnerable: Health Plan carried a debt of $14 million, and the guarantor of that debt was none other than Kaiser Industries. In addition, both men knew that Garfield's loose management style coupled with his casual approach to business matters was likely to scare away other potential lenders.

GARFIELD'S DILEMMA

Garfield had recommended that TPMG adopt the Kaiser name. He had supported the building of the Walnut Creek Hospital. Both stands had been unpopular with the physicians. Now, on the one hand, he found himself in conflict with his own Medical Group; on the other, his long-time champion Henry Kaiser was growing increasingly critical of Garfield's haphazard management style and his inattention to business matters. In another of his bold moves (one more example of his meddling in the eyes of the physicians), Kaiser hired Clifford Keene, Medical Director for the Kaiser Frazer Corporation automobile company at Willow Run, to administer the Health Plan. Kaiser's installation of Keene as assistant to Garfield was a screen; in fact, Keene was now Garfield's boss.

Resentful of Kaiser's intrusion in the affairs of their health care system, the Medical Groups in both Northern and Southern California refused to work with Keene. Exacerbating the tension, Kaiser immersed himself even more in the affairs of Health Plan. His growing personal involvement only increased fears among the physicians that they would become managed employees. When two of the founding partners resigned from the Medical Group, Bay Area newspapers pounced on the story, trumpeting the physicians' criticism of the program.

REFORMS

Garfield met with the executive committee to address the concerns that had led to the two resignations. The resulting reforms included these: TPMG was to be an independent entity—organized so as to recognize separate and equal status. Laboratory and x-ray services, physical therapy, and anesthesia were to be under the direction of the physicians. Contracts with membership groups were to be subject to approval by the Medical Group. No major expansion of membership was to occur without a corresponding increase in physician staff and facilities.

A "Statement of Fundamental Policies and Responsibilities to Provide Services for Kaiser Health Plan" was approved and ratified by TPMG and by Kaiser Foundation Health Plan in October 1953. Still, distrust lingered, and conflict flared a mere two months after ratification of the document when Kaiser Foundation Hospitals unilaterally appointed a hospital administrator. Never consulted in this appointment, hospital Medical Director Collen must have found this snub galling. Nevertheless, he continued in his role as a member of the Executive Committee and emerged as the chief strategist in the behind-the-scenes battle to prevent Kaiser's domination and control over the physicians.

THE TAHOE AGREEMENT: TEMPLATE FOR PERMANENTE MEDICAL GROUPS

The rejection by the Medical Group of Keene, its fading confidence in Garfield, and its perception that Kaiser wanted to treat physicians as employees caused the working relationship between physicians and administration to deteriorate still further. In April 1955, the organization suffered near paralysis. Expansion stopped. Membership growth stalled. Spending ceased. The Permanente experiment had reached a point of crisis.

TPMG called for a working council to resolve the conflict. On the council were Henry and Edgar Kaiser, Eugene Trefethen, attorney George Link, Garfield, Keene, and representatives from each of the three Medical Groups. May 12, 1955, the first of four sessions, was marked by hostility and confrontation. With some difficulty, Trefethen steered the discussion to agenda topics. At the second session, Henry Kaiser, used to having his way and impatient with those who opposed him, suggested that the doctors consider a buyout of the organization and proposed separate partnerships at each medical facility site. Dismissing these challenges as transparent bluffs, the council went on to discuss the pertinent issues: representation for policy-making decisions and management teamwork among Health Plan, Hospitals, and the Medical Group. The fourth and final session took place at Kaiser's mile-long waterfront estate at Lake Tahoe. It was here that the council made its far-reaching stipulations to preserve the medical program and to establish a permanent advisory council. This seminal event, thereafter known as the Tahoe Agreement, included representatives from Northern and Southern California Medical Groups, and Saward and Frink from the Portland-Vancouver physician group.

Unlike California's robust programs, replete with regional management teams, the Portland-Vancouver program was so small that Saward single-handedly managed all its affairs; Sam Hufford, Regional Manager in name only, followed Saward's instructions. Kaiser viewed the Portland-Vancouver program as insignificant. Still, he insisted that any agreement include all three regional areas. So, Saward and Frink attended the Tahoe sessions—though they were little more than bystanders, little consulted and largely unaffected by the resolutions made between California's Medical Groups and Kaiser. It would not be until the 1959 opening of Bess Kaiser Hospital in Portland that the Northwest program would be recognized as a success.

The terms of the Tahoe Agreement stipulated that Health Plan and TPMG were to remain separate and autonomous organizations. Collen was obliged to resign his position as hospital Medical Director in order to remain as TPMG Medical Director. Thus, his resignation was a formality, rather than a sign of protest, as some characterized it. Still another result of the Tahoe Agreement was the removal of Garfield from his previous positions and from day-to-day management. His new position better suited his recognized talents for facility planning, policy making, lobbying in Washington, and promoting Permanente to a national audience.

Subsequent advisory council meetings addressed capitation payments, minimal requirements for generating capital, incentive compensation, and a physician retirement program. In 1956 the council, deftly led by Trefethen, finally honed the Medical Service Agreement, the backbone for what would become longstanding cooperation between physicians and Health Plan. The Southern California Permanente Medical Group was the first to sign the agreement, effective January 1, 1957. Two years later, after much contentious negotiation, TPMG adopted the agreement. The Portland-Vancouver Medical Group did not adopt the Medical Service Agreement until 1961.

EXTERNAL PRESSURES: RESOLUTION 16 AND THE LARSON REPORT

At the June 1954 meeting of the American Medical Association in San Francisco, the New York delegation introduced Resolution 16—a challenge to Health Insurance Plan (HIP) of New York (later to become Health Insurance Plan of Greater New York), a prepaid group practice. The resolution cited as unethical those medical insurance plans that limited physician choice to a group practice panel. During these mid-century years, the AMA exerted enormous influence with the nation's physicians. If Resolution 16 were to pass, the Permanente Medical Groups would be seriously crippled in recruiting physicians. Permanente's Keene proposed an amendment to modify the resolution, which delayed a vote, thus sending the amendment to the judicial committee for deliberation. Given this additional time to oppose Resolution 16, Garfield, together with representatives of Health Insurance Plan of New York and the Palo Alto Clinic, prepared a brief to present to the AMA opposing Resolution 16. If unsuccessful, they determined to appeal to the Antitrust Division of the Department of Justice.

In 1955 the AMA appointed a commission on medical care plans, headed by Leonard Larson, MD, to study prepaid group-practice health care—specifically in areas of quality, differences among plans, and legal implications. The commission visited 22 health plans in New York City, St. Louis, Chicago, and Washington, D.C. On the West Coast, the commission studied the Palo Alto Clinic, TPMG in San Francisco and Oakland, and SCPMG in Los Angeles. The Larson Report, released in January 1959, found group practice to be ethical; moreover, it found the quality of care provided by these plans equal to and, in some cases, better than that found in most communities. Finally, the commission found group practice more likely to provide care to those who otherwise might not receive it than were physicians in private practice.

Later that year Garfield, Saward and Collen attended the AMA meeting in Florida, prepared to fight Resolution 16, and armed with recent rulings by the Washington State Superior Court that had found in favor of Group Health against King County Medical Society. To their delight, they learned that Resolution 16 had been withdrawn. Collen recalled in a 2005 interview, "Since we did not need to appear at the meeting, and we had reservations there for a few days, we did take the few days to celebrate and relax." The three promptly booked flights to Havana, where they savored their surprise victory in Cuba's warm sun.

PUBLIC IMAGE AND PHYSICIAN RECRUITMENT

By 1953 more than 600 Medical Group practices operated in the U.S., including Mayo Clinic, Cleveland Clinic, and Virginia Mason Clinic. Eighty-five million Americans were enrolled in medical insurance plans. Still, the established medical community considered the combination of prepayment, group practice, and comprehensive care for a single premium payment to be radical—verging on socialized medicine. Nevertheless, despite the staunch objections by fee-for-service physicians, the public was warming to the practical advantages of comprehensive care, prepayment, and group practice.

ABC's Chet Huntley, in a September 10, 1952 broadcast, praised the Kaiser Foundation Health Plan as an innovative way to provide health care to the American family. The June 20, 1953 edition of the *Saturday Evening Post* featured an article headlined "Supermarket Medicine," that began, "The biggest squabble in medicine today is over prepaid group practice." The article went on to describe several prepaid plans, including the HIP of New York, corporate-sponsored Endicott Johnson plan in Johnson City, New York, and the union-run Labor Health Institute in St. Louis. The article also featured the Kaiser Foundation Health Plans in California, Oregon, and Washington, with their combined membership of 345,000. The December 15, 1953 issue of *Look Magazine* included a four-page pictorial of Kaiser's Walnut Creek Hospital, describing "pampered patients" in a hospital providing care that "actually costs less than older hospitals."

Physicians and the public were drawn to the Permanente Foundation Health Plan. In a 2003 interview, Charles Varga's widow Jacqueline described Varga's path to The Permanente Clinic. After residency training, he set up a solo practice off Park Avenue in New York, but finding that business aspects of his practice interfered with the care he wanted to give his patients, he moved to Sheridan, Wyoming, joining a group practice. Not long thereafter, former classmate Gregory Slater told him about an opening with TPMG in San Francisco and an even more attractive offer as Chief of Pediatrics with The Permanente Clinic in Portland and Vancouver. He chose the Portland position and arrived in the city January 19, 1951—his wife's birthday. She recalled that their first home had a surprise in store. After weeks of typical Portland rain and mist, the weather cleared and they saw to their delight what had been hidden from them—a magnificent view of Mt. Hood from the windows of their new home.

Peter Hurst was a medic in the 11th Airborne Division serving in the Pacific during the war; he later graduated from University of Washington School of Medicine in St. Louis, Missouri. He was a co-discoverer of Maple Syrup Disease (Hurst-Merkle syndrome) when he was at Children's Hospital in Boston, Massachusetts. After reading about the Kaiser Permanente system on the West Coast he took a tour of the Northwest with his wife Lannie, visited Norbert Fell and Varga, and decided to stay. He moved into a tract home in Cedar Hills in July 1954.

Wisconsin native Lawrence Duckler's decision to become a doctor followed his experience as a combat medic in the Pacific during World War II. After medi-

cal school and a surgical residency, he deliberated between a surgical precep-
torship with The Permanente Clinic in Vancouver and a position in Boston. He
accepted the Permanente position in 1954, where he joined surgeon Gilbert
Rogers, a product of Chicago's Northwestern University.

Orthopedist Robert Rubendale, a poliomyelitis survivor who had participated
in naval medical service during the war, joined Permanente after completing orthopedic training in Schenectady, New York.

Surgeon Paul Trautman, a native of New Orleans, was another World War II
veteran. After his graduation from Tulane University School of Medicine, he
completed his surgical residency with Altan Ochsner at Charity Hospital and
Medical Center of Louisiana. It was Rubendale who persuaded Trautman to
leave private practice and join Permanente in Portland, which he did on his birthday June 1, 1955.

Internist Noah Krall, following
a stint in the U.S. Public Health
Service, looked at several group-
practice possibilities, including
Group Health in Seattle, where
his sister was a founding member;
TPMG in San Francisco; and The
Permanente Clinic. He chose The
Permanente Clinic and joined the
Medical Group in 1956.

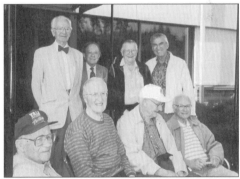

Within days of Krall's arrival,
internist Arnold Hurtado joined
the group as well, following a fellowship with hematologist Clementine Finch at the University of
Washington in Seattle.

Former 1950's staff of Northern Permanente Hospital
at final building closure August 2003. Back row (left to
right): Charles Grossman, MD; Laurence Duckler, MD;
James DeLong; Jack Hilbourne, OD. Front row: Noah
Krall, MD; Henry Kauitt, MD; Eckhard Ursin, MD;
Paul Trautman, MD. *From the author's collection.*

Eric Liberman, a 1954 Harvard Medical School graduate, left a private practice
in Connecticut for what he saw as a better way to practice medicine on the West
Coast. He joined The Permanente Clinic in April 1959—mere days before the
new Bess Kaiser Hospital (BK) opened.

Korean War veteran and Bronze Star recipient Charles Pinney tried private practice in Texas, then New York. Next, he worked at Fitzsimmons Army Hospital in
Denver, Colorado. As he was completing a pulmonary fellowship in Salt Lake City,
he learned about the Permanente program and moved to Portland in 1959.

Joseph Bilboa, who at age 17 contracted polio, was, despite his paraplegic condition, able to attend medical school at Columbia University College of Physicians

and Surgeons in New York and to complete residency training at Columbia University Medical Center. In the last year of his residency in 1959, he wrote to chambers of commerce in all 48 states for information about practice opportunities. He wanted a group practice in a geographic area with mild winters, and he narrowed his choice to California, Oregon, and Washington. Portland provided not only the group practice he sought but a radiology residency as well for his wife Marcia.

John Bondurant, whose Huguenot ancestors had fled to America in the late 1600s, decided with his wife Marjorie to move to the West Coast after residency training in Dayton, Ohio. They came to Portland and, against advice from contacts at Oregon Medical School, joined Permanente. Marjorie Bondurant later said in an interview that they were attracted by "… the opportunity to provide care without worrying about the patient's ability to pay." John Bondurant joined the Medical Group shortly before the 1959 opening of Bess Kaiser Hospital.

These physicians and others were attracted by one or all of the values of a system that featured medical economy, democratic treatment of patients, and group practice. All these features were solidly in place when the opening of Portland's BK ushered in an era of tremendous growth for KP in the Northwest Region.

BESS KAISER HOSPITAL

In 1955 Saward's concerns were far different from those expressed by the physicians of the California Medical Groups at the recently concluded Tahoe summit. If KP Northwest were to grow— if it were even to survive—a Portland-based hospital was an imperative. But how to finance it? Edgar Kaiser was sympathetic, but scarce resources were pledged to the robust California programs—specifically to a planned new hospital on Sunset Boulevard in Los Angeles. Few Kaiser executives were interested in the struggling, small Northwest program.

Then, circumstances intervened. Bess Kaiser's will had stipulated setting up a Kaiser Family Foundation. Largely through the influence of Edgar Kaiser and Clifford Keene, the foundation agreed to finance a Portland hospital. After a long search, during which a Lloyd Center site was considered and rejected, the foundation purchased a site in northeast Portland on a bluff overlooking Swan Island and the wartime shipyards for $25,000. But just when the long-held dream of a Portland hospital seemed imminent, Saward learned, to his dismay, that 60% of the funds earmarked for the Portland hospital—about 3.5 million dollars—would instead be diverted to the new Honolulu Medical Center. Disappointed but undeterred, planners arranged a loan with First National Bank.[1]

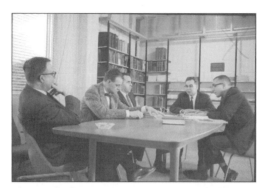

Physician leader meeting in Bess Kaiser Hospital library, 1960. (left to right) Noah Krall, Gilbert Rogers, Charles Varga, Ernest Saward, Arnold Hurtado.
Courtesy of Kaiser Permanente Heritage Resources.

During the construction phase, a large sign announced that the site was the new home of Bess Kaiser Hospital for members of the Kaiser Foundation Health Plan. Denounced as an impropriety by the fee-for-service medical community, the advertisement nevertheless drew 15,000 new members in the year leading up to the hospital's opening.

Garfield helped design the facility after a similar plan for the new Walnut Creek Hospital. As the first post-war Portland hospital, BK could boast numerous innovative design features. Its 130 beds occupied a 6-story inpatient wing. An adjacent outpatient clinic provided office space for 30 physicians. Inpatient nurses and physicians worked within a central core area. Patient rooms surrounded the work areas, giving clinicians easy access. Visitors, on the other hand, accessed each floor from the perimeter, walking along an outside corridor to approach patient rooms. All patient rooms were equipped with private telephones, television outlets, bedside cabinets with wash basins, electrically controlled window coverings and bed adjustments. The maternity unit's nursery was unique, designed with drawer bassinets that could slide from nursery to mother's bedside and back again. Built-in air conditioning was standard throughout the hospital and clinics, making BK the first fully air-conditioned hospital in the Northwest. A pneumatic tube system transported medical records, and an audio call system connected patients to the nursing station.

As construction progressed on the bright, white building, public interest mounted. Completion culminated in a dedication ceremony July 7, 1959, at which Garfield and his wife represented the Kaiser family. Ceremonies concluded with the unveiling of artist Virginia Saward's portrait of Henry Kaiser's

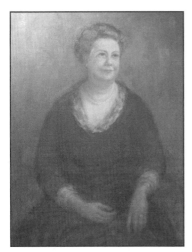

Portrait of Bess Kaiser by Virginia
Saward.

wife Bess. An imposing presence throughout
the 35-year life of the hospital, the painting
was relocated to Town Hall at the hospital's
1996 closure and to a permanent place at the
Center for Health Research for the anniversary exhibition of the Saward art collection.
During the first two days of the hospital's
grand opening, administrators and physicians gave guided tours to more than 30,000
curious visitors, creating traffic jams along
North Greeley Avenue. Saturday, July 11, saw
the transfer of patients from the old Northern
Permanente Foundation Hospital in Vancouver to BK.[2] And on that day, Lawrence Duckler performed the first surgical procedure at
the new hospital—on an infant with pyloric
stenosis, following a referral by pediatrician
Norbert Fell.

PART III:
PEOPLE, POLITICS,
AND PARADISE

CHAPTER 5:
VIENNA, VLADIVOSTOK,
AND VANCOUVER:
THE NORBERT FELL STORY

—ɱ—

Of all the journeys that brought physicians to Northwest Permanente (NWP), perhaps none was more compelling or more harrowing—with its elements of fear, courage, and luck—than that of the gentlemanly Norbert Fell. Born in Vienna in 1898, Fell was drafted into the Austrian army in 1916. Just 18 when he became a soldier, Fell quickly ascended the military ranks to become a lieutenant in charge of a company of Bosnian Muslims. Twice wounded at Trieste, once when he led his company to capture a hill and again when the bridge he stood on was destroyed by a dynamite blast, he recovered at a field hospital and made a pledge that should he survive his wounds, he would become a physician. Survive he did, and as a veteran he received the second-highest award of the Austro-Hungarian Empire. Returning home, he witnessed the awful aftermath of war: widespread poverty, hunger, and suffering. He resolved then to make good his promise, and he completed his medical training in Vienna in 1923. His eminent teachers included Clemens Pirquet, who introduced the tuberculin test and coined the word "allergy"; Karl Landsteiner, the developer of the modern system of blood group classification (A, B, AB, O); and the legendary Sigmund Freud.

By the late 1920s, Fell had a well-established practice in internal medicine and pediat-

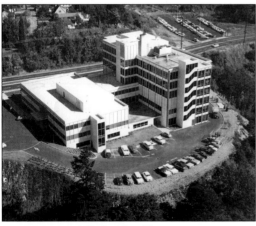

Bess Kaiser Hospital before the addition, circa 1960.
Courtesy of Acroyd Photography.

rics. During leisure hours he and his wife Jennie immersed themselves in Vienna's rich intellectual and cultural life. The family lived near Schloss Schonbrunn,[1] the magnificent Hapsburg summer palace west of Vienna; his son Alfred and daughter Alice played in its park and gardens. Later the Fells moved to Ausstellungsstrasse near the historic Prater with its landmark Ferris wheel and pleasure gardens. But ominous warning signs were there for those who were willing to see them; a calamitous bank failure, unemployment, and hyper inflation were causing political chaos in the provinces. The Nazi party was gaining a foothold among the Austrian citizenry, and its message attributing social and economic ills to Jews fueled the growing anti-Semitism. In 1934, Nazi conspirators assassinated Chancellor Dollfuss in an unsuccessful attempt to overthrow the government. By 1938 most Austrians, aware of neighboring Germany's economic and social improvements under Nazi leadership, were finding Nazi political messages increasingly attractive. On

March 12, Hitler moved his troops into Austria; that night thousands of Nazi thugs ran through the Jewish quarter of Leopoldstadt, looting shops and homes and beating hundreds of Jews.

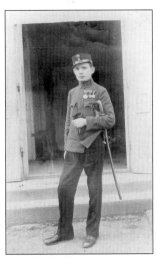

Norbert Fell in World War I Austrian Army uniform.
Courtesy of Alyce Fell Rene.

Fortunately for the Fells, they had an ally in a Catholic family, whose head—Leo—was a member of the Nazi party. When the government froze the assets of all Jews, Leo helped Fell recover his bank savings by telling authorities that the money had been a loan from Leo and therefore was rightfully his. Soon thereafter, on an otherwise ordinary day in July, Leo alerted Fell that Nazis intended to round up all Jewish physicians and dentists. Quickly gathering together his medical instruments, Fell said goodbye to his family and disappeared into the night. Traveling by train to Memel, Lithuania, Fell reunited with his family six weeks later. Then, fearful of a likely Nazi takeover of Lithuania, the Fells moved again in September—this time to Riga, Latvia. Two months later, Fell's wife learned that her father had been killed during the Nazi rampage of Kristallnacht.[2] In Latvia, Fell was unable to obtain a license to practice medicine, though he cared for numerous refugees and, through an intermediary in Sweden, surreptitiously obtained scarce sulfa drugs. Though he desperately wanted to emigrate, he lacked a sponsor and was thus unable to obtain visas for his family to the U.S.

Then, in 1939 came an announcement that visas were available for three teenagers; 15-year-old Alfred Fell obtained one of the three. Alone, the youth boarded a ship bound for the U.S. He spoke no English, knew no one in the U.S., and assumed he would never see his family again. He arrived penniless in New York. Years later, in an interview with the author, Alfred's sister Alice recalled her brother meeting with a Jewish farmer near Poughkeepsie, who offered Alfred work in an arrangement that provided the young Fell with room and board, though little else. Meanwhile, Fell continued his efforts to obtain visas to the U.S. Then Russia invaded Latvia in June 1940, further postponing the family's emigration plans. With the help of the American Consul, "an awfully nice guy," according to Fell, he and the rest of the family finally got visas and in August began their journey. They traveled by train to Moscow, then boarded the Trans-Siberian Railroad to Vladivostok, and from there traveled to Kobe, Japan. On their arrival in Kobe, the refugees were given a large single room, furnished with grass sleeping mats, and it was there that Fell experienced his first attack of Meniere's Disease. (Similar attacks would occur periodically for the rest of his life, though he would later control them with medication). After a two-week stay in Japan, the Fells joined a group of 21 other refugees and boarded a Japanese freighter bound for Seattle. Only later would they learn that this was the last group of Jewish refugees allowed to flee Europe via the eastern route through Russia, China, and Japan. It was a difficult voyage. Passengers endured severe seasickness and encountered a terrifying typhoon during the passage. Unlike the adults on board, the two children, 8-year-old Alice Fell and another girl of 4, remained remarkably well throughout most of the journey, succumbing neither to seasickness nor to the fierce assault by the typhoon. However, the girls did not escape entirely—both contracted severe cases of chickenpox.

Disembarking in Seattle, the refugees became wards of a charitable organization, the Hebrew Immigrant Aid Society (HIAS), that provided money, housing, and jobs to those in need. Fell wanted to go to New York, where he could take the medical board examinations; he was disappointed to learn that to receive HIAS aid, he would be obliged to move to Portland. Frustrated by the menial jobs they found in Portland, the family moved to New York where a relative made a meager living washing windows. Sleeping three to a bed in cramped quarters and demoralized by their reduced circumstances, they returned to Portland after six weeks and to an apartment on Southwest 2nd Street in what is now the downtown core area of the city. At the time, a bakery on the street sold rye bread, which marked the area as Jewish. The Fells hung on with menial jobs, Norbert sweeping floors and Jenny sewing in a local seamstress shop.

More bad luck followed: The Board of Medical Examiners would allow no refugee physicians to take the medical boards because of its previous experience with a refugee physician who was revealed to be a charlatan. Again disappointed, the Fells found work managing a small grocery store in an Italian neighborhood in Southeast Portland. Fell's wife learned English with an Italian accent and introduced cold-pressed coffee to Portland.

Two years went by, and at last Fell obtained a position as an extern at the Coffey Memorial Hospital (later Good Samaritan Hospital). In 1943, he secured a better paying job as night doctor for the Northern Permanente Foundation Hospital in Vancouver. After working for 18 months on the night shift, he finally earned a daytime office practice. The city of Vancouver had only two pediatricians at the time, and one of those had joined the Army. Because of the shortage, Fell was able to open a private pediatric practice, while maintaining his regular practice for Permanente members.

Years later, when Bess Kaiser Hospital opened in 1959, Fell remained at the outpatient department for the hospital as clinic leader for a group that included Ekhard Ursin,[3] Roger George, Mac Copeland, and Virginia Gilliland. Retaining two indispensable clerical employees and two top nurses, he was able to maintain an exclusively pediatric practice in Vancouver. Pediatrician Charles Varga provided the pediatric care for Health Plan members in Portland.

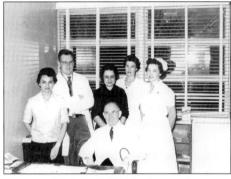

Vancouver Clinic Staff, 1961. Back row (left to right): Vi Mann; Ekhard Ursin; Roberta Arnold; Margaret Frederickson; Connie Sanders. Front row: Norbert Fell.

It was Fell who convinced Ernest Saward and Sidney Garfield that a church property for sale on Mill Plain Boulevard in Vancouver was an excellent site for a new medical office. With offices and exam rooms to accommodate four physicians, the Vancouver Medical Office opened in 1962. With its opening, the outpatient clinic at the Northern Permanente Hospital closed. Fell was consistently able to care for many more patients than was typical. Accordingly, the new medical office allocated him four exam rooms, two more than the standard two per doctor.

Fell was unfailingly genial and good humored, never displaying the underlying anger he felt because of the inhumanity he had seen and experienced. Known for the kindness and respect he showed to both patients and their families, he believed in the importance of caring for patients in their home surroundings and regularly made home visits.

Norbert Fell retired in 1973 but at the request of his department he continued to work part time for an additional year.

CHAPTER 6:
PARIAHS AND
PRESIDENTS

OPPOSITION TO PERMANENTE

On April 4, 1945 Sidney Garfield addressed the Multnomah County Medical Society at the University of Oregon Medical School auditorium, where he described the history and the principles of Permanente. Much of what he said that day was a repeat of a talk he had given the previous year at the annual meeting of the American Medical Association[1] before the Permanente plan opened to the public. He described his industrial medical care program as "applicable to the care of families of industrial workers and others." He tried to convince his audience that his plan was not socialized medicine at all but its opposite—a plan that would prevent government control of medicine. He told his listeners about a statement he'd heard the previous evening by John H. Fitzgibbon, MD, AMA delegate and reigning expert on medical economics, who had pronounced that "The most expensive thing in the hospital is an empty bed." Garfield told his audience that Fitzgibbon had been wrong. "He wasn't referring to our hospital. The most expensive thing in our hospital is a filled bed. This new economy is geared to the preventive medicine of the future. It puts the patient, the doctor, the hospital, the employer, and the insurance company all on the same side of the ledger. They all benefit by the patient remaining well."

Garfield went on to describe his health care program for workers in the Mojave Desert, at Grand Coulee, and in the shipyards in the Northwest and in California. In detail he explained the four principles: prepayment, group practice, prevention, and adequate facilities—physicians' offices, laboratory, x-ray, and hospital under a single roof. He explained to a wary audience that the salaried physicians of Permanente did not work for laymen, that Henry Kaiser did not dominate the Health Plan, and that The Permanente Foundation was a charitable trust whose accumulated funds paid for building construction, teaching, research, and rehabilitation of physicians returning from war service.

The next day, *The Oregonian*, under the headline "Socialized Plan Denied," quoted Garfield: "a chief aim of doctors everywhere is to prevent government medicine, and in our plan with its principles of group practice, prepayment, adequate facilities, and greater quality of medicine renders government control impossible." Despite his persuasive arguments, Society members remained unconvinced. Many years would pass before Permanente physicians would gain entry to Multnomah County Medical Society or to the influential AMA. Group practice continued to carry a stigma—one that extended even to those august institutions, the Mayo Clinic and the Mason Clinic.

ORIGINS OF THE AMERICAN MEDICAL ASSOCIATION

To understand the opposition by the AMA to prepaid group practice, one must examine its origins, growth, and eventual power. In 1846 a group of young physicians were determined to organize a national medical association. Meeting in New York, the group wanted to standardize the curriculum for medical training, create a code of ethics, and exclude sectarian practitioners who promoted Thomsonian (botanic) and homeopathic methods, including emetics, hot baths, and herbal remedies—treatments that the more educated physicians derided. This first attempt to influence medical practice failed, and sectarian practitioners continued to ply their remedies and to thrive. By 1900 the AMA had attracted only 8,000 members, whereas local societies could count 33,000. More galling still to those who wanted to elevate the practice of medicine, fully 77,000 practitioners were without any professional affiliation at all.

GROWING AMERICAN MEDICAL ASSOCIATION POWER

Near the end of the 19th century, university medical schools began to improve their curriculums.[2] A national association, to become known later as The Association of American Colleges, replaced the standard two-year medical degree with more stringent requirements of three or more years. The AMA joined the effort to improve medical education and, in 1904, created a Council on Medical Education to standardize and to improve medical training, requiring a four-year undergraduate degree and an additional four years of medical school. The Council then began to inspect and to grade these schools. As a result, many schools failed to meet new requirements. The 1910 Flexner Report, the work of Johns Hopkins educator Abraham Flexner, exposed inferior schools. An astonishing 100 of 130 medical schools closed their doors. The Federation of State Boards began to adopt the AMA's ratings of schools, and the AMA became the regulating body for the nation's medical schools. The growing power of the AMA was reflected in its membership; by 1910, 70,000—half of the nation's physicians—were affiliated with the AMA.[3]

Even as the AMA gained strength, however, competitors abounded. Patent medicine marketers were even more influential than sectarian practitioners. Not only did they advertise their nostrums in newspapers and magazines, but they freely dispensed medical advice as well, exhorting the public to avoid what they saw as harsh—even toxic—medicines and invasive surgeries performed by physicians. (To be fair, there was legitimacy in much of the criticism of the medical profession in the early years of the 20th century; doctors continued to rely on 18th-century methods like blood letting and purging. As late as 1917, the eminent Sir William Osler recommended blood letting as a treatment for pneumonia.) Hucksters of patent medicines touted "MicrobeKiller," a mixture of water, red wine, and traces of hydrochloric and sulfuric acids in the treatment of infectious diseases. "Lydia Pinkham's Vegetable Compound" (whose main ingredient was alcohol) was said to be effective for female illnesses. The gullible public swore by the benefits of hundreds of other concoctions, with names like "Turlington's Balsam of Life," "Steer's Genuine Opedelor," and "Hoodwink's Sarsaparilla."

To combat the proliferation of patent medicines, the AMA declared unethical the sale of medications whose formulas were secret. It demanded that the composition of all preparations be known and compounded by a pharmacist. These included the opiates morphia and heroin, strychnine, quinine, arsenic and even aspirin, which made its debut in 1900. Then the popular press joined the physicians to expose unregulated patented medicine. With its now considerable financial resources, the AMA established a Council on Pharmacy and Chemistry and published New and Nonofficial Remedies (NNR). Now manufacturers who wished to be listed in the NNR had to disclose a medicine's composition, defer false advertising, and engage in no direct marketing. (In 1912 the Portland Medical Society persuaded *The Oregonian* newspaper to ban advertisements by fraudulent practitioners and medicines.) In 1906 Congress passed the Pure Food and Drug Act—the beginning of federal regulation.

THE COMMITTEE ON THE COST OF MEDICAL CARE

In 1926 concerned about the availability and cost of medical care in America, 15 physicians, economists, and public health officials established the Committee on the Cost of Medical Care to conduct a five-year study. Ray Lyman Wilbur, Stanford University President and former AMA President, chaired the committee. The study published in 1932 reported that the nation's medical needs were not being met and recommended increased financing for medical care. Notable for its endorsement of prepaid group practice, the report also recommended that medical centers incorporate ancillary departments. These three principles— group practice, prepayment, and centralized medical facilities—were the very ones that Garfield was to advocate in the next decade. Despite the distinguished makeup of the committee, the now influential AMA opposed the committee's recommendations; and largely because of AMA influence, the extensive report languished in obscurity, its recommended reforms largely ignored.

AMERICAN MEDICAL ASSOCIATION CODE OF ETHICS

The AMA Code of Ethics published in 1934 took direct aim at prepaid, group-practice medicine. Its ten principles sought to regulate physician practice, the first principle stating, "all features of medical service in any method of practice should be under the control of the medical profession." The next insisted that institutions for medical care be an extension of the physician's armamentarium and that no third party come between patient and physician. Patients were to have freedom to choose their physicians; the private relationship between patient and practitioner was fundamental. The Code condemned as unethical a physician working for an organization; a physician employee whose services were a commodity would lead to poor-quality medicine. Principles 6 and 8 held economic implications: patients were to pay at time of service, and physicians were not to provide service for less than those fee schedules established by the local medical community. Despite the AMA Code of Ethics, various medical care programs—especially on the West Coast—disregarded the AMA code and continued to flourish.

THE COLD SHOULDER

Some physicians graduating after World War II were attracted to Permanente Medical Groups because they were scornful of local medical politics within established medical societies. Others who joined found painful their isolation and their exclusion from professional societies. Still others surmounted these barriers, finding ways around restrictions. Paul Trautman, prevented from transferring his membership in the New Orleans Parish Medical Society, attended the Portland Surgical Society meetings as a guest. Radiologist Henry Kavitt allied himself with an influential sponsor and thus gained entry to the local medical society.

In the main, though, Permanente physicians were ostracized, both professionally and socially. Moreover, the cold shoulder extended to spouses and children of Permanente physicians. One such snubbing occurred at a reception following a performance at the Fox Theatre when the President of the Multnomah County Medical Society's Women's Auxiliary approached Lanni Hurst. "I understand you are a doctor's wife. You must join our auxiliary. Where is your husband's office?" Told that Hurst's husband was a Permanente physician, the woman's face froze. She turned and walked away. Pediatrician Fred Colwell's children were taunted by schoolmates as communists and reds. Despite these rejections, Permanente physicians persevered. Peter Hurst gained entry in the local pediatric society and found an assignment as clinic instructor at the medical school. Paul Trautman recalled that on moving to Portland to join The Permanente Clinic, he contacted a classmate and close friend from medical school, only to be told that the friendship could not survive Trautman's Permanente affiliation. Another friend was more accepting; a former high school classmate, now a local surgeon, he welcomed Trautman to Portland and was eager to renew their old friendship. Permanente physicians could cite numerous examples where local physicians befriended them and encouraged their admission to professional organizations.

MEDICARE BATTLES

In 1958 the powerful AMA, mounting a massive campaign, prevented passage of a federal program to cover hospitalization costs for the elderly. But progressive change was in the air. The 1960s saw a groundswell of support for a national medical care program. Congress passed the Medical Assistance for the Aged Act—better known as the Kerr-Mills Bill—in 1960 to increase federal funds for state welfare programs to the aged poor. Oregon took advantage of the bill. President Kennedy, meanwhile, was promoting a more universal program linked to Social Security (King-Anderson bill S. 909 and H.R. 4222). Though organized medicine gave tepid support to the Kerr-Mills Bill, it vigorously opposed the expansive King Bill. The December 1961 *Multnomah County Medical Society Bulletin* announced newly formed national and state political action committees to fight the King-Anderson Bill. It quoted the Oregon State Medical Association Women's Auxiliary President, who warned, "Our husbands are in a political fight for their professional lives" and who urged readers to mount "… a vigorous program … to turn back the forces that would transform medicine from a free profession to a controlled trade." A subsequent *Multnomah County Medical Society Bulletin* announced a report to be given by internist Edward Rosenbaum: "The inside story of how so-called forces of liberalism prevailed with strong-arm tactics at the recent White House Conference on Aging will be unfolded in alarming detail at the March 7 general membership meeting of the Multnomah County Medical Society. Wives are urged to attend."

Actor Ronald Reagan joined the chorus of those opposed to federal funding for health care. Having recently produced a record, "I Speak Against Socialized Medicine," to be used, he said, by "medical auxiliaries to acquaint housewives of the dangers of federal intervention in medicine," he concluded a speaking tour in Oregon to deliver his message. Multnomah County Medical Society paid him tribute by making him an honorary member. Many Permanente physicians supported Medicare and indeed Saward was a member of the Physicians Committee For Health Care for the Aged Through Social Security.

Voices in support of Medicare appeared in a full-page endorsement of the program in *The Oregonian*. The list of supporters included 18 Permanente physicians. Arnold Hurtado advocated for Medicare in a public debate with Edward Rosenbaum. At the 1961 AMA annual meeting in Portland, Peter Hurst and Noah Krall stood at the entrance of the Coliseum, holding signs supporting Medicare. As the physicians' wives were passing to attend some AMA function a few spat upon Hurst and Krall. Hurst later recalled that at a reception at the Civic Theatre, he found himself in formal introductions with one of the ladies who had spat upon him.

FROM REJECTION TO ACCEPTANCE AND RESPECT

Restrictions of Permanente physicians from membership in the Multnomah County Medical Society were taking a toll. Permanente surgical specialists could not qualify for specialty boards unless they belonged to a medical society. Permanente urologist Luis Halpert submitted his application, sponsored by Portland urologist Arnold Rustin, on February 16, 1963. He waited in vain for a response. Twenty-two Permanente physicians then applied en masse and, when they received no response, they threatened legal action. At last the society replied that it would accept individually submitted applications. Byron Fortsch, formerly a probationary junior member in private practice, applied, together with orthopedist George Adlhoch and obstetrician Harold Cohen. All three were accepted. Gradually more Permanente physicians joined. A tangible sign of warming relations toward Permanente occurred when, in 1967, Multnomah County Medical Society President Louis Maclan attended a staff meeting at Bess Kaiser Hospital to solicit members. (That year, too, AMA President Charles M. Hudson paid a courtesy call to The Permanente Medical Group in Northern California.)

In 1972 irascible, outspoken Permanente internist Charles Pinney[4] won a two-year term as Multnomah County Medical Society trustee, and Permanente physicians secured six committee assignments. Harvey Klevit was one; his assignment was to the grievance committee. (Klevit would go on to serve successive terms as trustee, secretary, and treasurer.) Though he declined the traditional step of ascending to the presidency, he resumed his trustee position and served on both peer review and grievance committees.

In 1976 Marvin Goldberg left his position as Medical Director of the Southern California Permanente Medical Group in San Diego to become the Northwest Permanente Medical Director of The Permanente Clinic. On assuming the position, he urged Permanente physicians to become more active in the medical community and encouraged them to obtain leadership roles in local medical societies. To help achieve this goal, the Board of Directors authorized payment of medical society dues for Permanente physicians. By 1978 both Trautman and Klevit were trustees; both held committee assignments as well. Goldberg secured positions on the public relations and public policy committees. Maurice Comeau, a member from his medical student days, became active on various committees. Curiously, Comeau had not been identified as a Permanente physician. One day, he recalled, a society member suggested in a conspiratorial aside, "We've got to do something about these Kaiser doctors." When Comeau explained that he, himself, was a Permanente physician, his nonplussed fellow member struggled to recover from his gaffe: "You don't look like a Kaiser doctor," was all he could think to say.

Northwest Permanente physicians continued to be represented in local and state medical associations. In 1980, Goldberg, like Pinney, Klevit and Trautman before him, became a Multnomah County Medical Society trustee. The OMA included four Permanente delegates: Comeau, Duckler, Goldberg, and Trautman. That year, OMA President psychiatrist Guy Parvaresh, addressed the growing influence of HMOs in the community—most notably Kaiser Permanente. "Kaiser Permanente," he said, "is a formidable competitor about which many doctors know little .... Uninformed general comment, indiscriminate resolutions, and unfair legislation is not the appropriate way to address this competition." After these seemingly conciliatory opening remarks, however, he leveled his criticisms. He cited as unfair a federal government ruling, as well as pending legislation, that would exempt health maintenance organizations from obtaining a state certificate of need—a requirement for other hospitals.

This critical point of conflict between the medical societies and NWP culminated in an exchange of letters between Portland physician Ralph Crawshaw and Permanente's Goldberg published in the 1981 edition of the *Portland Physician*. In their debate, Goldberg pointed out that the Multnomah County Medical Society did not provide service to NWP. Crawshaw charged KP with not accepting its share of indigent care. In one letter, Crawshaw seemed to try to reach across the divide, reflecting that in Hippocrates' time, there had been a place for both fee-for-service and salaried physicians and for conceding the necessity for both approaches in modern societies.

In the end, however, these attempts at rapprochement were undermined by the Medical Society's continued lobbying against legislation beneficial to KP—the certificate-of-need exemption and the Medical Society's sponsorship of BestCare were central sticking points. A confrontation between the society's President and NWP Medical Director Goldberg at the Multnomah

Athletic Club brought the long-simmering conflict to a climax, after which NWP withdrew from local medical society activities and ceased its policy of subsidizing medical society membership dues for Permanente physicians.

PRESIDENTS

Attitudes toward NWP underwent a transformation in the late 1980s. In 1988 at the Multnomah County Medical Society began to eagerly court Permanente physicians. Overtures started with a call to BK Area Medical Director Allan Weiland from the Medical Society's Executive Director Brad Davis, inviting Weiland to serve on its Board of Directors. Interested but with his hands full because of the region's nursing strike, Weiland approached BK's Chief of Ophthalmology Ernest Aebi to assume the position on the Board.[5]

Aebi had previously enjoyed a private practice and had been a member of both the Multnomah County Medical Society and the OMA. Not surprisingly, he, like so many others, had held a prejudice against Permanente. He recalled that as a student working as an orderly at Physicians and Surgeons Hospital, he routinely heard disparaging comments about KP. It was his medical school classmate and friend Maurice Comeau who convinced him to try working within NWP. Thinking at first that his time would be temporary, he joined Bobby Nevill, Craig Sutton, and William Harris in the Ophthalmology Department. To his surprise, he found the organization impressive.

Weiland's choice of Aebi for the position with the Medical Society was politically shrewd. Aebi's time on the Board marked the beginning of improved relations between the Medical Society and Permanente. In 1993, he became treasurer; in 1995, secretary; and in 1996, the first Permanente President of what had now become the Medical Society of Metropolitan Portland (MSMP). In his inaugural address (Appendix 3), he gave a brief history of NWP. He reminded the group that in the not-so-distant past Permanente physicians had been barred from membership in the Society; that times had changed in that interim; and that physicians must come together to deal with challenges in the delivery of medicine. The medical society newsletter *Scribe* reported, "Aebi offered a historical and often times amusing perspective on KP's early years in the Northwest, recalling how the state of Washington tried to stop the HMO's development by charging Kaiser doctors with practicing medicine for a salary."

Other Presidents would come from within the ranks of NWP. Otolaryngologist Colin Cave was one. He had become interested in national and state politics during his medical school training. Joining the California Medical Association, his enthusiasm for that group lessened because of its sheer size. Moving to Oregon and joining NWP in 1994, he found that the smaller county and state medical societies were more cohesive and more relevant to problems in the community. With encouragement from Maurice Comeau, he joined the Medical Society, progressing quickly to leadership positions—both in the local society and in the OMA: a delegate to OMA, 1995; MSMP trustee from 1996 to 1998; OMA trustee 1998 to 2001; speaker of the OMA house of delegates 1999 to 2001. In 2001, the MSMP elected Cave President; his inaugural event at the 116th annual meeting was at the Portland Art Museum, where two Permanente physicians— pianist Ron Potts and violinist George Oh—were part of the entertainment. Following his term as Medical Society President, Cave turned his attention to the OMA, becoming President in 2004. In office, he made his top priority to reestablish caps on noneconomic malpractice awards, becoming chief petitioner for Oregon Ballot Measure 35; with help from Peter Bernardo,[6] he led a campaign that raised more than $6 million to bring about liability reform (the measure lost by less than 2% of the 1.72 million votes cast in the election).

Like Cave, anesthesiologist David Watt had gravitated to local medical politics even before he joined NWP in 1991. Watt's testimony in response to an anti-HMO ballot initiative was instrumental in defeating the OMA resolution in support of the measure. Then during Cave's tenure as President, Watt maintained NWP's involvement by becoming the local medical society trustee. He was installed as its 121st president in 2005.

Permanente physicians in Clackamas County made even earlier inroads into leadership roles in local associations. When Kaiser Sunnyside Medical Center opened in 1975, physician leaders encouraged involvement in local and state societies. Emergency Care physicians Dean Barnhouse and Michael Hoevet were elected Presidents of the Clackamas County Medical Society—Barnhouse in 1986 and Hoevet in 1988. In addition, gastroenterologist Charles Zerzan and Barnhouse were both delegates to the OMA for many years.

CHAPTER 7:
ISLAND PARADISE

—〰—

KAISER HONOLULU MEDICAL CENTER
AND PACIFIC MEDICAL ASSOCIATES

Most people, even those long associated with Kaiser Permanente, would be surprised to learn that Northwest Permanente played a significant role in helping to develop and stabilize the emerging Hawaii Region of KP. Henry Kaiser first visited Hawaii in 1940. Ostensibly on vacation with his wife Bess, he nevertheless managed to conclude some important business, arranging to supply cement to better fortify Pearl Harbor and to install storage silos for the cement that his California plant produced. Thus, Kaiser's economic ties with Hawaii predated 1945, when his Permanente cement helped rebuild Pearl Harbor. At one time, he had even considered establishing a shipping service to Hawaii. In 1950 he returned to the island, undoubtedly exploring the terrain for additional business opportunities. By now, he was well known for his successful entrepreneurial achievements and he was courted by local business leaders and local reporters.

In December 1953 he visited Hawaii again, this time with his second wife Alyce. Two months later, the couple purchased a spectacular house in the heart of Honolulu—a first step toward transferring Kaiser's personal head-quarters to the island. Next, noting the limited hotel accommodations for visitors to the island, in 1955 the restless industrialist bought the decrepit Niumalu Hotel and Waikiki beach property and began its transformation into the sumptuous Hawaii Village Resort. A new 100-room hotel sprang up in just 89 days; the complex would eventually feature a convention center with a 1,000-seat auditorium, 70 thatched-roof cottages and a 14-story residential building. Other ventures included a Permanente Cement Company plant (sporting pink cement trucks), radio and TV stations, and a tour-boat business. But his most ambitious undertaking was a 6,000-acre residential development, Hawaii-Kai, between picturesque Maunalua Bay and Kuapa Fishpond, and near his own estate on Portloch Road.[1]

Busy as he was with these entrepreneurial enterprises, Kaiser continued to nurture his long-held interest in health care. In January 1955 the Hawaiian

Medical Association (HMA) appealed to him not to introduce a health plan in Hawaii. Kaiser's response was to suggest that the HMA establish a health plan that offered prepayment and group practice; he even offered to cooperate in the venture. When he received no response from HMA, he decided to forge ahead with his plan. Ignoring a Stanford Research Center study that concluded that Honolulu's Queen's Hospital was adequate for the Region's existing and future needs and that the Hawaiian Medical Service Organization health insurance plan was doing a good job, in 1958 Kaiser broke ground on the 10-story, 150-bed Honolulu Medical Center at Ala Moana Boulevard on the waterfront overlooking Ala Wai Yacht harbor near Waikiki Beach. He began the project without first having organized a health plan, without having planned for medical services, without having obtained a full set of architectural plans, and without having gotten approval by the appropriate Honolulu authorities. To call the undertaking audacious would be a vast understatement. This single venture reveals the legendary Kaiser: the supreme self-confidence, the indefatigable energy, the fearlessness in taking on new challenges—often with little or no experience in the business that attracted his interest.

He began by approaching three socially prominent local physicians: orthopedist Richard Dodge, general surgeon Richard Durant, and pediatrician

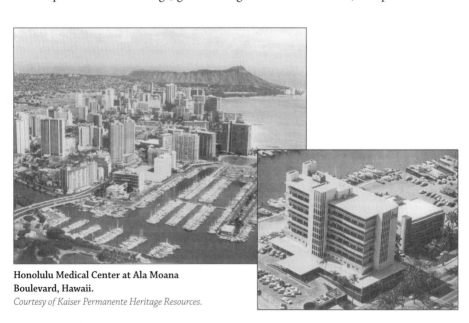

**Honolulu Medical Center at Ala Moana
Boulevard, Hawaii.**
Courtesy of Kaiser Permanente Heritage Resources.

W. B. Herter.[2] He proposed a partnership, whose features were to include prepayment and salaried physicians. Making his case to physicians long indoctrinated with a fee-for-service tradition might have seemed futile, but the three physicians were swayed, as one of them later said, by "the tycoon with unlimited resources" who seemed to be single-handedly changing the face of Hawaii. The new partnership, called Pacific Medical Associates, soon added general practitioner Homer Izumi and surgeon Samuel Yee. (It was thought that including Chinese and Japanese principals would attract more business in a multiethnic Hawaii.) Then, Kaiser flew Clifford Keene and Health Plan attorney Scott Fleming from Oakland's central office to teach the five partners the intricacies of prepaid group practice. Keene and Fleming delivered a series of evening lectures—a crash course—on the new practice model over the course of two weeks.

PROBLEMS

Problems arose quickly with the realization that Sidney Garfield's innovative hospital design—so effective in the Pacific Northwest and in California—was ill suited for Hawaii. The lava rock exterior failed to comply with city codes, and was an attractive haven for rats. Tropical storms battered the outside access to patient rooms, causing flooding to interior hallways. Elevators were too small to accommodate patients on gurneys, the kitchen was inadequate, and halls lacked air conditioning.

The Medical Group structure, too, became problematic, aggravated by the slow growth of the new Health Plan. Dissatisfaction arose among the nascent Medical Group. The newly employed physicians felt overworked and underpaid, and the 5 partners failed to enjoy the extra earnings they had anticipated. In 1959 at Edgar Kaiser's request, Saward visited the hospital and medical center. Meeting with the partners, Saward observed a Medical Group in trouble. He arranged to spend a month working as a practicing physician at the medical center. Though he publicly called the reason for his long stay a learning experience, in fact he was there to observe the physicians and to report his findings to Keene. During the month-long immersion in the day-to-day operation of the medical center, he assessed the capabilities among the employee physicians and tried to determine who among them could be groomed as future leaders. His overall conclusion was that the five partners were exploiting the salaried physicians. Primarily interested in their own private practices, they showed little interest in the views of the physicians in their employ.

SAWARD TO THE RESCUE

In July 1960 growing problems within the physician group erupted when the five partners demanded an increase in compensation. In response, Keene terminated their agreement, gave the partners notice to vacate the premises, and invited the 33 remaining salaried physicians to form a new Medical Group. Keene believed Saward was the right person to assume the position of acting Medical Director, given Saward's strong leadership of the Medical Group in the Northwest and his proven ability to deal effectively with problems. Attending a management course at Cornell in Ithaca, New York, Saward got a telephone call from Keene directing him to report immediately to Hawaii. During the next six months Saward and Bess Kaiser Hospital Administrator DeLong divided their time between the Portland and Hawaii operations, alternating between the two locations at two-week intervals, and camping on the ninth floor of the Honolulu Medical Center. Saward's principal role, he later recalled, was to advise the Medical Group regarding "how to run the hospital, how to promote the health plan and how to motivate the physicians." He and DeLong initiated a remodeling of the hospital, centralized the appointment center and reorganized the medical records system. Saward even suggested that the Hawaii and Oregon Regions merge, but that idea was unpopular with both the Hawaii and Oregon physicians. Bess Kaiser Hospital, opened the

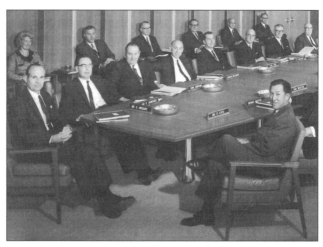

Kaiser Foundation Health Plan Board meeting, 1966.
Courtesy of Kaiser Permanente Heritage Resources.

previous year in Portland, was financially stable and the Northwest Region opposed taking on the risk of the Hawaii organization, beleaguered as it was with conflict and debt.

The reorganization effort increased tensions to a near boil. Some employees remained loyal to the five partners. One administrator, a close personal friend to one of them, opposed the changes and sabotaged them when she could. Keene himself took over the management of Health Plan and, together with Scott Fleming, sought a settlement with the fired partners who reacted with a lawsuit claiming damages. *The Honolulu Star-Bulletin* eagerly reported the dispute and ran headlines for seven nearly consecutive days in August 1960.[3] Its press releases brought unwanted media attention to the conflict until Kaiser, with his influence, including ownership of a television and radio station, managed to extinguish it. The dispute was eventually settled out of court.

Surgeon Phillip Chu, hired in 1959 by Pacific Medical Associates, joined the newly formed Hawaii Permanente Medical Group (HPMG) in 1960 as its first Medical Director.[4] Saward spent considerable time coaching Chu, borrowing from his own leadership model in the Northwest, which featured a strong, centralized authority. Under Chu's leadership, the Hawaii Region would achieve stability and growth and, although his tenure was cut short by his untimely death, he would become an icon for the HPMG.

The Southern California Permanente Medical Group sent physicians to Hawaii to provide temporary help during this time. The Permanente Medical Group, however, perhaps still smarting from Kaiser's earlier effort to establish a separate partnership at Walnut Creek, refused to support another health care project where Kaiser had acted unilaterally. Several of The Permanente Clinic physicians traveled to Hawaii to bolster physician services. Saward asked for volunteers who were willing and able to relocate to Hawaii for short periods to see patients in support of the Medical Group.

Like Saward and DeLong, their temporary living quarters were on the ninth floor of the hospital just steps away from Waikiki Beach. Pediatrician Fred Colwell, a swimming enthusiast, and internist Ekhard Ursin, hit the beaches after office hours ended at 4:00 p.m. Internist Noah Krall, after a day's work, mingled with others at the dinner party at Kaiser's magnificent Portloch Estate. Internist Arnold Hurtado found the multicultural city appealing. Surgeon Norm Frink recalled his scheduled visits to what seemed an island paradise; flying from Portland, he found a lineup of surgical cases awaiting him at the hospital. He spent a week performing surgeries, then returned to Portland.

HARD TIMES AND GOOD TIMES

Predictably, the established medical community viewed Permanente physicians with hostility. One local physician, incredulous that general practitioner William Dung had joined Permanente, asked him bluntly, "Why are you committing professional suicide?" Others made life difficult in more subtle ways. Permanente's only orthopedist, for example, Grant Howard, on call 24 hours, seven days a week, finally managed to schedule a vacation. A local orthopedist in private practice had agreed to cover Howard for emergencies in his absence. Under pressure from community physicians, the outside physician reneged on the agreement. Opponents of Henry Kaiser's plan, a veritable chorus, trotted out the old familiar epithets, calling prepaid practice socialized medicine and a communist conspiracy. Henry Kaiser's ownership of a pink Lincoln automobile and his pink cement trucks were emblems that incited Permanente detractors to blast its physicians as "pinkies."

The year Henry Kaiser died, 1967, was also the year that the Northwest Region again came to the aid of the struggling Hawaii program. Conflict had increased between the physicians and the administration, and Regional Manager Martin Drobac, Edgar Kaiser's son-in-law, resigned and returned to the mainland. DeLong assumed the position of Acting Regional Manager.[5] This time, however, instead of occupying spare quarters in the hospital itself, De-Long resided at the next-door luxurious Ilikai Hotel. In addition to myriad urgent challenges, DeLong had to wrestle with one very pressing problem: the Hawaii Region had become the chosen health care system for the 2,300 employees of the Ewa Sugar Plantation. For almost 100 years, Ewa had functioned as a paternalistic company town; with three churches, a primitive 30-bed hospital, a small clinic, a school, and a general store, it was virtually self-contained. The reorganization meant closing down the plantation hospital and orienting Ewa employees to a new and unfamiliar Kaiser Foundation Health Plan. The International Longshoreman Workers Union had provided complete care for its members, including a drug benefit—an element with which the Health Plan had had no previous experience. When DeLong called Oakland to determine how to charge for the drug benefit, he received no instructions. Left to work the formula out for himself, he contacted the pharmacy, determined the average prescription charge to be about $3.50, estimated the number of prescriptions per member at 12 per year, and simply multiplied $3.50 by 12 to calculate the annual prescription premium.

By 1969 the plan had grown sufficiently successful that the program extended service to the island of Maui. Phillip Chu's death, in 1970, left a leadership void. Chu had been a strong, skillful Medical Director. Replacing him posed another significant challenge. Keene's choice to replace Chu was cardiologist and Chief of Medicine Tung Kwang (T.K.) Lin, but Lin demurred, preferring his clinical practice to a major administrative role.[6] In an election between William Dung and obstetrician-gynecologist Hau Vu, Dung won the Medical Director position. His leadership style was not always popular. During the course of his 20-year tenure, a number of physicians would leave, including Chiefs of Medicine, radiology, urology, and anesthesiology: Lin in 1975 to join the University of Kansas; Vu to a practice in Stockton, California; Tom Lee, Chief of Anesthesiology to academic medicine on the mainland, though he would return to Hawaii and to private practice in the 1980s. Despite a disquieting exodus of physicians from Permanente, the Hawaii Health Plan grew steadily, and under Dung's leadership the Medical Group continued to attract a number of outstanding doctors.

CHANGING NEEDS

In the early 1970s the organization recognized the need to innovate and improve services and Health Plan dispatched an Oakland team to Hawaii to modernize the hospital in 1972. Team member Barbara Anderson's[7] mission was to improve the obstetrical service, establish an ICU and initiate team nursing. After her own research that showed a nurse who wore street clothes was more effective with children, she encouraged nurses in pediatric wards to replace their caps and white stockings for civilian attire. As membership grew, building infrastructures proved inadequate to meet the Region's needs. Accordingly, in 1983 a new facility replaced the original medical office on Maui. In 1989 an office opened on Oahu to serve members in the Kailua area; others followed, including one on the campus of Hawaii Pacific University. In 1985 the 202-bed Moanalua Medical Center, nine miles northeast of downtown Honolulu, opened. A demolition team imploded the old Honolulu Medical Center creating a huge cloud of pulverized concrete. The television series *Magnum, P.I.* used the destruction of the hospital as a backdrop in a segment featuring the popular series' star Tom Selleck. Portrayed as trapped within the collapsed building, Selleck's character managed to escape from the rubble. The 30-story Hawaii Prince Hotel now occupies the site.

In addition to the usual challenges that accompany the opening of a major medical center, behind the scenes at Moanalua a precedent-setting battle was taking place. For CEO of the medical center, those in power backed two less-than-qualified male candidates over the woman candidate whose qualifications were clearly superior. Finally, when threatened with legal action for gender discrimination and faced with the fact that Kaiser Foundation Health Plan President and CEO James Vohs backed the woman, the opposition retreated, and Barbara Anderson was named CEO of a KP medical center—one of the first women to achieve that distinction.[8]

—◊—

PART IV:
SPECIALTIES

—◊—

CHAPTER 8:
THE ER AND THE OR

―⟋⟋⟋―

EMERGENCIES AT NORTHERN PERMANENTE FOUNDATION HOSPITAL

A worn leather-bound logbook lying in the Kaiser Permanente Northwest archives shows visits to the emergency room (ER) of Northern Permanente Foundation Hospital from July 1944 to April 1946. Entries are surprisingly few, averaging just six to ten per day. Of these, most are for minor diagnoses like tonsillitis and bronchitis. The small number are, however, easily explained: a state-of-the-art first-aid station at Kaiser Vancouver Shipyard provided almost all the care for worker emergencies.[1] Consider this: in just 16 months, the shipyard's first-aid station and two substations recorded 430,098 visits. By contrast, visits to the hospital ER for the same period totaled approximately 3,500, or less than one percent of the total.

But Permanente physicians and nurses were not just taking care of emergencies. They were also busy providing care at Permanente's medical offices. The September 12, 1944 edition of *The Columbian* breathlessly reported, "the astronomical figure of 434,335 visits by Kaiser workers to the outpatient department of the Northern Permanente Foundation Hospital and outlying clinics in the past year."

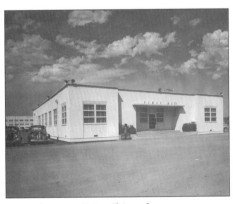

First Aid Station, Kaiser Shipyards.
Courtesy of Kaiser Permanente Heritage Resources.

When the shipyards, together with their first-aid stations, closed in 1945, visits to the hospital ER spiked, placing added pressure on the Permanente surgeons, who were responsible for all emergency cases. Surgeon Norman Frink's 1956 sabbatical leave in England to study cardiac surgery and the six-month illness of orthopedist Robert Reubendale only added to the strain. The remaining surgeons, Gilbert Rogers, Paul Trautman, and Lawrence Duckler, were obliged to serve 36-hour shifts on call for general surgical emergencies, in addition to treating fractures and pinning hips. It would be 15 more years before The Permanente Clinic would hire full-time ER physicians.

Permanente was not unique in this regard. At the time, few of the nation's hospitals had well-organized Emergency Departments. The Permanente Medical Group in Northern California was an exception. There, Cecil Cutting hired emergency medicine specialist Thomas Flint, Jr. in the late 1940s, and Flint designed protocols for emergency care in that Region's Permanente hospitals. In 1954, W.B. Saunders and Company published Flint's 645-page, *Emergency Treatment and Management*. The work addresses emergency treatment of specific conditions; a short section discusses administrative, clerical, and medical-legal principles and procedures. The comprehensive work gained national and international recognition and underwent several printings.

EMERGENCIES AT BESS KAISER
AND KAISER SUNNYSIDE HOSPITALS

The 1959 opening of Bess Kaiser Hospital drew increased attention to emergency services. The hospital unveiled a fully equipped Emergency Department, featuring a spacious treatment room with an operating table and a moveable overhead light. Two exam rooms were outfitted with gurney stretchers and oxygen outlets to treat medical emergencies. A small cast room complemented the area. A hallway adjacent to the treatment area led to offices and exam rooms of the Orthopedics Department; these doubled in the evenings as pediatric, internal medicine and surgical walk-in clinics.

Surgeon Duckler was appointed Emergency Department Director. One week before the opening of the new hospital, he orchestrated a dry run; nurses pushed him on a gurney into the Emergency Department, only to discover that they were unable to maneuver the wheeled conveyance into the minor surgery room. Workers quickly made the necessary adjustments to accommodate the gurneys.

In 1960 the Medical Group hired five residents to cover the ER and to attend hospital and clinic patients. With their relative inexperience, they were often overmatched, especially on the overnight shift; during those long hours, with no technicians to provide support, they were expected to do EKGs and to perform laboratory tests. Resident coverage lasted only one year; in 1961, internists, pediatricians and general surgeons resumed after-hours coverage of the ER, from 5:00 p.m. to 8:00 a.m. the following morning. In addition, they attended inpatients and outpatients during evening clinic hours.

In 1969, with emergency services still under the organizational umbrella of surgery, Chief of Surgery Frink hired surgeon Will Hage to focus exclusively on strengthening emergency services. At the time, Emergency Department staff comprised part-time physicians awaiting residencies and moonlighting Oregon

Medical School residents. Hage raised department standards and began active recruiting and, in 1970 he hired David Hale as the first full-time physician in the department. Hale had completed his tour in Vietnam, needed a job, and applied for the position without any long-term plan to remain with Permanente. His experience in a medical unit, similar to those depicted in the *MASH* feature film and TV series, was a fitting entry into emergency medicine.

Later that year, Josephine "Sunny" Colbach accepted ER work on an hourly basis; before long she, too, became permanent and full time. Not long thereafter, she was joined by Dean Barnhouse, a four-year Navy Veteran and Oregon Medical School graduate; Barnhouse would go on to become the Director of Emergency Care.[2] After three months of an unsatisfactory psychiatric residency, James Brodhacker became a full-time ER physician at BK for 15 months before entering a residency in internal medicine. He would later join Permanente as an internist. During a long career he would serve as Chief of Internal Medicine, a member of the Board of Directors, and Assistant Regional Medical Director for three regional Medical Directors. Others joined the growing department: Robert Miller, Albert Martin, Craig Dougan and Wilhelm Jawurek. Some on the executive committee had misgivings about hiring Martin, who at 51 was thought too old; fortunately, his supporters won over their hesitant colleagues. Martin would go on to enjoy an exemplary career in the Emergency Department and in the surgical trauma clinic and, in 1979 he would receive Permanente's Distinguished Physician Award.

Michael Hoevet and Oregonian Ron Potts both joined The Permanente Clinic in 1973. Potts' career path had taken him from an internship at the University of California Medical Center at Irvine, to the Public Health Service in the U.S. Coast Guard, to a practice with a Medical Group in emergency medicine before he returned to his home state and joined Permanente.

Nights in the ER were often chaotic. Patients packed the waiting room; the more seriously ill and injured arrived one after the other, through the ambulance entrance. At 11:00 p.m. the walk-in clinics closed; then one lone physician assumed responsibility for all ER admissions until the following morning at 7:00 a.m. That physician was fortunate to have a remarkably capable group of knowledgeable nurses and technicians, among them Peg Pemberton,[3] who managed to impose order on the wildly unpredictable ER. Helen Pike, with her years of experience, had more knowledge than most of the part-time doctors. Seeing a physician begin to droop after hours of duty, she would obtain a history and order x-ray and lab tests before calling the weary physician to see the patient.

Circumstances could test even the most resourceful and experienced of the staff. Martin recalled an evening when a man, furious at having been denied a prescription for Percodan, grabbed him by his necktie and lifted him from the floor. Hearing the altercation, Robert Miller emerged from the surgery room and, though a mere 5 feet tall, weighing only 120 pounds, he tackled Martin's attacker. A security guard helped to untangle the pair and escorted the patient, still spoiling for a fight, outside. In another remembered altercation, an ER physician disarmed a pistol-packing boyfriend who objected to the casting of his girlfriend's fracture—a fracture that he had inflicted.[4] When Kaiser Sunnyside Medical Center (KSMC) opened in 1975, Potts and Hoevet let a coin toss determine which of the two would go there.[5]

Winning the toss, Potts chose to remain at BK as Chief; Hoevet went to KSMC, taking with him Colbach and Hale.

In 1977 emergency care achieved department status, heralding a period of remarkable growth and excellence. Potts implemented a rigorous program to improve physician skills and, in 1980 Colbach, Hoevet, and Potts achieved board certification with the American College of Emergency Physicians—the first time that emergency physicians could obtain board certification. Thus, Permanente was at the forefront of the trend, still in its infancy, to grant board certification to emergency physicians.

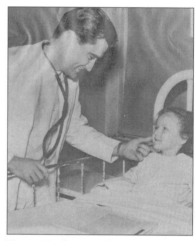

Norman Frink, MD, with young patient, circa 1946. *Courtesy of Norman Frink, Jr.*

SCALPELS AND SUTURES, HAMMERS AND SAWS

In 1942 Sidney Garfield hired Ernest Burgess, the Medical Group's first orthopedist, its first Chief of Surgery, and its first Medical Director. A bacteriologist before he entered medical school at Columbia University, Burgess interned at Swedish Hospital in Seattle, where he worked with leading Seattle orthopedist Roger Anderson. Burgess then obtained additional training at the Hospital for Special Surgery in New York, was appointed house surgeon for two more years, and then joined Northern Permanente. His tenure, however, was brief; Burgess resigned to join the U.S. Armed Forces the following year, creating a temporary leadership vacuum within the Surgery Department.

During the war years, Northern Permanente general surgeons were Frederick Bookhotz, William Armstrong, and Grand Coulee veteran Eugene Wiley. The three orthopedists were Fred Roemer, Lawrence Noall, and Patrick Dwyer. In 1944 the American College of Surgeons fully accredited the Northern Permanente Foundation Hospital and its surgeons. By contrast, the other two area hospitals, St. Joseph Community Hospital and Clark General Hospital in Vancouver, received only conditional accreditation.

In 1945 at war's end, Medical Director Wallace Neighbor and Ernest Saward recruited Frink to be Chief of Surgery. It was a shrewd choice: Frink would remain the department leader for the next 23 years, and he would dominate the Surgery Department through a period of major growth and development. The son of a general practitioner in the small South Dakota town of Wagner, Frink had grown up on the Yankton Sioux Indian Reservation. As Department Chief, Frink was both self-assured and demanding; his reputation for periodic outbursts earned him the nickname, "Stormin' Norman." Like Permanente pioneer Garfield, he had fair skin and red hair, and he was, at least most of the time, soft-spoken. Also like Garfield, he wore impeccably tailored suits.

During the upheaval years of 1949 and 1950, as the first partnership dissolved and the second partnership faltered, Frink's department lost surgeon Lucius Button and orthopedist Frederick Waknitz. Frink and recently hired Theodore Dillman were left to carry the full surgical load. That load included orthopedic, urological and some neurosurgical procedures. Frink got some relief in 1953 when Rogers joined the Medical Group. His arrival was followed by that of Duckler, who was hired as a preceptor before becoming a staff member, and Trautman in 1955. Members of the small department reverted to a private-practice model, eschewing the Permanente group-practice model championed by Garfield. They did not take responsibility for the patients of other surgeons and followed only their own patients in the hospital.

The 1959 opening of Bess Kaiser Hospital brought changes to the organizational structure. Duckler assumed responsibility for the ER and the operating room (OR). Rogers was to oversee the surgical inpatient services. The Permanente Clinic hired Lewis Hughes in 1960 and Louis Phillip in 1961. Two years later Ivan Altman arrived. In that decade, with the addition of Roy Sandvig, Augusto Bernardo, Richard Davis, and John Johnson,[6] the department grew to ten.

Meanwhile, iron-fisted nurse Marjorie Watters ruled the OR. She began working at the Northern Permanente Hospital and eventually rose to become OR supervisor. She continued in that role when BK opened. Respected and judged fair by those who worked for her, she accepted no nonsense from anyone in the OR. Her voice was distinctive and, when raised, commanded the attention of those within hearing range. If a surgeon was late to arrive for a scheduled surgery, she was known to call his home to be certain he was on his way. Any conflict between a surgeon and a nurse went directly to her for mediation. Though some might have viewed her as autocratic, the surgeons for the most part appreciated her management style, and found her surprisingly sociable outside the OR.

Frink resigned as chief of general surgery in 1969 and Lewis Hughes accepted the position. Judged impartial by his peers, he was a good choice to lead the surgeons, known for large egos and a collective disdain for authority. Within a year, however, Hughes was elevated to the position of Medical Director, and finding a replacement for Department Chief became a problem. Rogers tried the post for a time but quickly grew disillusioned and stepped down. The group next turned its attention to newcomer Robert McFarlane, hired in 1970.[7] McFarlane had acted as Hughes' Assistant Chief of Surgery during the short period when Hughes had held positions as both Medical Director and Chief of Surgery. The more the group thought about it, the more McFarlane seemed a likely choice. He carried no political baggage; he hit it off well with Frink; and he had the distinction of being the only member of the department who was double-boarded—that is, board certified in both general and chest surgery. Finally, and very important indeed, he got along well with the formidable Watters. The likeable McFarlane adapted easily to his role as Chief and continued the work already begun by Hughes to form a more cohesive group. In 1972, the department welcomed Edward Ariniello and two years later, George Chang.

After the 1975 opening of the Kaiser Sunnyside Medical Center, an expansion that necessitated a hiring surge of new physicians, Permanente leaders recognized the growing need for a medical education program for its physicians, now numbering 186, to serve approximately 200,000 members. (Official numbers showed 196,000 members in January 1975 and 208,000 members in January 1976.) When they tapped McFarlane to be the first regional Director of Continuing Medical Education in 1976, Edward Ariniello replaced him as Chief of Surgery. His strong advocacy for his surgeon colleagues made Ariniello a popular chief and almost certainly accounted for his long tenure as head of his department—a remarkable 26 years. Settling on a Surgery Chief at the new KSMC proved more problematic. A succession of physicians—Ariniello (before he returned to BK), Trautman and Bruce Huntwork—took a brief turn as Department Chief. Then, in 1978 George Chang assumed the position—acknowledged to be a difficult one. Remarkably, given the inability of his colleagues to find satisfaction in the role of department leader, Chang would retain the position for the next six years.

Surgery departments at the two hospitals were very different: longevity and stability characterized BK, whereas KSMC was noted for innovation. Both departments continued to expand. Chang and newcomer Michael Schiedler, hired later in 1989, performed vascular procedures at KSMC; Peter Feldman and James Nolte at BK. Chest surgery was the specialty of McFarlane at BK and of Ivan Altman and James Bisio at KSMC. Thyroid and parathyroid surgeries were performed by veteran Gilbert Rogers at BK and by more recently trained Louis Kosta at KSMC.

In 1979 McFarlane introduced a surgical residency program through the medical school at BK. As a result, Permanente surgeons obtained teaching affiliations at OHSU as clinical instructors, professors and associate professors. This first residency program started an extensive graduate medical education program that today comprises 15 residency, fellowship, and postdoctoral programs, and 6 student programs.

ORTHOPEDICS

Orthopedics within Permanente did not obtain separate department status until the mid-1960s. And until the 1952 arrival of orthopedist Robert Reubendale, the general surgeons helped carry the orthopedic load. Lewis Hughes, hired in 1960, split his practice equally between general surgery and orthopedics. With the arrival of George Adlhoch in 1961, the small orthopedics component began to coalesce. Still, surgeons Rogers, Trautman, Duckler, and Phillip were required to take orthopedic call.

The Permanente Clinic was at a significant disadvantage in attracting orthopedists. The reason was simple: they could command much higher salaries in private practice. A 1968 Permanente income schedule shows a starting salary of $30,000 for board-certified orthopedists, low by community standards, though 25% higher than the $24,000 paid to board-certified internists and pediatricians.

In 1965 orthopedic services gained separate status from general surgery and orthopedist Harry Nash arrived. His outsized personality (and frequent displays of temper) contrasted sharply with the low-profile demeanors of Reubendale and Adlhoch. His tenure as Chief was short-lived; he went to half time in 1968 and resigned from Permanente in 1976 after a dispute with the new Medical Director Marvin Goldberg. The arrival of orthopedists Edward Stark and David Long in 1971 was greeted with a collective sigh of relief.

Though Stark and Long had attended different medical schools and had trained at different hospitals, they became acquainted during their specialty training at Carrie Tingley Children's Hospitals in Truth or Consequences, New Mexico. Stark, raised in the coastal community of Coquille, Oregon, wanted to return to his home state but didn't relish the business aspects of private practice. He decided to join Permanente. Long had sought opportunities in Seattle, but that city was experiencing a downturn in its economy and job prospects were poor. Discouraged, he consulted Stark, who suggested that he join Permanente.

From the beginning of their Permanente careers, Stark and Long experienced an avalanche of orthopedic cases. They said they thrived in the environment. Long later recalled that, when attending orthopedic teaching rounds at the medical school, faculty members would present a single unusual case; Long, steeped in complex cases at KP, could often choose from five similarly complex cases. Orthopedists William Courogen and Yiichiang Khan joined the department in 1973. Osteopathic physician Harry Sironian, trained as an orthopedic surgeon, followed later that year.

In 1972 Frink asked new arrival Stark if a physician assistant (PA) could relieve some of the orthopedic workload. Stark remembers responding, "What's a PA?" Once informed, he quickly warmed to the idea and helped hire PA James Yarusso. Josiah Hill, the first formally licensed PA in Oregon, joined Yarusso shortly thereafter. Hill's previous experience included work on the medical team for the Minnesota Vikings.[8] PAs quickly proved themselves indispensable in the department. One asset among many was their availability to follow-up on fracture cases in clinic when an orthopedist was called to surgery for an unscheduled, urgent case.

The transition of the Orthopedics Department to the newly opened KSMC went smoothly, at least initially. Stark, Sironian, and recently hired orthopedic PA, Tavo Guthrie, moved their offices and occupied space near the hospital's small ER. But the smooth transition was short-lived; what followed was an unsettled period characterized by frequent resignations, transfers, and new hires. Sironian was the first to leave in 1976. Orthopedists Michael Marble and Stephen Thomas joined Permanente that year only to resign after just two years. The opening for an orthopedist drew Edwin Wright, a graduate of King's College London School of Medicine, whose formal training included a fellowship at Tufts-New England Medical Center in hand surgery. BK orthopedist Donald Tilson transferred briefly to KSMC, but within a year he returned to BK to become area Chief of Orthopedics when David Long stepped down from the post. Khan then transferred to fill Tilson's spot.

In 1982 Frink suggested another innovation for the Orthopedics Department— a podiatry service. Recruitment of orthopedists was lagging and, as a consequence, appointment waiting lists had grown. The Permanente Medical Group already had a podiatry service, as well as a teaching relationship with a podiatry college in San Francisco. Frink had been impressed with the California program and the vigorous training requirements for a podiatry degree: four years of university training with an emphasis on basic sciences, four years in a school of podiatry followed by a typical two-to-three-year residency. In some cases fellowship training followed. Though there were objections by some orthopedists, recruitment began for a podiatrist.

The first to be hired was Forrest Ligget, the son of a Portland podiatrist. Ligget had worked as a surgical assistant at KSMC before attending podiatry school. He was well-liked and familiar with the KP system. In 1982, he began working half time under the auspices of the Orthopedics Department; within a year, he achieved full-time status. Jeffrey Schoen, hired in 1987, was assigned to Health Center West in the BK area. Schoen had previously worked with orthopedist James Loch in the

Naval Reserve; and it was Loch who influenced Schoen to join Permanente. Tina DeMuth was the next addition; she had completed her residency at Kaiser Foundation Hospital in Vallejo. The expanding division added Joseph Neary, from the Dr. William M. Scholl College of Podiatric Medicine.[9] Neary would become both lead podiatrist and, when the department achieved department status in 1988, its first chief. In 1992, podiatry officially joined Northwest Permanente.

NEUROSURGERY

In 1959, Oregon Medical School neurosurgeon Harold Paxton received a late-night request for a consultation on a patient at BK with a questionable diagnosis of dissecting thoracic aortic aneurysm. Making the final diagnosis of epidural hematoma, Paxton performed a decompression laminectomy and evacuated the clot. This was Paxton's first collaboration with Permanente. In the next ten years, he would perform most of their neurosurgeries—until the Medical Group hired its own staff of neurosurgeons.

A graduate of Johns Hopkins Medical School, Paxton trained at Washington University School of Medicine in St. Louis before joining Portland neurosurgeon John Raff. Paxton had a previous connection with Permanente; he and Permanente's Noah Krall had taken the Arkansas basic science examinations together and had become friends. In 1966, Paxton became Chief of the neurosurgical program at Oregon Medical School and trained a number of neurosurgeons who worked for KP. Mian Tahir was one. Having completed his residency in 1970, he went on to join The Permanente Clinic, where, during a 30-year career, he would become a stabilizing influence in the Neurosurgery Department.

Tushar Nag, born and raised in Calcutta, India, got his medical neurosurgical training in England and Scotland. He joined The Permanente Clinic in 1970, the same year as Tahir.[10] From the beginning the two realized that they needed support staff. Accordingly, the Medical Group recruited neurosurgical nurse assistants. Jane Stradley, a hospital nurse in Minneapolis, had recently moved to Portland and learned about two open positions at KP—one in urology and the other in neurosurgery. She chose neurosurgery, with the understanding that she would assist Tahir. Another RN was hired to assist Nag. After a year of training and instruction from Tahir, Stradley easily passed the two-day examination as PA. Stradley performed a wide range of tasks: she arranged Tahir's OR schedule, communicated with his patients and their families, made hospital rounds with and without Tahir, saw patients in clinic, assisted in the OR and took after-hours call. Tahir and Stradley formed a striking pair as they strode together through the hospital and outpatient corridors—Tahir, in a dark suit and expertly knotted tie, Stradley in a tailored dress or suit suggesting the corporate board room.[11]

Neurosurgeons came and went over the years—Clifford Roberson, Edmund Frank, Richard Schwartz, Paul Amstutz, and Francisco Soldevilla. But Hirohisa Ono, a native of Japan and a graduate of Nagasaki University Medical College, joined NWP in 1982 and stayed. Like others he had received training by Paxton at Oregon Medical School where he became an associate professor. Together with Paxton, he developed the neurosurgical residency program at BK.[12] Medical Director Marvin Goldberg first hired Ono on contract; within a short time he achieved full-time status. Like Tahir, Ono would become a mainstay in the department, eventually assuming the position of Department Chief. Mitchell Weinstein, hired in 1991, had previously practiced in Rochester, New York. From 1988 to 1990, he was senior attending neurosurgeon in Tromsø at the University Hospital of North Norway, 250 miles above the Arctic Circle and the northernmost university medical center in the world.

"TURPS" AND STONES

Luis Halpert joined The Permanente Clinic in 1961 as its first full-time urologist.[13] After graduating in medicine from the University of Mexico, he completed the mandatory requirement of one year of public service by providing medical care in the jungles of Mexico. He recalls traveling by horseback, a .45 automatic in one pocket and stethoscope in the other. He and Army personnel were sometimes ordered to round up villagers to ensure they received government-sponsored immunizations.

Coming to Portland, Halpert established a relationship with the University of Oregon Medical School, joined the volunteer teaching staff and pursued his interest in pediatric urology. At the time, the medical school did not have a pediatric urologist. Occasionally a senior resident would rotate with Halpert to gain experience. Halpert also formed an important friendship with local urologist Arnold Rustin. Rustin had performed urologic surgeries referred to him by Permanente surgeons Rogers and Frink, and he was well-disposed to Permanente. He was to play a helpful role in the future of Permanente urologists.

Halpert's introduction to Permanente was inauspicious. He experienced maddening delays in obtaining his Oregon licensure. Without the necessary license, he could work only under the direction of other Permanente surgeons and was prohibited from writing prescriptions. Thus, while he waited for the elusive license, he performed general, urologic, and emergency surgeries as permitted in accordance with his status. Meanwhile, others were impatient as well. In 1962, Surgery Chief Frink hired another urologist, Walter Berlin, and appointed him Chief of Service. Halpert found these days difficult. Berlin and Halpert had their differences, both in substance and style. An Army Medical Corps Veteran of World War II in Africa and Europe, the 46-year-old Berlin was schooled in older methods and was bombastic in touting them. Halpert, young and soft-spoken, was nevertheless confident; his training was recent and founded on newer surgical techniques. For a time Halpert considered leaving Permanente, but he held on—largely because of Saward's encouragement. Saward advised him, "Don't worry; as long as I'm around you won't need to go anywhere—unless you want to go to Hawaii." (At the time Permanente in Hawaii had openings for urologists, and Saward had some say in matters of hiring.)

In 1970, the arrival of gentlemanly and experienced Ferenc Gabor helped dampen frictions. Gabor had been on the staff at the Portland Veterans Administration hospital and at the University of Oregon Medical School, where he had worked with the revered Clarence Hodges. A two-year teaching stint at a Louisiana VA hospital followed, after which he returned to the Northwest and joined Permanente. The addition of Iraqi-born and educated Matti Totonchy and Oregonian Thomas Carey in 1974 allowed Halpert to take a sabbatical leave to enhance his skills in pediatric urology.

Totonchy, a graduate of the University of Baghdad, had left Iraq in 1965 and obtained his urology training at the Medical College of Ohio at Toledo. Eager to leave the Midwest flatlands, he decided to move to the Northwest, choosing Portland over Seattle. Carey had obtained his MD at Oregon Medical School. He was enrolled in the surgery residency at the University of Minnesota Medical School, awaiting an opening in that school's urology residency when a resident in the Oregon Medical School urology program withdrew. Carey took the spot and returned to his alma mater to train under Clarence Hodges. During his training he obtained skills in pediatric urology from Edward Tank. Soon after, in 1974, Carey joined the Medical Group implementing a urology residency program at BK.

The 1975 opening of KSMC allowed Halpert and Totonchy to establish a separate department there. The Urology Department's ties to the local medical school and its residency program were to be hugely beneficial to KP. After the 1970s, most newly trained Permanente urologists came from the medical school program: Roger Wicklund, 1980; Stephen Lieberman, who later became Department Chief, 1982; Matthew Forsythe, 1988; Robert Skinner, 1991; Douglas Ackerman, 1994; Christopher Merson, 1994; Timothy Fleming, 1997; Jeffrey Johnson, 1999; Richard Burt, 2001; Edith Legg, 2003. With the 1996 closure of BK, the residency program made a seamless transition to KSMC. BK urologists relocated to Permanente offices at the Mother Joseph Plaza at Providence St. Vincent Hospital Medical Center.

HISTORY OF ANESTHESIA IN OREGON

The first anesthesia administered in Oregon by nurses took place in 1896 at Sisters of Providence St. Vincent Hospital in Portland. In 1909, St. Vincent introduced anesthesia training in its nursing curriculum. Until the 1940s, nurses administered virtually all anesthesia. Surgeons preferred a well-trained nurse to the inexperienced intern or resident-in-training. Physicians themselves had little interest in the discipline. It was underpaid and generally considered a nursing skill. Ether was the agent of choice.

The first nurse anesthetist for what was to become the KP program, Geraldine Searcy, had worked with Cecil Cutting at San Francisco General Hospital in the 1930s. When Garfield and Neighbor opened their hospital at Mason City to provide care for workers building the Grand Coulee Dam, Searcy joined them. When Garfield established the prepaid health plan for shipyard workers in Oakland and Richmond in 1942, she followed them there as well. Seven years later, in 1949, TPMG hired its first anesthesiologist, Carl Fisher. Fisher and Searcy thereafter worked closely together.

Like their Northern California counterparts, Permanente surgeons in the Northwest at first relied solely on nurse anesthetists to administer anesthesia. The first nurse anesthetists at the Northern Permanente Foundation Hospital in Vancouver were Dorothy Paulson, Olga Schieber, and Ann Gordon. Both Paulson and Schieber lived on the hospital grounds in the nurses' residence, which also housed medical residents and the occasional office worker.

Though anesthesia was generally thought to be the work of nurses, Portland surgeon Thomas Joyce had long advocated for the Oregon Medical School to include a division of anesthesia. Persuaded by Joyce to head this new division, Mayo Clinic-trained John Hutton introduced an anesthesia residency program in 1938, as well as a training program for nurse anesthetists. Still, many surgeons were cool to the idea of a physician-administered anesthesia. Surgeons were used to dictating the type of anesthesia; as captains of their OR ships, they disliked the idea of another physician in the OR who could challenge their decisions.

Ironically, Joyce himself was one of those who discouraged physician-administered anesthesia at the medical school.[14] But with his sudden death in 1947 of a heart attack in the faculty lounge at Multnomah County Hospital, a change occurred. Fred Haugen returned to Portland (he was an Oregon Medical School graduate) as chairman of the division of anesthesiology at the medical school. Unlike Joyce, Haugen, an advocate of physician-administered anesthesia, developed a strong, progressive medical residency program. As a result of the growing physician interest in anesthesiology, local hospitals discontinued their nurse anesthetist programs: University of Oregon Medical School in 1950 and St. Vincent Hospital in 1956.

ANESTHESIA AT NORTHWEST PERMANENTE

It wasn't until 1959, after BK opened, that The Permanente Clinic hired Jack Edwards, its first anesthesiologist and chief of the anesthesia service. A 1949 graduate of the Oregon Medical School, Edwards served his residency in anesthesiology.

After his military service in the Navy, he returned to the medical school, joining the teaching staff there until 1958, after which he devoted his time to a practice at St. Vincent Hospital. An active member in the Oregon Society of Anesthesiologists (OSA), he was elected incoming President in 1960. But discrimination against Permanente physicians among community physicians was still rife. A delegation from OSA came to his home and asked him to resign. Angered and disappointed, Edwards nevertheless felt he had little choice and resigned as President but continued his membership in the OSA.[15]

In 1967 Edwards hired Rex Underwood, who was willing to leave his position at the University of Oregon Medical School.[16] Underwood had trained under Edwards a decade earlier and respected him as a superb physician; he had been disappointed when Edwards left the medical school. Underwood had a rich and varied training experience. As a medical student, he externed at Holladay Park Hospital where he administered open-drop ether to slow the labor of obstetric patients until the obstetrician arrived. He gained experience in the polio ward as well, managing iron lung respirators. During an occasional power failure, he learned to use manual pumps—a terrifying experience for patients. Underwood recalled a previous association with Permanente: as a medical student he had started the preoperative IV for his father, under the supervision of surgeon Frink. Later, as a staff physician at the medical school, he had moonlighted at the Northern Permanente and Bess Kaiser Hospitals, where he was Frink's preferred anesthesiologist.

Underwood knew and liked anesthesiology resident Bhawar "Bo" Singh. At his urging, Singh joined Permanente in 1968, just months before Edwards died of a myocardial infarction. According to Underwood, "Bo was a real catch."[17]

A side light to the evolution of anesthesiology in the Northwest and throughout most areas of the country was the conflict that arose once physicians adopted the subspecialty of anesthesiology. Nurse anesthetists now posed an economic threat to their physician counterparts. This conflict within the greater medical community never affected KP, where, with its unique team approach, certified registered nurse anesthetists (CRNAs), have long had an integral role, with supervising anesthesiologists, in administering anesthesia.

Singh eventually became Chief of Anesthesia at BK, and Underwood Chief at the new KSMC, which opened in 1978 on an empty stretch of land at the SE corner of Interstate 205 and SE Sunnyside Road, now the busiest intersection in Portland. Both groups optimized the model of a supervising anesthesiologist with a CRNA in the OR, and the CRNA as primary provider for labor and delivery.

Growth dominated the anesthesia work of the next decade with Steven Forrest following Underwood as Chief at KSMC and Singh continuing as Chief at BK. It was Underwoods' position that Tom Janisse filled in 1989 on completing fellowships in cardiac anesthesia and pain medicine. Suzanne Zarling, also from a pain management fellowship, joined Singh at BK. Janisse and Zarling started acute postoperative pain services and opened chronic pain management clinics. Janisse became Chief of Anesthesia at KSMC in 1990, and hired Randy Kreps after a pain management fellowship, and appointed him Director of the Pain Clinic, and eventually the Director of the Regional Chronic Pain Management Clinic, when the two clinics combined in 1977, and were located at the site of the previous BK. Both Kreps and Marilee Donovan, PhD, an Advanced Practice Nurse with expertise in pain and group education classes, created the next-state Multidisciplinary Chronic Pain Management Program, which later included a Pain Board of content experts from physiatry (Paul Jacobs), neurosurgery, psychiatry, neurology, internal medicine, surgery, social work, and pharmacy. The group won the national James A. Vohs Award for Quality in 2002 as the KPNW Integrated Pain Management Program, which included primary care, specialty care consultation, group visits, and group education.

What characterized anesthesia evolution over this time, more than new drugs and medical devices, was the use of "regional anesthesia": to control pain at a location or a region. Infusions of morphine and local anesthetic pumped through a paraspinal epidural catheter to significantly improve intraoperative and postoperative pain. An alternative process, called Patient-Controlled Analgesia (PCA) allowed intravenous infusion of morphine by the patient to meet the need for pain relief. Anesthesiologists and CRNAs at both hospitals managed these through Acute Post-Operative Pain Services requiring daily rounding. Anesthesia work outside of the OR, also a mark of this era, grew more routine and with more significant interventions—conscious sedation for pediatric MRIs, adult cardioversions, dental procedures, and electroconvulsive therapy. Anesthesia even managed a Medical Procedures Unit in the medical office. A triple advance came in the area of thoracic surgery—a preoperative high-risk assessment clinic, analgesic infusions through thoracic epidural catheters, and a dedicated thoracic team.

The most dramatic event of the nineties, however, was the social and emotional trauma deeply experienced by the entire staff with the closure of BK, which severely disrupted lives, relationships, and the community-like working environment when required to dislocate to the west side Providence St. Vincent's Hospital.

The next major anesthesia advance occurred in 2009 with the start of cardiac anesthesia to support open-heart surgery in the new Cardiac and Cardiovascular Care Service at KSMC. At that time, the original two anesthesia departments at KSMC and BK finally regionalized under one chief.

CHAPTER 9:
PEDIATRICIANS,
OBSTETRICIANS, AND QUINTS

PIONEERING PEDIATRICIANS

When the Permanente Health Plan debuted in 1942, enrollment was limited to ship-yard workers. Then, in August the following year, the coverage expanded to include dependants. The cost was 15¢ per week per child, 30¢ per week for each adult, and a flat $25 maternity fee. With its decision to include dependants, Permanente needed pediatricians and hired Paul Patterson as the Region's first full-time pediatrician. A Chicago native, Patterson arrived wearing a brilliantly colored bow tie, suggesting a taste for style. Shown his makeshift office in a coatroom that doubled as the physician lounge, Patterson must surely have been taken aback at his less-than-impressive quarters. Two more pediatricians, Cire Scheer and Katherine Van Leeuwen, arrived soon thereafter, necessitating a move of the pediatric clinic to the west end of the hospital outpatient offices. By 1944 the busy children's ward averaged 40 patients a day. Murals of Porky Pig, Donald Duck, and Mickey Mouse decorated its walls. A visiting counselor made regular visits to help families who needed guidance or reassurance.

The unavailability of antibiotics undoubtedly accounted for the relatively high hospital pediatric census. In those years, general surgeons regularly performed tonsillectomies—45 in a single July week in 1944. To keep pace with the needs of members, the Pediatric Department offered special pediatric clinics at outlying Ogden Meadows and McLoughlin Heights housing developments. Pediatrician Margaret Ingram worked in the clinic at McLoughlin Heights.

Post-war years brought new pediatricians to Permanente: Edward Bradley[1] in 1946; Joseph Schaefer, 1947; and Virginia Gilliland, 1948. Gilliland had completed an Ear Nose and Throat residency under Ullman and was able to perform some of the many scheduled tonsillectomies. The pediatric team established its Portland presence in an old house on NE Weidler Street next to the property that later became the site of the Broadway Clinic at 2606 NE Broadway. Together, pediatrician Earl Pearce and Mary Gulley, RN, set up an allergy clinic in the Weidler Street house.

In 1951 Charles Varga joined the Medical Group as Chief of Pediatrics[2] and in 1954 he hired Peter Hurst. Hurst would enjoy a 33-year career with Permanente over the course of which he would attract stellar pediatric talent to the Medical Group.

At the time, polio, meningitis, complicated otitis media and whooping cough were all too common in pediatric practice.[3] But the scourge of polio was about to end with the 1955 release of the Salk vaccine. Long lines formed at Permanente immunization clinics as anxious parents presented their children for the long-awaited immunization. The 1959 opening of the new Bess Kaiser Hospital, with its attached medical office building, was to alter the nature of the pediatric practice. Thereafter, an on-call hospital-based pediatrician saw patients throughout the day during clinic hours; covered the delivery and emergency rooms, the nursery, and the pediatric ward overnight; and resumed regular office hours the following day.

THE NEW PEDIATRICIANS

In 1961 pediatricians Morton Eleff and Fred Colwell, residents together at Rainbow Baby and Children's Hospital, in Cleveland, Ohio, left private practice in Cleveland to join Permanente. Colwell's disenchantment with private practice had its genesis early. As a medical student, Colwell had steered toward pediatrics, influenced by Frederick C. Robbins. The 1954 recipient of the Nobel Prize in Physiology or Medicine, who at the time was professor of pediatrics at Case Western Reserve University. When Colwell began his Cleveland practice, his junior status meant a grueling schedule of continual night call and house calls, but little financial reward. As a way to introduce Colwell to the community, the owner of a neighborhood pharmacy and Colwell's office landlord, hit on the idea of offering free polio vaccination clinics each Sunday with Colwell in attendance. Advertised Sabin on Sundays (SOS), the program drew an immediate reaction from local physicians, who accused him of unethical practice and threatened to isolate him from the local medical community. Stung by the hostility displayed by his peers, Colwell determined to look elsewhere for a practice. He contacted Eleff, who had preceded him to Permanente. The Cleveland connection drew two others after Colwell: pediatrician Lloyd Johnson and obstetrician Sheldon Spielman. (Spielman was Eleff's former college roommate. Dissatisfied with private practice in upstate New York, he would join Permanente in 1966.)

Pediatrician Mark Butzer, a Minnesota native and graduate of Marquette University Medical School, joined the Medical Group in 1964. His exposure to the West Coast and to Kaiser Permanente had occurred during his pediatric residency at Children's Hospital in Los Angeles, where he moonlighted at the KP Fontana Medical Center. It was a Children's Hospital staff physician who told Butzer about an opportunity for a pediatrician in Oregon and, after consulting the *World Book Encyclopedia* to determine the location of the state, he traveled to Portland for an interview with Northern Permanente.

Peter Hurst's appointment as Chief of the Pediatric Department led to the recruitment of a spate of talented pediatricians. Raymond Blair was one.[4] A graduate of Queens University Belfast School of Medicine in Northern Ireland, Blair accepted a pediatrics residency at the prestigious Hospital for Sick Children in Toronto, Canada. The residency completed, he returned to Ireland for a time, but, having developed a liking for Canada, he decided to settle there instead. He considered a residency in internal medicine until he learned of the surplus of internists in Canada, so he moved to Edmonton, Alberta, becoming senior resident in pediatrics at the University of Alberta Hospital. There, the Department Chair asked if he would be interested in a two-year endocrinology fellowship in Portland. "Where's Portland?" Blair remembers asking. "Oregon," was the reply. "Where's Oregon?" asked Blair. It was with some misgivings that Blair left behind Canada with its vestiges of a familiar British heritage for the unknown U.S. Still, he received reassurances that he could always return to Edmonton and to the medical school staff should he find the U.S. not to his liking. His Oregon fellowship began under the tutelage of Harvey Klevit, head of pediatric endocrinology at the University of Oregon Medical School.

Nearing the completion of his fellowship, Blair received offers from small pediatric group practices in Eugene and Portland, and from the medical school, but he was looking for something different. Meanwhile, Hurst was attending Klevit's and Blair's weekly endocrine clinics. Liking what he saw in Blair, Hurst determined to woo him to Permanente. Together, they toured the sparkling new BK, and the two-year-old Division Medical Office. Hurst offered Blair an office with two exam rooms, an on-site laboratory and x-ray services, and his own office nurse. Permanente was the something different that Blair was looking for. He happily accepted Hurst's offer to join The Permanente Clinic.

Hurst's recruitment efforts didn't stop with Blair. When he heard reports of Klevit's unhappiness at the medical school, he set about luring him to Permanente. Harvey Klevit obtained his MD from Temple University School of Medicine in Philadelphia, interrupted his training for a tour of duty in the U.S. Army, and completed his pediatric residency at the University of Colorado Hospital. His chief resident was Oliver Massengale,[5] who, after a stint in private practice in Portland, also joined Permanente. Returning to Philadelphia for a three-year pediatric fellowship, Klevit received offers from Columbia University, Chicago, and Oklahoma, as well as from his Temple Medical School Professor Richard Olmsted. Olmsted had been hired as Chair of the Department of Pediatrics at the University of Oregon Medical School. Klevit came west and brought with him considerable resources from National Institutes of Health grants, but his expectations to have his own well-equipped laboratory were not fulfilled. Disillusioned, he considered returning to

Philadelphia, but after talking to Hurst he decided to give Permanente a try. Thus, Klevit and Blair joined the Medical Group in 1966 within days of each other.

Still later that year, the Medical Group recruited pediatrician Dallas Hovig. Born in Prosser, Washington, not far from Hanford, Hovig obtained his pediatric training in California and completed an infectious disease research fellowship at the University of Southern California. Realizing that academic medicine wasn't sufficiently compelling to him, and wanting to return to the Northwest, he joined Permanente and began working at the Vancouver Medical Office. He became the pediatrician for a Mr. and Mrs. Anderson and their two children. Neither the Andersons nor their pediatrician could have foreseen the circumstances that would bring them international fame within a few short years, when in 1973 Karen Anderson would deliver quintuplets (see page 100, section: "And Then There Were Five: The Quints").

With his rugged features and luxuriant, well-groomed beard, Gunnar Waage resembled the prototype of a Norwegian seafarer. He comes by this resemblance honestly, for he was born on Norway's West Coast on the tiny island of Hitra, population 800, where his ancestors had settled at the mouth of a fjord. Most of Waage's forebears were fishermen, though his own father departed from family tradition by choosing another seafaring career as captain of an oil tanker. Born in 1938, Waage grew up under German occupation (the family home at the mouth of the fjord was strategically located near a vital mining facility, which the Germans zealously protected). Waage did not see his father until he was seven; together with an older brother, he was raised by his mother who sustained the family on a small farm. After completing high school on the mainland, Waage attended medical school in Basel, Switzerland. He returned to Norway for an internship and that country's mandatory rural medical service, where he routinely made house calls by skis or by boat. In 1966 six U.S. medical centers accepted him for a pediatric residency. Richard Olmsted reached him by phone at 11:30 p.m. Norwegian time, as Waage was working up an acute abdomen case. Despite the lateness of the hour and Waage's attention to his urgent task, Olmsted convinced him to come to the Oregon Medical School. Once there, he met Hurst and Klevit, from whom he learned about practice opportunities at Permanente. Convinced by Hurst to join The Permanente Clinic, he began as a general pediatrician, though his real interest lay in establishing a neonatal program. By 1974 he devoted half his time to neonatology. By 1980 he enjoyed a full-time neonatology practice. Pediatrician Fred Nomura was another talent Hurst recruited to Permanente. His story and his later leadership roles are told in Chapter 18: "The Eighties: New Directions."

In 1970 the Pediatric Department began to separate into two distinctive groups: those who favored hospital and nursery work and those whose primary interest lay in outpatient pediatrics. All department members took night call, but those who specialized in neonatology worked more daytime hours in the nursery. Waage established a neonatology consultant group, with Hovig overseeing a hyper-alimentation program and Blair contributing his endocrinology expertise. Respiratory therapists developed intubation skills, and nurses learned neonatal intensive care procedures.

Californian Phillip Brenes obtained his MD and completed his pediatric residency and neonatology training at the University of California, San Francisco. It was during this training that he participated in the delivery of triplets—an experience that would serve him well at Permanente. Having completed a tour of duty in the Navy during the Vietnam era, he decided that the Northwest was a desirable place to raise his children. As nothing was available at the time at Permanente, he entered private practice with two other pediatricians in Parkrose, a district just outside the city limits. On his days off, he volunteered as faculty at the University of Oregon Medical School, where he became acquainted with Klevit, who was still overseeing the endocrine clinic. Klevit alerted Brenes when a position opened at Permanente. Hired by Hurst, Brenes began his Permanente career at the Vancouver Medical Office in 1972.

INNOVATIONS

In addition to recruiting top-flight pediatricians to Permanente, Hurst encouraged innovation within the department. In the early 1970s, he trained well-baby practitioners, including RNs Lois Grufke in Portland and Connie Sanders at Vancouver to provide the service. At the same time, Hurst implemented a program for Oregon Medical School students to preceptor with Permanente pediatricians and offered pediatric residents at Good Samaritan Hospital a rotation with Permanente physicians. Specialization began in the Pediatric Department in 1968, when newly hired Max Yao began to provide neurology consultations. In 1971 Clarence Morgan was hired away from the University of Oregon Medical School to add cardiology expertise.

Not all of Hurst's ideas met with approval. Though he proposed developing a teenage clinic,[6] the Executive Committee turned the idea down. He did, however, convince the Executive Committee to extend the age for pediatric patients to 18, at the same time securing two additional pediatricians to support the added patient population. This change was followed by an increased interest in adolescent medicine, including prevention of teenage pregnancies and nutritional education.

In June 1973 Fred Nomura succeeded Hurst as Chief of the Pediatric Department, whereupon he hired pediatric nurse practitioner Sally Weise to develop a nurse practitioner program for pediatrics. He and other pediatricians designed a training program, taught by Permanente pediatricians as well as by physicians at the Crippled Children's Division of the University of Oregon Medical School (now the Oregon Health and Science University Child Development and Rehabilitation Center and Doernbecker's Children's Hospital). In September, he enlisted three staff nurses in the four-month training program: Anna Chapman, Christa Spaltf-holz and Sandy Uhlig. At the end of the course, the three, now the Region's first pediatric nurse practitioners, had the special skills to counsel and examine teenage girls. They were promptly assigned to work in the medical offices.

In 1973 James Powell joined Permanente and Gunnar Waage's neonatal team. Two years later, Virginia Feldman followed Powell, her former chief resident at the Oakland Kaiser hospital. Like Powell, she joined the neonatal team beginning a career that would span 30 years, including 17 years as Pediatric Department Chief for the Bess Kaiser Hospital area. A passionate advocate for vulnerable children, Feldman worked tirelessly and ceaselessly to end child abuse. She launched a program to educate physicians, started an evaluation clinic to which physicians could refer at-risk children, and promoted a citywide, centralized child-abuse program that extended to other medical centers, community social workers, and police. She also focused on prevention, leading a successful lobbying effort for mandatory seat belts for children. And to ensure that KP supported the safety message, she made certain that the organization's pharmacies made car seats available to members.

Pediatrics continued to specialize. Two years after his arrival at Permanente, Richard Cohen was sent to Children's Hospital and Regional Medical Center of Seattle, Washington, to learn the new specialty of pediatric intensive care. On his return he organized a pediatric intensive care unit at BK. Mary Lynn O'Brien joined the Pediatrics Department in 1978; her expertise was developmental behavior pediatrics, a specialty that Powell, after a sabbatical leave, would also pursue. John Pearson joined the department in 1979, bringing consulting expertise, including muscle biopsy procedures for pediatric neuromuscular disease.

EARLY OBSTETRICIANS

During the early war years, mothers enrolled in Vancouver Permanente Health Plan were served by Raymond Gillette and Dudley Wiley, both veterans of Grand Coulee, and by obstetricians David James and George Stollwerck. Obstetric Department activity increased significantly when, in 1943, the Health Plan expanded to include families. And on June 2, 1944, Edgar and Sue Kaiser's fifth child and second son Henry Mead became the 259th baby delivered at the Northern Permanente Foundation Hospital.[7] In 1946 the program hired

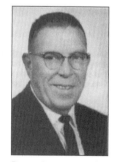

Roger George, MD, first Chief of Obstetrics. *Courtesy of Kaiser Permanente Heritage Resources.*

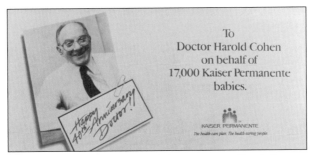

Billboard on North Greeley Avenue below Bess Kaiser Hospital.
From the author's collection.

Roger George as Chief of Obstetrics.[8] An experienced obstetrician, George was a good choice to join the pioneering Medical Group. Easily recognized for his crew cut and short, athletic body, he was rarely seen wearing a tie. He combined a sense of humor and an affable manner with a sense of professional self-assurance, instilling confidence in his peers and his patients.

Harold and Charlotte Cohen, medical school classmates who married in 1943, graduated together from the University of Illinois College of Medicine in 1945. Together they applied for internships at Los Angeles County General Hospital where Charlotte's aunt was a nurse. They were dismayed when only Harold was accepted in the program. Then the couple read about the Northern Permanente Health Plan in the *American Journal of Industrial Medicine*, were impressed by the article's illustrations of the hospital and the description of the program, and decided to intern at the Northern Permanente Foundation Hospital. They arrived in Vancouver in October 1945. Having never before ventured north of San Francisco, they had envisioned Vancouver, Washington, to be much like Vancouver, British Columbia. They were taken aback to find their new city a small town of just 60,000. Together the couple began their rotating internship with nine other interns; they were assigned living quarters—just two rooms—in the nurses' residence. At the time, Permanente trained residents in internal medicine and in surgery but not in obstetrics. When the Cohens completed their internships, Charlotte dropped out of the training program to raise their children. Harold began an obstetrics residency with Roger George, joining the medical staff in 1949.

Throughout his 48-year career at Permanente, Cohen was perhaps the most endearing, productive, and influential member of the Department of Obstetrics. He loved babies and women; it is said that when he entered a new mother's room he carried an aura of one supremely at home in his profession. A favorite of the other physician's wives, he drove one of them to the hospital for her delivery (after first dropping his own children at school along the way). In 1957 he delivered Selma and Larry Duckler's daughter, Mary Dawn; 27 years later he delivered Mary Dawn's son at BK. During his astonishingly long career, Cohen delivered more than 17,000 babies.

In 1963 Cohen was named Chief of the department, a position he held until 1974. During his tenure as chief, he recruited 16 obstetricians to the department: William Coburn, William Knox, and Sheldon (Shelly) Spielman, 1966; Daniel Pletsch, Barbara Manildi, Gordon Devilliers, 1968; Jess Dishman, Mark Hanschka and Stephen Sandor, 1971; Robert Broselow, 1972; Michael Axman, Brigitte Mengelberg, Nicholas Frattaroli, Robert McDowell, William Davolt, and Raju Sarda, 1973.[9]

In 1969 the continually short-staffed department delivered 2,372 babies. In 1970, Cohen contacted the American College of Nurse-Midwives for information about introducing a midwife program to KP. The Oregon Medical Practice Act had no provision for midwives; the executive secretary of the Board of Medical Examiners ruled that only a licensed physician had "the right to deliver a baby." Cohen was undeterred by the cautious, even negative, response to a midwife program. He readjusted his plan, proposing a program that would not involve deliveries but would instead feature prenatal office visits and postpartum home visits after early discharge. Carolyn Stadter began a career as the first midwife with KP Northwest at the Vancouver Medical Office in August 1971.

In time, the State of Oregon certified nurse midwives with the CNM certificate. Requirements included a master's degree in nursing, licensure by the Oregon State Board of Nursing, and certification by the American College of Nurse-Midwives. In 1989 obstetricians and midwives at Kaiser Sunnyside Medical Center began to manage patients jointly and midwives attended routine deliveries by 1996 nurse midwives delivered an estimated 50% of births at the hospital.

Cohen innovated in other ways. Always interested in new technology, Cohen studied the new diagnostic technique ultrasound. Convinced of its potential, he developed competency in its use. Knox learned the technique as well; he and Cohen proposed purchasing the equipment and hiring a technician. The Executive Committee resisted, uncertain about investing in a technique still not standard in the community. The committee also questioned the wisdom of designating personnel for ultrasound in a short-staffed department. Cohen and Knox persisted, however, and in 1972 became the first obstetricians in Oregon to use the new technique. Because ultrasound technicians were a rarity, they performed their own procedures until they were able to train a technician.

AND THEN THERE WERE FIVE: THE QUINTS

In February 1973 Karen Anderson visited midwife Carolyn Stadter[10] for a routine prenatal examination. Roger George, her regular obstetrician, was on vacation. Anderson seemed large for her estimated gestation time and Stadter spent many minutes listening with the then-standard head-mounted fetal scope. She listened until her neck began to ache. Thinking that she heard two fetal heart sounds, she ordered an x-ray, which revealed twins. When George returned from vacation, Stadter reported that his patient was carrying twins. During Anderson's next visit in March, George repeated the x-rays before examining her. Entering the exam room with the x-ray films, he placed them on the view box and showed the stunned Anderson that she was carrying four babies, rather than the two that had been identified during the February visit. Based on the new fetal count, George advised hospitalization, and the following day Anderson reported to BK for an ultrasound study to assess her condition. The ultrasound study took 45 minutes and showed a baby already within the birth canal, indicating the risk of labor at any time. The mother-to-be was immediately hospitalized for bed rest and observation.

Word soon spread about the imminent birth of quads. In the next two months much preparation was necessary. A special pediatric group formed—Brenes, Colwell, Hovig, and Waage—to coordinate protocols with obstetricians, as well as with respiratory therapists, laboratory personnel, and nursing staff. Brenes assumed the role of group spokesman, overseeing a 30-member team that became known as "the Quad Squad." George and Cohen were assigned to deliver the infants, and each baby was assigned a pediatrician, respiratory therapist, and nurse for care after delivery. Seven on-call blood donors remained on standby to ensure desirable fresh blood at delivery. Four isolets were transported from the intensive care nursery. Essential members of the team carried pagers 24 hours a day, a practice uncommon at the time.

Anderson went into labor April 25. The next day, her birthday, she was taken to the labor room. After laboring 12 hours, she was wheeled to the delivery room, and the Quad Squad went into action. The first baby, delivered by George and promptly named Roger George, was handed to Brenes to place in an isolet. Next came Owen, followed quickly by Audrey. It was then that the astonished team discovered that two more babies, rather than the expected one, were to be delivered. Baby Scott appeared next, followed by baby Diane, who, in major distress, required mouth-to-mouth resuscitation. After an anxious six-and-a-half minutes, Diane began to breathe on her own and was quickly taken to the neonatal intensive care unit. In the ensuing hours, reporters and TV cameras from local network television stations: KATU, KGW, and KOIN, together with newscasters from Seattle's KING and KOM, descended on the parents and hospital staff. This was only the fourth

time a set of surviving quintuplets had been born in the U.S.

The tiny infants required oxygen amid concern by physicians
and staff about how to and how
much to administer to avoid ret-
inopathy. The team monitored
blood gases frequently. Chief of
Anesthesia Rex Underwood and
pulmonologist Albert Vervloet
had discussed trying to avoid
intubation for respiratory support. At the time, injury to the
respiratory tract was a very real
threat; physicians lacked the so-

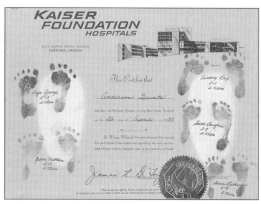

Multiple birth certificate presented to pediatricians attending the Anderson quints birth. *Courtesy of Fred Colwell.*

phisticated equipment that make intubation in today's health care settings almost
routine. Baby Diane remained sluggish and developed hyaline membrane disease
of the lungs. As her condition deteriorated, Hovig delivered to the parents the grim
news that Diane might not survive. Nevertheless they would try a new method, devised by Vervloet, to deliver oxygen without intubation. Twin tubes were inserted
short of the larynx to deliver adequate oxygen without injury, and the procedure
improved blood oxygen levels. Though her pulmonary function improved, Diane
now showed cardiac distress because of a patent ductus arteriosus, a complication
that required digitalis.

The neonatal intensive care unit remained the quints' home for many weeks until
gradually, one by one, they were discharged to the Anderson home. The exception
was the fragile Diane. Her mother had understood that she would be allowed to
bring her baby home when she reached five pounds. Now, however, the attending
pediatrician, worried about Diane's cardiac condition, strongly advised against discharge. Against the advice of the pediatrician, Anderson insisted on bringing Diane
home, and in preparation for the infant's discharge, she learned how to suction,
how to monitor Diane's heart rate, and how to give medication. Thus, with careful
supervision by Hovig, the Andersons were finally reunited—the parents, their two
older children, and the five quints.

In December, Diane's heart failure showed significant worsening and, in January, she was evaluated by specialists at the Oregon Medical School, who advised
urgent surgery. On January 16, surgeons successfully closed Diane's patent ductus
arteriosus. Five days later, baby Diane rejoined her parents and her six siblings at
the Anderson family home.

CHAPTER 10:
OPHTHALMOTORHINOLARYNGOLOGY

—⚮—

ULLMAN, MOSSMAN, AND HILBOURNE

In 1946 the Medical Group hired its first eye-ear-nose-and-throat (EENT) physician—Egon Ullman. In 1927 Ullman emigrated from Vienna where he had earned a reputation as a distinguished faculty lecturer at the University of Vienna. But he had become disillusioned, believing that Austria's socialist predilections were damaging the medical profession. And so he came to Oregon, accepting a position as special lecturer in biology and physiology at Oregon Agricultural College (now Oregon State University). An article in *The Oregonian* on April 10, 1927, quoted the newly arrived Ullman: "Vienna, a city that might be said to have a scientific proletariat, is under a complete socialistic government [where] a professional man is taxed so heavily that regardless of his income he is unable to keep more than enough for bare living." Interestingly, both Ullman and Norbert Fell fled Vienna, but for very different reasons: Ullman because of Vienna's socialism in the early part of the century, and Fell (see Chapter 9), a decade later, because of Austria's embrace of socialism's ideological opposite, fascism. During World War II, Ullman served as a colonel in the U.S. Air Force. At war's end, he sought an organized practice in Oregon. Although a man of science, Ullman, a dedicated bibliophile, was a lover of the arts, literature in particular. His considerable book collection included an autographed Mark Twain. Erudite and worldly, he loved Mozart, fine food and wine, and had a raconteur's talent for delighting friends and colleagues with stories. But Ullman was no effete; his wide-ranging interests included professional wrestling, whose heroes he likened to Roman gladiators. The day a friend introduced him to wrestler Gorgeous George was a cherished memory.

Frank Mossman came to Permanente the same year as Ullman, in expectation of a thoracic surgery residency with Norman Frink. Told on his arrival that the thoracic residency was no longer available, he trained instead with Ullman in EENT. Thereafter he joined the medical staff and was a member of the short-lived first and second partnerships. He left Permanente for private practice in 1953.

In its early years, Permanente's Health Plan was the only medical insurance program that included a covered benefit for refraction exams and for eyeglasses. (In the community, optometrists and ophthalmologists competed for this lucrative business.) Ullman and Mossman were hard-pressed to accommodate all those who clamored for vision appointments. Waiting lists grew unmanageable and, with only two to provide care, the service was poor. Relief came in 1953 when Health Plan hired its first optometrist, Jack Hilbourne. A second optometrist, Jennings Grebstad,[1] joined Hilbourne the following year. But by now Mossman had resigned, and once again EENT was down to one physician. The situation remained untenable until 1956 when ophthal-

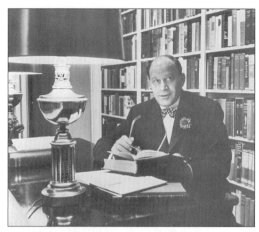

Egon Ullman, MD, first Northwest Permanente ophthalmotolaryngologist, circa 1959.
Courtesy of Jack Hilbourne.

mologist Donald Deering joined the department. (Deering could claim a brush with fame; while training at Cedars of Lebanon Hospital in Los Angeles, he had looked after and into the eyes of film beauty Elizabeth Taylor.)

OPHTHALMOLOGISTS

On February 27, 1962, Grebstad found Ullman slumped over his desk in his second floor office at Bess Kaiser Hospital. Cardiologist John Wild tried to resuscitate him without success. Again, Permanente found itself reduced to a single ophthalmologist. In 1964 Deering, like Mossman before him, resigned for a more lucrative private practice. Recruitment efforts intensified, and later that year, Permanente hired Bobby Nevill, formerly a flight surgeon in the Air Force. Three years later in 1967 James Sutton joined the department. Both Nevill and Sutton had obtained their ophthalmology training at University of California, Los Angeles—Sutton at the Los Angeles County Harbor General Hospital. In 1970 two more ophthalmologists were hired: Duane Diller and William Harris. Harris, formerly an industrial engineer, had been troubled by inefficiencies in the delivery of medical care. He decided to become a physician with the hope that he might contribute to change. He completed his medical education at University of Pennsylvania School of Medicine and his residency at Wills Eye Hospital in Philadelphia. Seeing no opportunities in the East with a health maintenance organization, Harris was drawn to the West Coast and to Permanente. By 1971 the department had grown to four and, with the hiring of Ernest Aebi in 1972, the department number rose to five. Thus, when Kaiser Sunnyside Medical

Center opened in 1975, the Ophthalmology Department was large enough to staff both hospitals. Aebi became Chief at BK, Nevill at KSMC.

During his residency training, Aebi had acquired a mistrust of optometrists and their competencies from his academic colleagues. This perception evaporated during his military service when he worked closely with optometrists. On joining the Medical Group, he began to collaborate more and more with the organization's optometrists, trusting them with procedures previously within the scope of practice of an ophthalmologist. One change he promoted, incorporating routine tonometry into the optometrist's regular refraction exams, was not popular with the optometrists, for it shifted to them more of the workload, which had to include the extra service in routine appointment time.

Aebi introduced other changes, among them a new, experimental cataract treatment called phacoemulsification.[2] At the time, the procedure was not yet available to Kaiser Permanente members, but when U.S. Senator Robert Packwood (R–OR) underwent the procedure in 1973, it attracted public interest. Aebi learned the technique at Good Samaritan Hospital where equipment was available and then began to perform phacoemulsification on KP patients. The established protocol called for an overnight hospital stay. But after one of his patients questioned the necessity of admission to the hospital, he made it an outpatient procedure at the hospital. Aebi trained his BK colleague ophthalmologist Christina West, and for a time they were the only two at KP who performed phacoemulsification. When West moved her practice to KSMC, both Nevill and Sutton, their competitive instincts aroused, learned the technique and began to incorporate the procedure into their own practices.

THE EARLY OTOLARYNGOLOGISTS

Ullman's untimely death in 1962 necessitated additional ear-nose-and-throat reinforcements. Otolaryngologists Eugene Petroff and Nolan Tanner, each building a private practice, contracted to work part-time for the Medical Group. Petroff knew Byron Fortsch from their residency training days. Having maintained communication with him. He knew that Fortsch was finding his private practice unmanageable. He bore the responsibility for covering Emanuel Hospital and Good Samaritan Hospitals, as well as emergencies at Gresham Hospital. Petroff suggested to Fortsch that he inquire at Permanente. At a lunch meeting with Executive Committee member Peter Hurst and Chief of Surgery Norman Frink, Fortsch was hired on the spot, making him Permanente's first full-time otolaryngologist and a one-man department. He began in March 1963, and immediately ordered new surgical instruments and endoscopy and bronchoscopy equipment.

Additional help arrived in 1964 in the person of Donald Hawkins. The Alabama native had completed two residencies, one in pediatrics, and one in ENT.

Hawkins' primary interest was in pediatric otolaryngology, and he left the Medical Group after only five years to pursue that interest. After Hawkins' arrival, Permanente hired brothers-in-law Lester Bergeron and Edward Korn. After Hawkins' resignation, Oregonian Charles Emerick joined the department. Born in McMinnville, Oregon and raised in Philomath, Bandon, and Tillamook, Emerick and his family finally settled in Gresham. A quarterback for his high school football team, he wanted to play college ball at one of the state universities but thought he was too small to make the cut. Instead, he attended the United Brethren College in Nebraska on a scholarship. Intending to become an engineer, he switched his major to medicine with the intention of doing mission work. At Creighton University School of Medicine, he ran out of money just one year before he could graduate. He joined the Navy to finance the rest of his training, graduated in 1956, and completed an ENT residency. His Navy service completed, in 1964 he traveled with his wife and three children to India where he served a five-and-a-half-year tour with the Presbyterian Ministries before joining Permanente.

Maurice Comeau came to The Permanente Clinic in 1971, two years after Emerick. Though he was born on his grandfather's farm in northern Saskatchewan, he was, like Emerick, essentially an Oregonian. He started attending school in a rural, two-room schoolhouse but his mother's illness later necessitated his attendance at a French-speaking boarding school run by nuns. He was still a child when his father, an American citizen, decided to return to the U.S. The family settled in Westfir, Oregon, a lumber town on the North Fork of the Willamette River. Two years later the family moved to another Willamette Valley lumber town, Oakridge, where Pope & Talbot, Inc., the lumber company, reigned as the major employer. Comeau graduated as valedictorian from Oakridge High School, went on to the University of Oregon and then to the University of Oregon Medical School. ENT Chief David DeWeese chose Comeau as his chief resident at the medical school and held a position open for him while he served his term in the Air Force. He was awaiting the results of his application for a UCLA fellowship when Bergeron offered him a temporary assignment at Permanente. Undecided, Comeau took care to weigh his choices, even making a visit to UCLA to see the program and campus for himself. After some deliberating, he decided against UCLA and joined Permanente instead. Comeau has reflected that two things probably influenced his decision to pursue a career in surgery: one was a three-week hospitalization as a child for a ruptured appendix; the other was his interest in anatomy, learned from his father, a master meat cutter.

Comeau became influential, not only within his department, but throughout Northwest Permanente and in the greater medical community. Over the years, he was elected to leadership positions with the Foundation for Medical Excellence, the Oregon Medical Association, the Multnomah County Medical Society, and the Oregon Board of Medical Examiners.

His 1971 introduction to Permanente and to his department must have given him cause for concern; expecting to be one of four, he learned instead that the small department comprised only three. Korn had departed, Bergeron was working only part time and preparing to leave (both resigned in 1971) and Emerick was leaving shortly for another year of missionary work in India.

Even after Emerick's return from India in 1972, ENT was still a three-person department. Meanwhile construction was beginning on the new KSMC, and when it opened in 1975, Emerick became ENT Department Chief. His tenure as chief lasted 14 years, during which a number of physicians passed through the department on their way to private practice. Still, despite the turnover, the department grew, and Emerick assembled a strong group of ENT physicians, including Sharon Higgins,[3] Geoffrey Lawrence, Jeffrey Israel,[4] and Clee Lloyd. In 1989, Emerick relinquished his position as chief to Sharon Higgins, who went on to hire additional ENT specialists, including Dieter Hoffman and Larry Demas.

The ENT Department at BK endured a rather more complicated coalescing. In 1972 the four-person department included Chief Fortsch, Comeau, the newly hired Richard Hendricks, and the returning Emerick. Looking for a leadership change, members of the department elevated the reluctant Comeau to the position of chief. More physicians joined the department during the next few years: Damianos Kyriakopoulos, David Chate, and William Knox. Individuals within the small department had strong personalities, held rigidly to their own ideas regarding practice styles, and could not seem to find common ground. Unwilling to be guided by Comeau, they asked Chate to replace him as chief. But the change of leaders did little to bring about cohesion. Chate stepped down as chief and resigned from NWP. Next Kyriakopoulos took a turn as department leader, apparently with no better success, for after a year Area Medical Director David Lawrence took over the leadership of the troubled department. By now, Comeau was physician-in-charge at the Interstate Medical Office, and when Lawrence solicited him to accept the position of Department Chief, he at first declined. Eventually, Lawrence prevailed on him to take the seemingly thankless job. To his relief and surprise Comeau's second term as chief went much more smoothly. When Fortsch transferred to the Beaverton Medical Office, Comeau hired two experienced otolaryngologists Hans Behrens and Jay Kent. Behrens gradually assumed increasing leadership responsibilities, first as assistant chief, then in 1990, as acting chief during Comeau's sabbatical leave, and finally, as department chief.

THE OPTOMETRISTS

When optometrists Jack Hilbourne and Jennings Grebstad were hired in 1953 and 1954, the ophthalmologists welcomed the two, including them in staff dinner meetings and in social activities. Still, recruitment of additional optometrists was painfully slow for nearly a decade; local optometrists, both recent graduates and those with experience, were slow to warm to the idea of working within a prepaid system. Hilbourne reported feeling isolated from his peers outside Permanente in those years.

With Aebi's encouragement, optometrists' scope of practice expanded to include prescribing contact lenses, screening for disease, and managing laser surgery patients both pre- and postoperatively. Many among a new crop of optometrists, like Steven Van Hee who joined in 1971, had broad experience. Van Hee, for example, had served in the U.S. Armed Forces, including tours in Vietnam, and had worked closely with an ophthalmologist at a military base hospital.

Optometrists in the Northwest Region were employees of Health Plan, though they reported to the Medical Group. By contrast, their counterparts in Northern California were employees of The Permanente Medical Group. In 1975 the Region appointed two optometry Chiefs: Van Hee at KSMC and Hilbourne at BK. Hilbourne stepped down in 1985, to be replaced by Grebstad, who in turn relinquished the position in 1990 to Charles Samuels. In 2000, the department would decide on a single regional Chief and elect William Borok[5] as its leader.

In 1985 NWP and Health Plan leaders decided to reorganize optometry services under Health Plan, with the goal of integrating optical services, aligning staff, and increasing revenues. An advisory board that included both ophthalmologists and optometrists was to assure quality of care. The reorganization was not popular with optometrists; they saw in the move a diminution in status and a weakening of their position with the physicians. Increasingly dissatisfied with their status whereby Health Plan imposed budget restrictions but physicians exercised administrative control, optometrists nevertheless decided against joining Allied Health Professionals when that group decided to unionize in 2000. Optometrists had resisted several earlier efforts to unionize, fearing such a decision would damage their professional status. They were happy when, in 2001, they were allowed to affiliate with NWP, where today they enjoy the benefits of the Medical Group.

CHAPTER 11:
PATHOLOGICAL NEEDS

—ᜠ—

THE EARLY PATHOLOGISTS

During the war years, Permanente had the good fortune to employ pathologist Lucy Hacker in a specialty that the Medical Group lacked. Internist Charles Grossman convinced Hacker to leave Yale University and New Haven and to accept the challenge of a new and innovative prepaid practice. Her arrival coincided with that of laboratory supervisor John Neufeld, also a newcomer to Permanente, and responsible for eight laboratory technicians and four assistant technicians. Trained at the College of Medical Evangelists in Los Angeles, Neufeld came from Portland Sanitarium Hospital where he had been laboratory director.

In 1946 as post-war membership plummeted, the struggling program scaled back. Both Hacker and Neufeld left (Hacker later joined the Kabat Kaiser Institute in Vallejo and pursued a new career in rehabilitation medicine). In these lean times, Permanente had to do without a formally trained pathologist for about two years. Physicians in other disciplines were obliged to fill the gap. Internist Joseph Kriss assumed the role of laboratory Director; internist Walter Noehren took charge of clinical pathology and autopsies. Even Chief of Surgery Norman Frink spent time at the microscope examining surgical specimens.

In 1948 pathologist William Lehman from Good Samaritan Hospital began providing part-time service at Northern Permanente Foundation Hospital. In 1959 after Bess Kaiser Hospital opened, he went into private practice but continued to provide service to Permanente on a per capita basis until 1969. During this time, pediatrician Peter Hurst served as Director of Laboratories, except for a period between 1962 and 1963, when he took a sabbatical leave. In his absence internist Arnold Hurtado was Acting Director.

Entrepreneurial Lehman founded the Physicians Medical Laboratories. But though he was engaged in a new business enterprise, he and associates Eugene Bogaty and John Hoffman continued to rotate duties at BK and to take call for cases needing onsite biopsies with frozen sections.[1] As technologies in the field grew, so Lehman's medical laboratories grew as well. He was now able to provide cytology screening and nuclear medicine services to his Permanente clients and to the community.

Unlike many community physicians, Lehman had a good relationship with Permanente; he socialized with the physicians and was helpful in many ways. On one occasion, he helped Paul Trautman prepare for his surgical specialty board exams by reviewing pathological slides with him. Lehman's interests revealed a restless energy. He had already demonstrated his entrepreneurial talents with a successful medical laboratory. He was a shrewd land investor as well and in 1968 he sold his 60-acre farm in Clackamas County to Kaiser Permanente.[2] Of little interest to others at the time he purchased it, the property would become suddenly valuable when the nearby Interstate 205 freeway opened. Today Lehman's former farm is the site of Kaiser Sunnyside Medical Center, Mt. Scott and Mt. Talbert Medical Offices, the Sunnybrook Medical Office and Surgicenter, and the 40-bed inpatient Brookside Center for the Departments of Mental Health and Addiction Treatment. Regional supply and process centers also occupy the site.

Meanwhile, two pathologists from Portland Providence Hospital, Daniel Baer and John Smith, met with BK Administrator James DeLong to discuss contracting their services. Baer was board-certified in both anatomic and clinical pathology, his primary interest. The Baer-DeLong discussions were not conclusive, and Baer moved on, accepting positions at St. Francis Hospital in Honolulu and at the University of Hawaii. But DeLong had not forgotten Baer, and on a visit to Hawaii, he contacted Baer again, this time with a firm offer: Director of Laboratories and Clinical Pathology, with the added bonus of planning the new regional laboratory to be located on the KSMC campus.

Baer began his new role in February 1970 and hired Richard Gourley as Assistant Director and Chief of Anatomic Pathology. (Gourley had been Associate Professor of Pathology and Director of the School of Cytotechnology at the Oregon Medical School.) With an eye to expansion, Baer hired pathologists with expertise in specialty fields. Ronald Jones was one. Jones had developed an early interest in microbiology and pathology. Seeing a unique opportunity with Permanente, he joined in 1974.

THE NEW CADRE

The 1975 opening of the new regional laboratory drew two more pathologists— Sushma Chawla and Walter Froelich. With the addition of Froelich, board certified in nuclear medicine, KP could establish its own Nuclear Medicine Department. George Chan replaced Gourley later that year, and Kathleen Holahan joined the department in 1978, attracted by the opportunity to pursue her specialty in hematopathology.[3] Still, despite these additions, the department remained short-staffed, so its members welcomed pathologists Neal Olson and David Scott in 1981. Olson knew Holahan from their training days at University of Minnesota Medical Center. Answering an ad in the *New England Journal of Medicine*, Olson flew on a January morning from Minneapolis, where the temperature was minus 20 degrees, arriving in Portland to mild weather and complaints by Mt. Hood skiers about the lack of snow. The addition of Olson helped lessen Holahan's work load and the reading of an increasing number of bone marrow examinations.

Montreal native David Scott graduated from McGill University School of Medicine with plans to become a family practitioner. Two months into a family practice residency in Michigan was all it took for Scott to change his mind. He then worked in an emergency room in Midland, Michigan before determining that pathology was his career choice. Pathology training included two additional years at McGill, another two at the Oregon Medical School, a staff position at Portland Providence, and a one-year fellowship in surgical pathology at Stanford. Permanente internist Arthur Hayward, a neighbor and friend of the Scott family, recommended Scott to Permanente pathologist Holahan.

Permanente now had a new cadre of talented pathologists and, in the 1970s Baer came under increasing scrutiny for performance issues within the department. In 1982 he stepped down as director and soon thereafter he accepted a position as director of pathology for the Portland Veterans Administration Hospital.

Assistant Department Chief Ronald Jones assumed the leadership position vacated by Baer. Jones was accorded near star status by his colleagues—at least for a time. In 1979 he was the first recipient of Permanente's Distinguished Physician Award. Two years later, *Oregon Magazine* included Jones in its list of "Super Doctors: the Best and the Brightest of Oregon MDs." He served on numerous journal editorial boards, was associate editor, editor, and editor-in-chief of others. He served as well on various committees and chaired at least one: the National Committee for Clinical Laboratory Standards.

In 1982 the year Baer resigned, pathologist John Thompson completed a fellowship at University of Pennsylvania. His wife sought a pediatric residency in the West and found one at Oregon Health and Science University. Their destination determined, Thompson viewed his options in the Portland area. He was already familiar with a group-practice model (his brother was practicing at Group Health Cooperative in Seattle), and he was delighted to find a position with Northwest Permanente.

Meanwhile, as he received more and more external funding, Jones spent an increasing amount of his time responding to the demand for microbiological services to support drug trials and for research on antibiotic resistance and susceptibility. In 1984 alone, Jones published 32 professional articles and presented his research findings at seven major national and international scientific meetings. Inevitably, these claims on his time left no time for department administration. Area Medical Director Stuart Bowne appointed Thompson Chief of Pathology in 1984.

TURF BATTLES: JONES VS. GREENLICK

Jones, meanwhile, expanded his clinical research activities employing three nurse practitioners for a study of preoperative prophylactic antibiotics. His work was increasingly encroaching on the turf of the Center for Health Research and placed him at odds with its director Merwyn (Mitch) Greenlick. It was inevitable that Jones would run into trouble.

Though Jones had received prior approval for his independent research from Medical Director Marvin Goldberg and from Permanente legal counsel Roger Miyaji, Greenlick was determined to rein him in. The Center for Health Research raised concerns about lack of oversight in Jones' activities, noting in particular deficiencies surrounding informed consent. Consequently, the Board of Directors performed an audit, which revealed some minor irregularities, and Jones was formally chastised.[4] By now internationally known in the field, Jones was not without options, and he resigned from the Medical Group. For a time he worked at the Clinical Microbiology Institute he had founded in Tualatin and retained his position as Associate Professor of pathology, microbiology and infectious diseases at OHSU. In 1989, Jones accepted a position as Professor at the University of Iowa Carver College of Medicine.[5]

AUTOMATION

An era of automation in clinical pathology, begun some time earlier, was gathering speed. The autoanalyzer[6] could provide multiple chemistries on a single specimen; the Coulter Counter could determine white and red blood cell concentrations using an electrical sensory zone method for sizing and counting particles. Gone was the day when a technician had to do a blood cell count by looking through a microscope.

As Department Chief, Thompson recognized the potential of automation for cost savings to the laboratory. That year he presented a paper at a conference of the College of American Pathologists entitled, "Potential Use of Computer Systems in Proving Cost Efficient Care." Forward-thinking though he was, Thompson could hardly have envisioned the explosion of technology and automation that would occur during his 23-year tenure as Department Chief. Together with administrative Director of the Laboratory Dixie Penwarden, Thompson and his team of pathologists and PhDs would implement startling and profound changes.

One of these was the 1988 introduction of a computer-tracking-and-reporting system. Now when a test was completed the computerized reports went directly to the physician's office; hand delivery was a thing of the past. Now when a physician called the lab for test results, they were instantly available. By 1992 automation could process two million tests a year. And the automation juggernaut continued:

the Bactic machine allowed pathologists to detect the presence of bacteria in blood without waiting for cultures. The Microscan Walkaway apparatus quickly identified bacteria and susceptibility without reliance on the lower disc diffuse method.

Moreover, automation extended beyond clinical pathology to anatomic pathology. Pathologist Olson remembers that his early work to differentiate difficult-to-diagnose tumors relied on morphology alone. With automation, immunohistochemistry with antibody and antigen techniques could distinguish malignancies. With its sophistication, efficiency, and high volume, by 1996 KP was a leader in the pathology community. That year the lab contracted to perform microbiology and nonemergent chemistry for OHSU.

Nor was the laboratory to be left behind in the field of cytogenetics. Jacob Reiss had served a one-year fellowship at OHSU in medical genetics. There he had met pediatricians Peter Hurst and Harvey Klevit and had provided genetic consultations to the NWP Pediatric Department. Though he was allocated just one hour per week to practice genetics when he joined Permanente as a pediatrician, Reiss gradually was given more time in his specialty, obtaining board certification in medical genetics. In 1982 Reiss took a sabbatical leave in Australia at the Children's Hospital in North Adelaide. There he met Northwest native, Peter Jacky, PhD who was also completing a training program in genetics. It was Reiss who persuaded KP to provide its own cytogenetic service. Reiss hired Jacky and a cytogenetic technician; together, Reiss and Jacky became Co-Directors of the cytogenetic laboratory under the Department of Pathology and undertook chromosomal studies on blood, bone marrow, and amniotic fluid. A year later the department achieved separate status, and the service grew until Reiss was able to confine his practice to clinical genetics.

As the scope and sophistication of laboratory work increased, the physical plant became woefully inadequate. The organization's leaders drew up plans for a new facility with a process-based design. Funds for the capital to build a new facility proved to be a stumbling block. The next best solution was to revamp an existing facility. Leasing agents found a 47,000 square-foot building, formerly a high-compression washer factory, east of Portland on Airport Way near the Columbia River. Starting with a shell, laboratory leaders hired Toronto-based Alcon, a laboratory design company, to supervise construction. The organization was breaking new ground. Few laboratories of the sophistication sought by KP had been attempted. A laboratory with this degree of automation required an area the size of a basketball court. Today the KP Northwest laboratory can be viewed from above through a glass partition. Robotic arms silently fill conveyor belts and automated workstations. Only rarely does one see a human presence in the cavernous space.

CHAPTER 12:
RADIOLOGY

—ᴍ—

The 1943 Radiology Department at Northern Permanente Foundation Hospital in Vancouver included just three members: Warren Zager, a roentgenologist; one technician; and one assistant. By 1944 the department had grown, and Zager, together with five x-ray technicians, four clerical workers, and two assistants processed an average of 4,500 x-ray exposures each month for 1,700 patients. In November of that year, Morris Malbin replaced Zager. (Malbin was one of seven pioneering physicians who elected to remain with Permanente after the closure of the shipyards and the exodus of workers after the war.)

In 1951 Henry Kavitt completed his training in Minnesota and applied for an Oregon license. The Permanente Clinic's Medical Director Ernest Saward learned through his secretary about Kavitt's application and promptly wrote him a letter, describing an open position. Unfamiliar with Permanente, Kavitt wrote an old friend, Portland internist Edward Rosenbaum,[1] to ask his opinion. Rosenbaum suggested Kavitt give Permanente a try and as an inducement offered him a part-time job in his own small group practice. At a lunch at Henry Thiele's restaurant on the corner of NW Burnside and 23rd streets, Saward offered Kavitt a salary twice that offered by a recruiting Minnesota group. Kavitt accepted the job offer. He was to replace Malbin and to work, half time at first, at the Broadway Clinic. He would be the sole radiologist for the next ten years.

Radiology equipment at the Northern Permanente Foundation Hospital and at the Broadway Clinic was World War II vintage; the fluoroscopy machine at the Broadway Clinic had a hand-cranked table and a screen with a precarious spring-balance mechanism. Wooden tanks used to develop films lacked a temperature regulator, and technicians routinely dipped their elbows in the solution to ascertain the proper temperature. Kavitt recalls an incident during the fluoroscope exam of the wife of Health Plan Manager Hufford when the screen loosened and fell on Mrs. Hufford's head. Fortunately, the patient escaped injury, but in less than a week a new fluoroscopy screen appeared. (Kavitt's request for a thermometer to measure the temperature in the developing tank, however, languished for three months.) The Broadway Clinic X-ray Department was tiny and cramped; the radiologist's office measured a mere six by seven feet, with a curtain for a door. A desk supported two tabletop view boxes.

The 1959 opening of Bess Kaiser Hospital brought a long-awaited modern radiology suite, which Kavitt would later describe in a 1991 publication, *From X-rays to Imaging Service*. New equipment included two state-of-the-art GE fluoroscopes, motor-driven tables, and counter-balanced fluoroscopy screens. The department lacked space for the bulky automated film processors. A smaller unit was installed in 1964—one that could develop film in just seven minutes and a huge improvement over the wet-tank system that required a 90-minute processing time. Attracting radiologists to Permanente remained problematic. Two who were recruited in 1961 resigned after only one year. Fortunately for Kavitt, Oregon Medical School radiologist James Haworth was looking for a career change and joined Permanente in 1962. Experienced and accustomed to high-volume work, Haworth proved a welcome colleague for Kavitt.

The acquisition of state-of-the-art equipment made recruiting for radiologists easier. Beginning with the hiring of Robert Vann in 1968, the decade of the 1970s attracted younger, recently trained radiologists eager to demonstrate their skills. Larry Renshaw came in 1971. He was followed by William Kadner in 1972, Alvin Graham in 1973, and Anthony Kostiner and Jerry King in 1974. This new breed, called interventional radiologists, began to extend their scope of practice, performing procedures previously done only by surgeons: myelograms, arthrograms, and cerebral angiographies. Graham specialized in femoral artery catheterization, a technical advance over the more risky aortogram, whereby a surgeon injected a long needle into the aorta. Frank McKowne, hired in 1978, began to perform ultrasound procedures in 1979. Peter Krook, trained in computerized axial tomography (CT), came in 1979. He coordinated the purchase of the Region's first CT machine, installed at Kaiser Sunnyside Medical Center in 1983. Four months later, radiologist Ben Brown, with a fellowship in CT, joined the Medical Group. Brown had sought a position in the Northwest and was attracted to Kaiser Permanente as a progressive group with state-of-the-art equipment.

CHAPTER 13:
INTERNISTS AND THE EARLY
MEDICAL SUBSPECIALISTS

HISTORY OF INTERNAL MEDICINE IN THE U.S.

Internists historically defined themselves as an elite hospital-based specialty with expertise in diagnosis and the use of the clinical laboratory.[1] As early as 1885, William Osler, together with seven other physicians, formed the Association of American Physicians (AAP) to distinguish internists, with their superior training in pathology and the laboratory, from generalists.

The 1910 Flexner Report required medical schools to provide training in basic sciences and, in 1913 the education council of the American Medical Association recommended two postgraduate years after internship as a requirement for specialists. Two years later, the American College of Physicians (ACP) formed, which, though it floundered for a time for lack of interest by academic physicians and medical leaders, in time became the major organization to represent internists.

In Osler's era, notable advances in surgery had helped bestow more prestige on U.S. surgeons than on their physician counterparts, and the American Surgical Society was already well established. As President of the American Academy of Physicians, Osler was determined to elevate the status of the internist. In an address to the Tennessee State Medical Association in August 1919, Osler exulted, "The surgeons have had their day—and they know it. The Mayo brothers have made their clinic as important in medicine as it ever was in surgery. Wise men! They saw how the pendulum was swinging."

Encouraged by the AMA, specialty boards began to grant certification in the 1930s (though non-certified physicians were still not prevented from practicing specialties). And in 1936 the American Board of Internal Medicine, with support from the ACP but not from the elitist AAP,[2] became the 12th specialty board. Osler would have been pleased.

More complexity arose when general practitioners, desiring commensurate recognition, in 1947 established the American Academy of General Practitioners. Residencies in family practice were introduced and, in 1969 the American

Board of Family Practitioners formed, adding to the shifting permutations within primary care. (The growth of family practice within Northwest Permanente is discussed more fully in Chapter 17 "The Seventies.") In response, primarily to achieve economic parity with other specialists, internists in 1956 established the American Society of Internal Medicine, which merged with the ACP in 1998.

EVOLUTION OF MEDICAL SUBSPECIALTIES AT NORTHWEST PERMANENTE

As advances in medicine increased in the last half of the 20th century, U.S. physicians increasingly sought additional training and specialization. Permanente reflected the national trend, one that evolved in roughly three phases. In the earliest phase, clinicians who had trained as internists who had an interest in a more specific aspect of medicine informally assumed responsibility for subspecialty work—often after their scheduled office hours. In the next phase, internists with formal residency training or certification in a subspecialty were relieved of primary care responsibility to devote all their time to the subspecialty practice. And finally, these internists attained official status as subspecialists and formed separate departments. And, as more fellowship-trained specialists joined Permanente, the organizational structure of the medical practice grew increasingly complex, with both medicine and surgery expanding to include an ever-growing number of subspecialties.

In the 1960s, young internists began to abandon internal medicine in favor of subspecialty training. Figures from 1970 show the change: that year 80% of internal medicine residents chose subspecialty training, and six more subspecialty boards came into being. Not surprisingly, recruitment of internists became increasingly difficult, even for Permanente, where the medical practice allowed far more flexibility to pursue one's subspecialty interests.

In 1974 Permanente adopted the traditional multispecialty model, which excluded general practitioners, and recruited family practitioners to the medical staff. The rationale for including these generalists was their ability to treat both young and old—a physician for the whole family—and a seeming reversal from the trend toward more and more specialization. As the Family Practice Department expanded, the dominance of the internists receded. Alarmed at the shortage of internists, residency programs have since tried, with little success, to popularize general internal medicine. In 1978 the ACP funded a Society for Research and Education in Primary Care, later to become the Society of General Internal Medicine, a professional organization to strengthen and promote internal medicine.

Permanente's history reflects the dual roles that many of its physicians brought to their practice and how various subspecialties developed within the Medical Group. As medical practice grew more sophisticated, Permanente adapted, hiring more fellowship-trained subspecialists and providing the new technologies and staff to support them. This chapter chronicles the increasing sophistication of physician training over time.

DEPARTMENT OF MEDICINE AT NORTHWEST PERMANENTE

Ernest Saward, hired as internal medicine Chief in 1945, held the position for 15 years until he relinquished it to Noah Krall in 1960. In 1964 Arnold Hurtado succeeded Krall as Chief. When, in 1975, Hurtado was promoted to area Medical Director for the new Kaiser Sunnyside Medical Center, the growing Region had two department chiefs: Perry Sloop at Bess Kaiser Hospital and Ian MacMillan at KSMC. Sloop's tenure of three years was interrupted by sabbatical leave in 1978, and a series of chiefs succeeded him in the BK area: James Brodhacker, John Emery, John Bakke, and Richard Olson. MacMillan enjoyed 14 years as Chief. Arthur Hayward replaced him in 1989 and served as Chief until 1996. Much of the period was marked by rivalry, sometimes friendly and sometimes not so, between the two departments for a dwindling number of top applicants for internal medicine positions.

CARDIOLOGY

The specialty of cardiology was still in its infancy during World War II. Treatment for cardiac disease was still the stock and trade of the internists. In the early 1940s Edward Steiner supervised the four-lead electrocardiogram machine at the Northern Permanente Foundation Hospital, averaging seven to eight readings per day. When Steiner left the Medical Group in 1944, no one else had the formal training to interpret the "graphs," which meant sending them to local cardiologist Harold Gillis for interpretation.

In 1961 Permanente hired internist John Wild, who brought significant training and experience in cardiology. Born in England, Wild spent five years of his childhood in India where his father was a British Army physician. His activities were restricted in medical school when a chest x-ray showed a tubercular lesion; during internal medicine training at the Royal Postgraduate Medical School at the Hammersmith and St. Mary's Hospital in London, he received periodic pneumothorax treatments for his tuberculosis. Rather than take a consultant posting in Liverpool, Wild emigrated from England to the University of Iowa, which accepted him as a senior resident. There, despite an essential tremor present since his childhood, he was invited to join the cardiac catheterization team and the Department of Cardiology. He joined Permanente as an internist in 1961.

It wasn't until the arrival of John Grover in 1968 that the evolution of the cardiac service really began. After serving an internal medicine residency at the U.S. Public Health Service Hospital in Seattle, Grover pursued his interest in cardiology, training for a time with a Seattle cardiologist. It was then that he observed the care of endocrinologist Robert H. Williams, hospitalized for a myocardial infarction. Grover recalls that Williams' colleagues remained at the bedside 24 hours a day to monitor his cardiac rhythm. Such close monitoring was unusual at the time, and Grover remembers thinking that continuous monitoring should be the standard of care in managing myocardial infarction. Consequently, on joining Permanente, Grover began to lobby for a small coronary care unit (CCU) and, in 1969, a two-bed CCU with monitoring equipment opened at BK on the fifth floor of the medical unit. John Wild was appointed Director and a cardiology call schedule was implemented. Shortly after an expanded CCU opened in the hospital's new south wing, a CCU nurse successfully defibrillated a patient who had suffered a cardiac arrest—the first such independent nurse action at BK.

In 1972 Wild and Grover, assisted by local Portland cardiologist Wayne Rogers, performed cardiac catheterizations at St. Vincent Hospital on NW Westover Road to evaluate patients for cardiac surgery. Permanente continued to insist, however, that its cardiologists devote some of their time to internal medicine and to carry a panel of patients. This insistence made the retention of cardiologists difficult; two physicians hired the following year resigned in quick succession, disaffected with the requirement. Inevitably, with the 1974 hiring of cardiologist George Baker, Permanente changed its ruling, and thereafter cardiologists practiced their subspecialty exclusively.

As the department grew more sophisticated, Permanente cardiologists began to perform cardiac catheterizations at BK. Grover's primary care duties included supervising Trudy Zeller, physician's assistant, whom he trained to perform treadmill exercise EKG testing; thus, Zeller became the first cardiology PA. (In 1989 Mary Sanders would become the first cardiac nurse practitioner at KSMC.) In 1974 Permanente contracted with Albert Starr and his cardiac surgery team to operate on Kaiser Permanente patients at Providence St. Vincent Medical Center. A result of this unique collaboration featured a weekly conference at one of the KP hospitals, with Starr or one of his associates consulting with Permanente cardiologists to determine candidates for surgery. The weekly conferences have been a staple of the Permanente-Providence St. Vincent collaboration.

In 1975 Wild moved to the newly opened KSMC, and four years later Permanente hired its first fellowship-trained cardiologist, Dale McDowell. The 1980s brought five additional cardiologists to Permanente, including Phillip Au in 1987, who joined Permanente as a coronary interventionist. Au was a dream candidate for the slot Permanente had in mind. His credentials were impressive. He had followed a three-year cardiology fellowship with additional training in coronary angioplasty at the KP Sunset Hospital in Los Angeles where he had enjoyed a high volume of cases within a well-managed program.

For his part, Au was attracted to the 290,000-member KP program, which at the time referred 100 angioplasties per year to Providence-St. Vincent, an exciting prospect for a beginning interventionist. He was to be based at the Providence-St. Vincent Medical Center, and he, rather than the Providence-St. Vincent cardiologists, was to perform these delicate procedures for KP patients. Not surprisingly, this decision and Au's integration within the medical staff at Providence-St. Vincent was far from smooth, for although the administrative staff supported the plan, the physicians did not. During his introduction at a medical staff meeting, Au remembers the grilling he endured by the Chief of the medical staff about his qualifications. Fortunately, the hospital administrator intervened during the increasingly hostile inquisition.

At his debut angioplasty procedure, Au recalls "20 people in dark suits" silently observing him from the control room; no Permanente physicians were present. (The "dark suits," he later learned, were from Providence-St. Vincent and included the Chief of the medical staff, the Chief of Cardiology, cardiac surgeon Albert Starr, angioplasty cardiologist Henry Garrison and various administrators.) The watchful audience found no fault with Au's inaugural performance. By 1990 performing 300 angioplasties and 250 coronary catheterizations a year, Au was the busiest coronary interventionist in the Northwest. When Au requested the support of a PA, the Providence-St. Vincent medical staff, long opposed to PAs on staff, strenuously objected. Au prevailed, with the support of the Providence-St. Vincent administrator, and Terry Glickman the first PA dedicated to cardiology on the Providence-St. Vincent medical staff joined Au. Much has changed since then. Today nine nurse practitioners and PAs perform various procedures, including cardioversion.

The 1990s would see the retirement of the pioneer cardiologists: Grover, in 1996, and Baker, in 1999 (Wild had retired in 1986). With the 1996 closure of BK, its cardiologists relocated to Providence-St. Vincent Hospital.

HEMATOLOGY

When hematologist Virgil Fairbanks joined the Medical Group in 1963, he and Hurtado had to make do with a single microscope located in the hospital clinical laboratory. Fairbanks resigned to join the staff of the Mayo Clinic, and when internist and fellowship-trained hematologist Norman Birndorf replaced the departing Fairbanks in 1971, he was confronted with the same lack of equipment. He was obliged to purchase his own microscope. During the next three years, Permanente recruited two more internists with fellowship training in hematology: Eldon Anderson and Stephen Chandler, both from Oregon Health and Science University. These two, together with Birndorf, would later join the Oncology Department to form a combined hematology-oncology service.

ENDOCRINOLOGY

Having developed an interest in diabetes management and endocrinology during his residency training at Beth Israel Hospital in Boston, Eric Liberman joined Permanente as an internist in 1959, after a stint in private practice. Eventually, though not fellowship trained, he was allowed to limit his practice to endocrinology. Like Liberman, Harold Nevis joined the Medical Group as an internist, but unlike Liberman, Nevis had completed an endocrinology fellowship.

A native of Chicago, Nevis traveled at age 16 to Israel for a planned six-month visit. The visit extended to seven years, during which time Nevis served as a pilot in the Israeli Air Force. A life-long goal to become a physician prompted his eventual return to Chicago, where he completed both his medical school and fellowship training at University of Chicago School of Medicine. While pursuing his goal and to help finance his long medical education, he put his pilot's experience to good use. Working for a local advertising firm that handled the Doublemint chewing gum account, Nevis flew the famous Wrigley family to their residences on the north end of Lake Michigan. At Permanente, Nevis eventually concluded that he was a general internist at heart and dropped his endocrinology specialty.

An early advocate of computerized record keeping, in 1983, more than a decade before KP Northwest adopted a computerized system, Nevis developed a computer-assisted pilot project, allowing the five physicians in his module to enter, retrieve, and share clinical information. Though reliance on the paper record remained the norm, Nevis's small project was a precursor to the electronic medical record that supplanted the paper record at NWP after 1996.

Harry Glauber came to Permanente in 1987, as its first full-time endocrinologist. He had earned his MD at the University of Witwatersrand in Johannesburg, South Africa and was at Baragwanath Hospital in Soweto during the June 1967 uprising that resulted in 500 deaths and 1,000 injuries—many youths in their teens. After residency training in Seattle, he took an endocrine fellowship at University of California, San Diego. His discovery of NWP was somewhat serendipitous when he was visiting friends in Portland. Once settled in at Permanente, Glauber recalled his pleasure and surprise when Chief of Internal Medicine John Bakke asked him to develop a systemwide approach to diabetes care. Glauber later credited the beautifully written, well-organized clinical notes of the retired Liberman for providing a kind of supplementary text for endocrinology. Claudio Lima, PA, whose Permanente career began in primary care at the Salem Medical Office, became increasingly interested in the management of diabetes. Beginning in 1984, he shared a Beaverton office with Glauber and took increasing responsibility for evaluating and managing diabetes.

In the following years Glauber received recognition for various innovative projects related to diabetes. He helped create a registry to track diabetic patients in the Health Plan membership. In 1989 he and a partner from the Center for Health Research received the first Sidney Garfield grant for a study to screen and assess diabetics and to generate reports to attending physicians. Three other fellowship-trained endocrinologists joined Glauber during the next decade: Michael Herson, 1991; James Prihoda, 1999; Laurie Hurtado Vessely, 2001.

RHEUMATOLOGY

As part of a three-year internal medicine fellowship at the Mayo Clinic, Ian MacMillan received training in rheumatology and, after joining Permanente in 1961, he provided rheumatology consultations and developed a small subspecialty practice. But it wasn't until the 1968 arrival of internist Perry Sloop that rheumatology acquired greater visibility as a subspecialty. Sloop had become interested in rheumatology at University of Oregon Medical School; later, both he and MacMillan took sabbatical leaves in England for additional training: Sloop with well-known pediatric rheumatologist Barbara Ansell, and MacMillan at Royal Postgraduate Medical School at Hammersmith Hospital. In the BK area, Sloop was assisted by PA Rodney Hooker.[3] At KSMC, Nurse Practitioners Mary Horton and Kevin Probst assisted MacMillan. Sloop and MacMillan expanded rheumatology consultations to members in outlying areas: Sloop at Longview-Kelso and MacMillan in Salem. Sloop earned board certification in geriatrics and, in 1996, left his rheumatology practice to assume directorship of the growing Geriatric and Long-Term Care Department. MacMillan retired later that year. By 1996 Permanente had added four more rheumatologists, and in the late 1990s the rheumatology group, formally recognized as a separate department, relocated to centralized quarters at the Interstate East Medical Office under the leadership of Lee Anna Jones.

GASTROENTEROLOGY

Vincent Chiu's odyssey began during the early years of World War II. His Chinese family lived in Japan, where his grandfather ran a small business in Kobe. After the 1942 bombing of Tokyo and other Japanese cities by the Allied Powers, the Chiu family relocated to Canton in Japanese-occupied China. Chiu's brother was killed there when the Americans bombed the area. Again the family moved, first to

PERMANENTE IN THE NORTHWEST

neutral Macao and, at war's end, to Hong Kong. In 1949 Chiu left his family behind and came to the U.S.

Chiu received his MD from the St. Louis University School of Medicine in 1956. Nearing the end of his internal medicine residency at Salt Lake City in 1957, he rotated on the pulmonary service with Charles Pinney as his instructor. (The two would meet again as Permanente physicians.) Chiu went on to acquire fellowship training in gastroenterology (GI) and joined Permanente as an internist and GI consultant in 1968.

Henrik Porter joined Chiu in 1970. After a four-year GI fellowship at University of Washington, Porter decided against an academic career in favor of a prepaid group practice. Like Chiu, Porter was hired as an internist with the understanding that he and Chiu would share GI consultations. But when flexible endoscopy became available in the late 1960s, Chiu and Porter were increasingly called on to perform GI procedures. The first flexible endoscopies took place in the BK operating room, with Chiu and Porter assisted by their office nurse. When an endoscopy suite was procured, hospital attendant Dale Fossati was assigned to look after equipment and assist at procedures. Porter learned of a federally funded program in Seattle to train GI assistants and arranged for Fossati to attend the program and obtain PA certification to perform sigmoidoscopies.

In 1973 gastroenterologist Charles Zerzan joined Permanente where he began a third career. Born in Portland and raised in Salem, Zerzan joined the National Guard as a college student. Three years later in 1940, his unit was mobilized. After officer's training he served three years as captain in an anti-aircraft unit in Northern Burma. After receiving his MD, he reenlisted, beginning a career in the U.S. Army Medical Corps reaching the rank of lieutenant colonel. During the 1962 Cuban Missile Crisis, his unit was activated for combat, with landing craft loaded, in anticipation of a planned invasion of that country. As Chief of Medicine at Fort Gordon, Georgia, he was awakened in the middle of the night by a phone call from his commanding officer: "Eisenhower is on his way in with chest pain." Zerzan found himself charged with the care of the former president and with responsibility as official spokesperson for reporting on Eisenhower's condition during his recovery. Zerzan's second official encounter with a prominent public figure took place in 1965 when, stationed in Jordan, he provided care to Jordan's King Hussein.

After retiring from the military in 1968, and receiving the Legion of Merit, Zerzan joined the faculty of medicine at the University of Oregon School of Medicine as teacher, consultant, endoscopist and Director of continuing medical education program. In 1973 he joined Chiu at BK, and two years later he moved to the newly opened KSMC. David Clarke, after completing his GI fellowship at Harbor-UCLA Medical Center, joined Zerzan in 1984. Both Zerzan and Clarke, like other medical subspecialists at the time, were required at first to devote half their time to general internal medicine.[4] By 1986, both were allowed to restrict the practice to their subspecialty.

In 1989 Robert Shneidman, whose GI fellowship at OHSU included time at KSMC, joined Porter and Chiu at BK. That year, Herb Salomon, following GI fellowship training at KP Sunset Medical Center in Los Angeles, joined the Medical Group to provide service at Salem. As with other specialties, requests for GI services increased. Nine more gastroenterologists would join Permanente in the following 19 years.

NEUROLOGY

Internist and neurologist Eberhard Gloekler joined Permanente after two years in private practice, where he labored in the shadow of neurosurgeon John Raff and neurologist Robert Dow. Dissatisfied with his position and with the fee-for-service world of diagnostic testing and billing, he was attracted to Permanente by its offer of a dual practice as an internist and a neurologist. Gloekler was born into a medical family: both his father and grandfather had been general practitioners in their small town near Stuttgart, Germany. At the start of World War II, Gloekler was 11 years old. He remembers listening to the BBC with his crystal set in the attic—at the time, an offense punishable by death. His entire class was drafted into the army in 1944, where he trained as an anti-aircraft gunner. Stationed at an airfield near Strasburg, he lived through the bombing that destroyed the airfield and killed many of his classmates. Next he was transferred to a unit protecting a dam in the Black Forest. In 1945 he deserted the army and lived in the woods near his home until the war's end. When local schools reopened he enrolled in a geology course and then, at his father's urging, entered medical school. At Permanente, Gloekler enjoyed dividing his time between internal medicine and neurology and later resisted the opportunity to limit his practice to neurology alone.

George Barton came to Permanente in 1973, following neurology training at Good Samaritan Hospital in Portland. Like Gloekler, he had worked with Dow and Raff and, like Gloekler, he had grown dissatisfied in his role, much of which was limited to determining disability status. Other neurologists followed: Nelson Stevland in 1979 and Nathan Blank in 1984.[5] Blank's tenure was short-lived, a mere two years, but requests for neurology services steadily increased. Today 11 physicians make up the Neurology Department.

INFECTIOUS DISEASE

The effectiveness of antibiotics in the 1950s led some physicians to doubt the need for specialists to treat infectious diseases. Attitudes shifted as evidence mounted that infectious agents were adaptable and capable of resisting treatment. Mark Gurwith was the first internist hired within Permanente to provide subspecialty expertise in infectious disease. He resigned in 1974 to accept a position at University of Manitoba Medical School. Jerry Slepack replaced Gurwith shortly thereafter. In the interim, veteran internist McCague Copeland, having spent a six-month sabbatical leave with the Infectious Disease Department at OHSU, provided infectious disease consultations to Permanente. After serving as a battalion surgeon with the fourth infantry division in Vietnam, Slepack completed an internal medicine residency and a fellowship in infectious diseases at the University of Cincinnati. In 1981 Joseph Kane resigned from his staff position at OHSU to cover Slepack during his sabbatical leave. Seven years later, infectious disease specialist Keith Riley joined Permanente to work half time in the AIDS clinic with Robert Lawrence and to provide infectious disease consultations at BK. Infectious disease specialist Freda Kerman joined the BK-area Department of Internal Medicine that year. In 1996 the group became a department separate from internal medicine.

NEPHROLOGY

The development of artificial kidney machines in the 1940s and 1950s opened a new era in the treatment of kidney disease. But the first machines were cumbersome, and the procedure itself expensive and unavailable to patients with chronic renal failure. Then in 1960 Belding Scribner and his Seattle co-workers developed a teflon-coated shunt (the Scribner Shunt) through which patients could tolerate repeated hemodialysis. Two years later Scribner introduced the world's first outpatient dialysis facility. Demand exceeded capacity, necessitating the formation of a committee to establish medical and social criteria to determine eligibility for maintenance dialysis.

In 1964 local nephrologist Richard Drake of the Northwest Renal Nephrology Group introduced a more efficient machine to provide dialysis. Drake's group provided dialysis for Permanente patients at Good Samaritan Hospital, where he and those in his Medical Group established a cordial working relationship with Permanente physicians. Internist and nephrologist Sam Miyatake joined Permanente in 1968, staying less than three years. In 1971 internist Jan Collins joined the Medical Group. Having received nephrology training as part of his residency under Drake at Good Samaritan Hospital, Collins provided consultations for his Permanente colleagues, and also performed kidney biopsies and an occasional acute peritoneal dialysis as part of his internal medicine practice.

Marvin Harner was introduced to nephrology somewhat by chance when, as an intern, he was advised by a staff physician to "learn kidney disease." Taking the advice to heart, Harner organized a renal clinic at the University of Iowa Hospital. His introduction to Permanente came when, just beginning a pediatric nephrology fellowship and needing extra income, he took a job working weekends at BK in the pediatric walk-in clinic. He joined Permanente in 1975 with the understanding that he would provide adult as well as pediatric nephrology services. Harner's hiring coincided with the opening of KSMC. Thereafter, Harner and Collins divided nephrology duties, Collins at BK and Harner at KSMC.

As the need for nephrology services grew, the Northwest Region, in 1984, established an inpatient unit for hemodialysis at KSMC. Collins, Harner and internist Michael Shanahan, who brought previous dialysis experience from private practice, were the unit's attending physicians; their nurse was a former dialysis instructor at Good Samaritan Hospital. The following year a position for a nephrologist at KSMC opened. John Solters and Susan Kauffman applied for the spot. Permanente chose Solters, who, with six years as Chief of Nephrology at Letterman Hospital and some time in private practice, was a seasoned nephrologist. Kauffman, more recently trained and like Solters an Army veteran, must have been undaunted by the selection of Solters. She simply readjusted her objective and accepted a position as an internist in the BK area.

To pay for her education Kauffman had joined the military in her teens and had earned her nursing degree at Walter Reed Army Institute of Nursing, graduating with a rank of second lieutenant. She went on to serve with a MASH unit in Vietnam and recalls harrowing experiences reminiscent of those depicted in the TV series M*A*S*H, starring Alan Alda as Hawkeye Pierce. On one terrifying occasion at Quong Tri her unit was overrun by the enemy and evacuated by air to Chu Lai south of Da Nang. It was only after her Army discharge that Kauffman set her sights on a medical education, earning her MD at OHSU in 1981. Her experience in Vietnam fostered a growing interest in managing renal failure. She continued her OHSU training with a nephrology fellowship.

On joining the BK medical staff, the hard-working Kauffman quickly drew favorable notice for her nephrology consultations. The nephrologist who had once been passed over for a nephrology position ultimately became Chief of the department. Along the way she expanded the scope of nephrology service in the greater metropolitan area. In 1999, KPNW contracted with an outside service, Fresenius Medical Care, at its 21-bed outpatient dialysis unit in suburban Milwaukie, Oregon. Kauffman became Medical Director of the unit where KPNW members make up 80% of the patients. She also established a renal center in the building, with offices for six Permanente nephrologists. In 2006, when Fresenius was sold, Kauffman convinced the new owners to open a nocturnal dialysis program so as to administer dialysis at a slower, more efficient rate while patients slept and thus help them avoid a day's absence from work. The program, the first of its kind in Oregon, was featured in a 2006 edition of The Oregonian. Today, under Kauffman's direction, six Permanente nephrologists make periodic visits to KPNW patients at 11 other dialysis units in the Portland metropolitan area. The program serves approximately 400 dialysis patients, 400 kidney transplant patients, and over 1,000 other patients in its chronic renal disease program.

INTENSIVISTS

Until 1977, the day-to-day on-site management of patients in the intensive care unit (ICU) remained the responsibility of the internist on call for the day. The continual rotation of internists through the ICU resulted in inconsistency in the continuity of care—particularly for those postoperative surgical patients with medical complications. To remedy the problem, four internists—George Feldman, Paul Jacobs, Kenneth Jones and Charles Newton—formed a team; each week one of the four rotated through the unit, assuming responsibility for all ICU patients. In addition, the designated intensivist was on call 24 hours a day and present in the ICU during the morning hours. The four were assigned offices on the KSMC campus, close enough to the ICU to respond to emergencies. The team approach worked remarkably well. In 1977 pulmonologist Robert Richardson, formerly on staff at the University of Iowa Medical School, joined Permanente and assumed leadership of the ICU team. Internist Arthur Hayward joined the Medical Group and the ICU team in 1978.[6] The following year internist David Zeps rounded out the roster of the early ICU team.

The ICU evolution at BK occurred later and took a different course. Anesthesiologist Bhawar Singh and surgeon Peter Feldman had been Co-Directors of the ICU from its inception until 1982, when BK internists organized an ICU team under the Department of Medicine. Pulmonologist Kyle Fuchs, formerly Director of critical care at Providence St. Vincent Hospital, accepted a position with Permanente in 1998 and assumed leadership of both the critical care and progressive care units.

PULMONOLOGY

In 1941 internists interested in pulmonary disease who treated tuberculosis separated themselves from other internists by obtaining specialty certification in tuberculosis. Saward's training is a case in point: following his residency in internal medicine, Saward was named chief resident at a tuberculosis sanitarium as part of a program to groom him as a pulmonary expert. The advent of chemotherapeutic agents revolutionized treatment for tuberculosis, decreasing for a time the demand for pulmonologists. Then, beginning in the 1950s, with the advent of new tests and techniques—pulmonary function testing and ventilator support—pulmonology regained its former specialty status. The arrival of fellowship-trained Charles Pinney in 1959 added expertise to Saward's considerable experience. In 1964 the newly introduced bronchofibrescope added to the pulmonologists' armamentarium and, by the 1970s and 1980s, technical advances for monitoring and treating patients in the ICU expanded the specialty into critical care medicine.[7]

Albert Vervloet joined Permanente in 1968, and he and chest surgeon Robert McFarlane performed fiberoptic bronchoscopies.[8] Vervloet organized and directed a state-of-the-art pulmonary function laboratory at BK and in 1969 he was joined by pulmonologist Jerry Reich. Reich became Director of the pulmonary function laboratory after Vervloet's departure in 1975. In 1977 Robert Richardson left academic medicine at the University of Iowa to bring his extensive experience in fiberoptic bronchoscopy and critical care medicine to Permanente, where he joined the Department of Medicine at KSMC. Chong Lee[9] joined the department in 1985, Thomas Stibolt in 1989. In the most recent 15 years, demands for pulmonary specialists have steadily increased. Today there are 13 pulmonologists in NWP.

HOSPITALISTS

The 1988 nursing strike, which forced the closure of all KSMC beds and reduced the number of beds at BK, necessitated innovation to ensure care for Health Plan members referred to community hospitals. As a temporary measure, Permanente physicians devised schedules whereby those assigned to a hospital for a one-week tour of duty were relieved of scheduled clinical appointments. In this way, internists experienced providing exclusively inpatient hospital care.

At the conclusion of the strike, and as normalcy returned to the organization, BK internists, led by internist Manuel Karlin, devised a plan to increase consistency of care for hospitalized patients. Members of the department each took a two-week rotation to provide hospital care. During this rotation, the hospital physician was relieved of outpatient responsibility.

In 1990 the Internal Medicine Department at KSMC went one step further: it established a core group dedicated to inpatient care, with the goal of improving patient access in the outpatient department. (Because of their hospital responsibilities some physicians had reduced their office hours to as few as two days a week.)

Not everyone liked the proposed change. In fact, many were opposed to the idea of not being able to follow their own patients. They argued that patients were almost certain to be dissatisfied at not being able to see their own familiar physician when they were hospitalized. Too, they foresaw that in limiting their practice to outpatient office visits, physicians were certain to lose crucial inpatient skills. To complicate matters further, the group had no models from which to adopt work schedules. (The Hawaii Permanente Medical Group designated physicians whose sole job it was to round on and care for hospitalized patients, but these were moonlighting physicians and residents in training rather than staff physicians.)

Thomas Lorence, a Permanente internist since 1981, provided the leadership to develop a job description and work schedules. Administration leaders approved four positions dedicated to inpatient care, later known as hospitalists. Lorence, Donald Venes, Terry Morrow, and Maureen Wright were the pioneers in the new field. Their small department may have been the first of its kind in the country.

The hospitalist movement, begun in 1990 by these Permanente physicians in the Northwest, has since been widely adopted throughout the country.[10] In 1993 KP CEO David Lawrence hired McKinsey and Company to assess the Region's inefficiencies.[11] An inadvertent finding in its assessment revealed that hospitalists help reduce average length of a hospital stay. Thereafter, the hospitalist program drew increased support. In 1995 Permanente physicians in Colorado introduced a hospitalist program at St. Joseph's Hospital in Denver. Later that year The Permanente Medical Group implemented a hospitalist program in the South Sacramento Medical Center. The following year physicians Lee Goldman and Robert Wachler at University of California, San Francisco Medical Center proposed the term "hospitalist" in the August 1996 issue of the *New England Journal of Medicine*. In 1997 the National Association of Inpatient Physicians was founded and later became the Society of Hospital Medicine. The estimated number of hospitalists that year was 1,000; a decade later that number has virtually exploded to approximately 20,000. Today hospitalists represent the fastest-growing number of specialists within internal medicine. Medical journals that advertise for hospitalists now also seek to fill positions for ever-more specific niches, including such esoteric positions as nocturnists and weekendists.

GERIATRICS AND LONG-TERM CARE

The origins of the Continuing Care Department began in 1967 as a research project designed to show how home health services could care for the sick and the frail where they lived. The department's history is an ongoing story of innovating to deliver medical care to members outside clinics and hospitals under direction of Health Plan Manager Linda Van Buren and her successor Andy Kyler, in serial partnership with internists and geriatricians Perry Sloop, David Zeps, and Arthur Hayward.

Whereas formerly all Permanente's primary care physicians visited patients in 70 intermediate care nursing homes, Sloop recruited a small group to see all patients in all facilities and hired staff with particular interest in geriatrics. Fellowship-trained, board-certified geriatricians Sally Rosenfeld and Patrick Fitzgerald were the first to join the department, called geriatrics and long-term care (GLTC). Zeps and Marshall Goldberg gave up internal medicine practices to join.

Attention also focused on how patients were managed in skilled-nursing facilities. As the department developed, its members took a more active role as skilled-nursing facility rounders or "SNFists" well before that term was coined or the importance of that role was widely recognized. Working with KPNW-affiliated clinicians and nurses, these "SNFists" rounded in nursing homes to improve quality and shorten excessive length of stay. Today, Permanente "SNFists" manage a census of 80-90 patients in five Portland and Vancouver skilled-nursing facilities. At any one time 350 or more KPNW members live in 1 of 750 or more of these adult foster homes in the Portland metro area. Expanding services again in 2004, the department inaugurated a home visit program for members residing in foster homes.

In 2008 the department expanded its scope yet again, launching a new program to include home visits to Clark County members living in Alzheimer's units, assisted-living facilities, and in private residences. KP Cares (CAres in RESidence) offers panel enrollment; the visiting physician becomes the patient's primary care physician. In its first year, by intensifying services at home, department geriatricians and clinicians cut hospital stays and trips to the emergency room by nearly 10%.

Today GLTC Department physicians are Patrick Fitzgerald, Sally Rosenfeld, Helen Duewel, See Woo, Mary Bodie, Megan Thygesen, Karen Kruse and Arthur Hayward. Eight NPs and two PAs round out the staffing model in GLTC.

NWP physicians showed the value of palliative care for both hospital inpatients and outpatients. Robert Richardson contributed findings from KSMC hospital to a multisite study of inpatient palliative care consultations. Louise Clark joined the GLTC Department as a hospice physician and started a pilot program of outpatient palliative care. She later recruited Virginia Sytsma, who succeeded her as Medical Director of the Hospice and Palliative Care Program. The two recruited four other physicians: Lori Siegal, Margo McGehee-Kelly, Jan Guziec, and Andrew Frank.

Palliative care is a relatively new subspecialty that offers hospice-like care. Whereas hospice is federally funded and limits enrollment to patients with a prognosis of six months, palliative care has no such eligibility restrictions. Extending geriatric and palliative care services has helped upgrade and shift the site of medical care for the frail and elderly to familiar and less costly settings. As one patient's daughter said during a home visit in her mother's living room, "This is the right place for her."

CHAPTER 14:
SPECIALTIES OLD AND NEW

—ɯ—

SYPHILIS, SKIN, AND SURGERY

Because of the numerous skin manifestations of syphilis, traditionally dermatologists were specialists in syphilis as espoused by the titles of the *American Journal of Syphilology and Dermatology* in 1870 and the present-day *Austrian Dermatology and Venerology*. As late as 1950, the University of Oregon Medical School included a Department of Syphilology and Dermatology. The availability of penicillin eventually eliminated that part of the specialty.

During World War II, Viennese-trained dermatologist Ernest Spitzer was Permanente's skin specialist. But the dramatic decrease in Health Plan membership after the war necessitated a reduction of his schedule to just two days a week and Spitzer resigned within the year. In 1953 Martin Weitz joined the Department of Internal Medicine as a dermatologist. His on-the-job training in dermatology as a medical officer in the U.S. Army during the war led him to prescribe unusual ointments and lotions that only a pharmacist could recognize and compound. Here are some examples:

For scabies:	For psoriasis:
Rx Sulph. Praecip 4gm Balsum, Peruviami 2gm Adipis 32gm Sig: apply locally	Rx Chrysarobini 1.3gm Aelheriset alcholis aa qs Collodi 30cc Sig: apply to patch with camel-hair brush after removal of scale

Weitz's clinical notes, extensive and always neatly written, occasionally belied his impatience; they traveled to the bottom of the page and, nowhere else to go, ascended vertically along the margin. Both his diagnoses and treatments were sometimes a mystery to those who had not had the benefit of studying Latin.

Paul Contorer introduced a new era to Permanente dermatology when he joined the Medical Group in 1966, shortly before Weitz retired. For a time, the shortage of office space forced him to adopt a kind of itinerant mode, rotating among offices at the Bess Kaiser outpatient clinic and keeping his records and equipment together on a rolling cart. Contorer had served with the U.S. Air Force and had requested assignment to the Northwest. His request resulted in a posting to Alaska, and there he met Richard Romaine, also posted in Alaska and formerly general medical officer at the Eielson Air Force Base in Fairbanks, Alaska.

Romaine had been considering dermatology as a career and his acquaintance with Contorer influenced his decision to pursue that course. After his discharge, Romaine lost no time in leaving Fairbanks, where the temperature could dip to 70 degrees below zero. He began a residency in dermatology at Wayne State University in Detroit, Michigan. He and Contorer periodically corresponded. Romaine returned to Portland, his home town, and went into private practice. Five years later, weary of the business requirements of private practice, he joined The Permanente Clinic and reunited with his friend Contorer.

Tennessean Lee Allen joined the small department in 1970. Then in 1977 and 1981 he took successive sabbatical leaves at France's leading hospital for skin disease, Hôpital Saint-Louis in Paris. Having spent an undergraduate year at the Sorbonne University some years earlier, Allen easily assimilated among the other French-speaking students and instructors. Angelito Saqueton, the next to join the department, had, like Romaine, a previous acquaintance with Contorer. Contorer had been senior resident at the University of Chicago where Saqueton trained. Saqueton returned to his home in the Phillipines after completing his residency. There he struggled in his practice, for many of his impoverished patients lacked the means to purchase the prescribed medications. After four years, Saqueton and his wife relocated again, this time to Connecticut, at the invitation of two dermatologists in private practice. But the small New England town could not support three dermatologists and, after four years, Saqueton began to look elsewhere. He contacted Contorer and joined him at Permanente in 1975.

In 1984 the restless Allen took another sabbatical leave, this time to learn Mohs surgery.[1] Dermatologist Clark Sisk was hired to replace Allen during his absence. During his residency, Sisk had trained in Mohs surgery, and he had incorporated the procedure when he joined his father's dermatology practice in St. Louis. Then, during the course of a dermatology seminar at the Salishan Resort on the Oregon coast, he learned about an opportunity at Permanente and he contacted Allen. Allen had been the attending physician during Sisk's residency training at Oregon Health and Science University. He thought Sisk would fit in well at Northwest Permanente. Before returning to St. Louis from the seminar, Sisk submitted an application and interviewed for the position. Back home in St. Louis, Sisk had the painful task of telling his father of his decision to leave their private practice and to join Permanente.

During Allen's absence the two corresponded about providing Mohs surgery at NWP. They approached administrators with a proposal, but the idea languished. Disappointed when he learned on his return from sabbatical that no action had taken place on the plan, Allen resigned from Permanente and entered a private practice in Memphis, Tennessee. Sisk, more patient than Allen, began to perform Mohs surgery at OHSU. His patience was rewarded; four months later, he was able to perform surgeries in a procedure room at the new Mt. Scott Medical Office. His team included an assigned nurse and a technician from the Pathology Department. At the time, he was one of only three physicians in the Portland area performing the Mohs surgeries.

During the 1980s five dermatologists joined and departed from the Medical Group—each to private practice. But Richard Romaine, Angelito Saqueton, and Clark Sisk remained, to be joined in 1986 by Mary Lyons.

In 1986 Health Plan administrators retained architects from Giffen Bolte Jurgens and asked Sisk to help plan a dermatology suite in what was then the regional administrative office building, Central Interstate, on Portland's North Interstate Avenue. Sisk envisioned a modern dermatology facility to include separate, well-equipped rooms for surgery and for phototherapy. Having received no assurances that the project would move beyond the planning stages for some time, he thought no more about it. To his surprise and delight, Health Plan approved the plans two years later and renovation began.

In 1995 Contorer, who had served as department chief for a remarkable tenure of 29 years, retired. Lyons replaced him as chief and took on the leadership of the department. In the next ten years the need for treating skin diseases, primarily cancer, continued to grow. Today, 13 dermatologists, including two Mohs surgeons, make up the Dermatology Department at NWP.

INDUSTRIAL MEDICINE

Before Medical Director Marvin Goldberg assigned surgeon Larry Duckler to organize a Department of Industrial Medicine in 1977, internists, general surgeons, orthopedists, and emergency medicine physicians billed for care of workers' injuries, each in his own way. Accustomed as they were to the Kaiser Permanente system of prepayment, they sometimes failed to bill at all. Compounding a haphazard billing system, the medical records for injured workers were inconsistent and often difficult to trace. In 1976 the Oregon State Workers' Compensation Board informed Kaiser Foundation Health Plan that the Board would no longer accept billing unless it dramatically improved its documentation of initial treatment, follow-up management, and disability determination.

Duckler, together with Health Plan administrator Mildred Durgan, rolled up his sleeves and began to organize a system that would satisfy the state. First, Duckler established a centralized Department of Industrial Medicine with its own billing office. Then he devised a color-coded green form, easily identifiable from the standard blue or white medical record, to be used for all work-related injuries. Finally, he met with insurance companies and the Medical Director of the Worker's Compensation Board to explain improved methods for tracking treatment for workers' injuries. These representatives, no doubt relieved to see some efforts to improve, readily accepted the changes.

In 1976 Donald Tilson, a 21-year veteran of the U.S. Army Medical Corps, joined the Permanente Orthopedics Department and quickly assumed a major role in the industrial medicine service for orthopedic evaluation and care. Meanwhile, Duckler continued his efforts and improved access to physical therapy, physiatry, and orthopedics. The service began to run like a business and Permanente physicians, accustomed to prepaid medicine, adapted to this segment of the fee-for-service world. Still, despite significant improvements, primary care physicians (who provided most of the initial care) were unable to keep up with changing legal requirements and state regulations in handling claims.

In 1983 and 1984 two catalysts demanded additional changes to industrial medicine. The first was the decision by KP to expand its territory to Longview-Kelso, a community dominated by the lumber and paper mill industry. Another was the growing number of complaints by employers who insisted on a more efficient service for their injured workers in Portland and in Salem. Family practitioner Thomas Syltebo, based at the Vancouver Medical Office, began to devote half his time to industrial medicine and workers' compensation cases. He developed expertise in the field and, together with his nurse and administrative staff, effectively dealt with the frustrating details of such a practice. Syltebo also made time to visit the local paper mills and industrial sites.

When the Longview Medical Office opened, a local physician was hired half time to provide industrial medicine services. Later family practitioner Joseph Davis took over the department, improving services to Longview and Kelso workers. For a time a succession of physicians rotated in the position at Longview. When the last of these left, Permanente physicians from Vancouver and Portland rotated at Longview until permanent replacements, family practitioner Vernon Harpole and internist Theresa Laskiewicz, were hired in 1996.

Responding to employer complaints about service for workers in the Portland and Salem areas, David Lawrence, Area Medical Director at Bess Kaiser Hospital, took action. He hired physician David Nelson, experienced in industrial medicine, who established a small, well-run clinic at Health Center West. His tenure, however, was a mere 14 months before he resigned to pursue a career in epidemiology. In 1984, retired orthopedist James Wilson joined the Medical Group as the sole industrial medicine physician at Kaiser Sunnyside Medical Center. Named Regional Chief of the department in 1986, he assumed the job just as employer complaints were again on the rise. Freightliner, with 1,800 members, and Intel Corporation both threatened to disenroll. And at least one employer, FMC Manufacturers with 400 members, did more than threaten, the company took its business elsewhere. Employer complaints were numerous but boiled down to an inescapable fact: the program was poorly run. In 1985 25% of industrial claims by KP Northwest were denied, in contrast to the denial rate in the greater community of just 10%.

Despite concerns about the cost effectiveness of revamping the entire program, Kaiser Foundation Health Plan provided $500,000 in seed money to fund a pilot project at KSMC. Wilson gathered a team, including two physicians, an administrative manager and claims and billing clerks, designating an empty hospital ward for the nascent department. The successful model was extended to other medical offices.

The medical staff came from varied disciplines[2]; some came from within the Medical Group and others from the local community. Eventually they assimilated with formally trained industrialists. Many would obtain their specialty boards in the discipline. Joan Browning, hired in 1987, was the first board-certified physician in industrial medicine to join Permanente. She was joined one year later by Adrianne Feldstein. In 1990 Feldstein was appointed Department Chief of what was now officially called occupational (rather than industrial) medicine. She would be instrumental in planning and managing a far-reaching innovation of care for the injured worker.

Feldstein, raised in New York City, attended George Washington University School of Medicine and Health Sciences and was one of the founding members of the Washington, DC chapter of Physicians for Social Responsibility. Even before graduating, she knew she wanted to work in public health. She trained in internal medicine at OHSU, completed an additional two-year residency in occupational medicine, and then went to work for the Virginia Garcia Memorial Health Center in Cornelius, a farm community in Oregon's Willamette Valley. There she provided primary care to migrant farm workers, improving systems for providing prenatal care and for managing diabetes, hypertension, and tuberculosis. It was at a journal club meeting for occupational medicine that she met Donald Tilson, who suggested she come to work for KPNW. In 1988, she was hired jointly by the Medical Group and by the Center for Health Research.

In 1990 the Oregon legislature changed the state's workers' compensation and employment laws, creating a new entity, a Managed-Care Organization (MCO). An MCO was defined as a health care provider, or group of medical providers, who would contract with an insurer or self-insured employer to provide a wide variety of managed health care services to workers. KP considered the many regulations and requirements for MCO certification,[3] which included offering chiropractic and naturopathic services and decided against applying for MCO certification. But two months later, just 24 hours after Legacy Health announced that its new MCO had an exclusive contract with SAIF, the State Accident and Insurance Fund, in the tri-county area, Regional Medical Director Fred Nomura and Kaiser Foundation Health Plan Regional Manager Michael Katcher, hastily reversed their earlier decision. Without meeting with the Permanente Board of Directors to gain approval for their decision, the two leaders applied for MCO status.

Feldstein was appointed Medical Director for the new MCO, called Kaiser-On-The-Job, which won the 1996 National James A. Vohs Award for Quality. She and her Health Plan counterpart George Marino created an exemplary program for occupational health and preventive medicine. Other KP Regions—Northern California, Southern California and Hawaii—adopted similar programs. SAIF data, for 1994 and 1995, showed claims costs significantly lower (21%) than other MCOs. Moreover, 90% of patients who responded to surveys reported satisfaction with their experience with KPNW care. The success of the program led to the creation in 1996 of a for-profit management holding company called Kaiser Works, Inc. Jointly owned by Kaiser Foundation Health Plan Northwest and Medical Group, the company named Feldstein President and CEO. In its first two years, Kaiser Works, Inc. provided consultation and other services for six KP Regions and two other non-competing organizations. Despite its commendable record, however, the program proved financially unsustainable. It ceased activity in 1999, though it remained a registered corporation until 2007.

Since 1999 Permanente veteran Curtis Thiessen[4] has led the Department of Occupational Medicine through an era of continued growth. Though the economic benefits to KP of Kaiser-On-The-Job remain unclear, for Oregon employers and workers, the program has continued to garner praise.

ONCOLOGY

Andrew Glass, KPNW's pioneering oncologist, served his pediatric residency at the Massachusetts General Hospital and his oncology fellowship at Dana-Farber/Children's Hospital Cancer Care Institute in Boston. During his fellowship years he met Permanente Clinic pediatrician Arthur Oleinick, and Oleinick encouraged Glass to consider Permanente, which could offer opportunities to practice oncology. Glass joined Permanente in 1970, though he received no specific offer of an oncology practice. But just as Oleinick had predicted, Glass almost immediately found opportunities to pursue his interest. Pediatrics Chief Peter Hurst welcomed Glass as a regular attendee at tumor board meetings, where Glass quickly demonstrated his knowledge in oncology and his interest in research. Within three years of joining Permanente, oncology made up 50% of his total practice at the Permanente Broadway Clinic. In addition, he became a principal investigator in the Western Cancer Study Group and secured a grant from the National Cancer Institute to fund a research assistant.

In 1976 Glass recruited Ivan Law as a full-time oncologist and established a separate Department of Oncology. Law resigned after just two years but pediatric oncologist David Tilford joined the Medical Group in 1979. Tilford, a junior member of the faculty of medicine at the University of Michigan, had not found academic medicine to his liking and he welcomed a chance to pursue oncology in a community-based practice. His agreement with Permanente called for him to provide general pediatric services at the Vancouver Medical Office. Glass, increasingly involved in research on both breast and prostate cancers and with cancer registries, gradually turned his own pediatric patients over to Tilford.

Thomas Leimert joined Tilford and Glass at the Broadway Clinic in 1980. Trained at the University of Iowa in both internal medicine and oncology, Leimert had concluded that opportunities in academic medicine and clinical research would be difficult to find. It was about this time that Leimert heard an eloquent speech by Glass at a National Surgical Adjuvant Breast and Bowel Project meeting. When an advertisement appeared in the *New England Journal of Medicine* for an opening with KPNW, he quickly contacted Glass. To his disappointment, the job had been filled. When another position opened, however, Leimert was hired. It came as a pleasant surprise when, months after joining Permanente, he learned that pulmonologist Robert Richardson was already a member; Leimert had admired Richardson at the University of Iowa for his combined skill with, and compassion for, patients in the ICU.

The Broadway Clinic was becoming an oncology center, though it still shared space with the Allergy Department and with one lone pediatrician, Fred Colwell. It housed a small laboratory and a pharmacy; across the parking lot the small, vintage Weidler House offered a cancer counseling service. Weekly oncology team meetings also took place at Weidler House. The three oncology nurses became adept at improvising. They mixed their own chemotherapy solutions without the benefit of overhead protective hoods. The basement of the Weidler House accommodated two beds where patients received blood transfusions; they were instructed to bang on the water pipes to signal that the transfusion was completed. Those on the first floor then alerted the oncology nurses at the Broadway Clinic. Glass remembers another instance in which he had to make do. One winter day a patient arrived at the clinic during a snow storm. Because she refused to leave her vehicle for fear of falling on the ice, Glass left his office and administered IV 5-FU to the patient while she remained in her car.

To the frustration of the centralized Medical Records Department, the oncology personnel retained their own records on site, believing that records were not always delivered to them on time.

Leimert described the Broadway Clinic years as "idyllic." He and Tilford were able to walk to work. The small department enjoyed a superb team spirit and viewed themselves as somewhat apart from the rest of Permanente. Nevertheless, Leimert enjoyed a cordial relationship with the physicians with whom the oncology group worked most closely: primarily surgeons, urologists, pathologists, gastroenterologists and pulmonologists.

In 1982 a long-planned oncology clinic opened at Health Center East, a dramatic change from tight quarters and make-do circumstances at the Broadway Clinic. The new clinic contained three infusion beds, an office for each oncologist, a centralized glass-enclosed nurse's station, a cancer-counseling suite, and a research suite. Despite the acknowledged luxury of the spacious new quarters, internal conflicts increased. One reason may have been Glass's increased interest in, and attention to, his research activities. In 1984 the department members elected Tilford, whose organization skills were widely recognized, as the new chief.

The department continued to expand. New standards of care and an increasing volume of patients mandated a renovation and in 1985 the clinic added six infusion beds and an oncology pharmacy with a dedicated pharmacist to mix solutions. Leimert then replaced Tilford as Chief in 1986, and the department added hematologists Stephen Chandler, Norman Birndorf and Eldon Anderson, all previous members of the Internal Medicine Department. The increase in staff exacerbated existing tensions: so many patients, so little office space for physicians and staff. Nevertheless, the department expanded yet again, and in 1992 three additional oncologists joined the staff.

By now the physical space at Health Center East could no longer meet the department's needs. Leimert who had anticipated the growth, met for months with regional administrators and finally got approval to design an oncology center, with three times the previous space, to be housed at Central Interstate Medical Office. Designed by a team of department members in conjunction with a local architect, the state-of-the-art facility opened in December 1993. The department moved from the old location to the new one in a single morning. By afternoon patients occupied all infusion beds and full service resumed. Today the oncology center has 21 beds or chairs for infusion treatment in a spacious open area with a view looking north toward KPNW's Town Hall on North Interstate Avenue. Five private rooms are set aside for new patients and their families. Adjacent to the treatment area is a pharmacy dedicated to oncology, an advice nurse station, the cancer counseling center, and offices for 11 oncologists.

CANCER COUNSELING AND EDUCATION

Oncologist Glass wanted to engage counselors to help his patients. In 1976 he heard about a person who, with a master's degree in both education and counseling, seemed a likely prospect. Marilyn Friendenbach had expressed an interest in starting a cancer counseling service with KP. She had one stipulation, however, and that was that her friend Ruth Bach assist her. Both women had been involved with support groups at Good Samaritan Hospital; Bach's son had been successfully treated there for Hodgkin's disease. Glass agreed to Friendenbach's wishes and the cancer education center opened its doors at Weidler House in March 1977. Services offered were an introductory workshop for cancer patients and their families to include communication skills and relaxation techniques. Those who participated in the workshops organized several smaller support groups. Bach led a separate parent group. Theirs was the first such cancer counseling center in the Portland metropolitan area.

Two years later Friendenbach developed breast cancer, which led to her resignation. The center's services continued under Bach. In 1983, she too developed breast cancer. Ironically, Bach would benefit from the counseling and support group that she and her friend Friendenbach had developed.

In 1989 David Spiegel, a pioneer in the field of psychoneuroimmunology of cancer, reported in *The Lancet* dramatic benefits, including extended survival rates for metastatic cancer patients in support groups.[5] Spiegel's results helped highlight the importance of counseling, and services expanded with the 1993 opening of the Oncology Center at Central Interstate. The new counseling center offered a separate waiting room, meeting facilities and additional offices for counselors and social workers Nancy Tilford and Vicki Romm. When Tilford retired in 1993, she was replaced by nationally recognized grief therapist Izetta Smith,[6] which enabled the center to provide additional counseling for children with cancer and their parents.

CHAPTER 15:
PSYCHIATRY AND PHYSIATRY:
HEALING THE MIND
AND THE BODY

—⚍—

POST-WAR PSYCHIATRY

A 1947 Northern Permanente Health Plan brochure listed premiums of $2.50 per month per employee, $2.00 per month per spouse and an additional $1.35 per month for the first child. Coverage explicitly excluded "insanity," tuberculosis, alcoholism, venereal disease, congenital conditions, and suicide. Psychiatric disorders would not be covered for another 19 years.

In the 1940s treatment for mental disorders was generally limited and often ineffective. The realm of psychiatry seemed to have two paths: individual psychoanalysis or custodial care and drug treatment. Psychoanalysis was on the ascendancy and winning the battle against psychiatry and drug therapy. Psychiatrists who believed in the biologic origins of mental illness favored drugs and other techniques such as insulin coma and electroconvulsive therapy (ECT), accused psychoanalysts of stifling scientific progress.

In 1946 Congress passed the National Mental Health Act in response to a national scandal over conditions in state mental hospitals. From 1948 to 1962 the Act provided funds for research and training in psychiatry as well as extra stipends to encourage resident training in psychiatry.

The drug chlorpromazine (Thorazine) revolutionized psychiatry when it became available in 1953. It enabled patients to better deal with hallucinations and to function more normally. As a result, the bedlam within mental hospitals was transformed into environments of relative calm and newly tractable patients were discharged into the community for outpatient treatment. In 1955 the first tranquilizer, meprobamate (Miltown, Equanil), was quickly adopted into the country's culture (within a year, 1 in 20 Americans was taking a tranquilizer) until physicians realized that the drug produced dependency. The first antidepressant drug imipramine (Tofranil) was made available in 1958, followed in 1961 by Merck's amitryptiline (Elavil). Thereafter, a flood of rival antidepressant drugs hit the market.

PERMANENTE PSYCHIATRY
AND THE FIRST THERAPISTS

The first Permanente Psychiatry Department opened in Southern California in 1961 after Joe DeSilva, President of the Retail Clerks Local 770, lobbied for a mental health program for his union members.

Health Plan in the Northwest was slower to adopt a mental health program. Until 1966 the Region's physicians had to refer severe psychiatric problems to non-plan facilities and to psychiatrists in private practice. Inevitably, internists tried to manage myriad mental disorders as part of their clinical practice, frequently searching for a community psychiatrist willing to accept the patient or for a hospital bed at Dammasch State Hospital in Wilsonville, Oregon. Social workers were not yet available in outpatient departments to help physicians address these problems.

Permanente's Medical Director Ernest Saward often referred mental health patients to the Delaunay Center, a private mental health clinic on the campus of the University of Portland, where psychologist Stanley Abrams cared for Permanente members. In 1966 Abrams approached Saward to discuss a more formal arrangement between the Delaunay Center and Health Plan. During the course of a lunch meeting, Saward suggested that Abrams join Permanente and implement a mental health program for the Northwest Region. Abrams voiced interest in the idea and, before any discussion took place about salary, Saward announced, "You're hired."

After military service as a combat medic in World War II and after medical school, Victor Gregory started a general practice in Portland in 1952. Later he enrolled in a psychiatric residency at University of Oregon Medical School, after which he opened a private practice in his new specialty. He joined Permanente at age 48 and became the first Chief of the Mental Health Department in 1966.

Gregarious and experienced, Gregory fit in well with his Permanente colleagues. Abrams, with both an MA and a PhD in clinical psychology from Philadelphia's Temple University, was aggressive and innovative. With their complementary training backgrounds and experience, Gregory and Abrams teamed well together to oversee the fledging department. As Chief, Gregory represented the department on clinical matters, and Abrams organized the department and performed most of the administrative work. In 1967 they hired psychiatric social worker Tom Goff. Later that year Arnold Hurtado, Chief of Medicine at Bess Kaiser Hospital, hired Eugene Nordstrom, PsyD, to supervise a federally funded demonstration project sponsored by the Center for Health Research to integrate a home and extended-care service and to study the program's impact on hospital utilization. At its start the Social Work Department assumed responsibility for discharge planning from the extended-care facility. Soon Nordstrom immersed himself in day-to-day operations of the program, participating in weekly small-group discussions, social gatherings, church services and psychotherapy. At the end of the two-year project, Gregory hired Nordstrom as the fourth permanent member of the department.[1]

By 1969 Kaiser Foundation Health Plan membership had grown to 125,000 and demands for mental health services were straining the resources of the four-member department. On weekends, from Friday noon to Monday morning, call was assigned to a single clinician, who might take dozens of phone calls during the 72-hour period and travel hundreds of miles to attend to Kaiser Permanente patients. The small department welcomed the arrival of Martin Levine,[2] whose considerable experience and quiet demeanor was to be a stabilizing influence within the over-taxed department.

Medical social worker Albert Fuller learned from colleagues about the Permanente Foundation Health Plan and its prepaid group practice while he was working toward his doctorate at the University of Southern California in 1962. His PsyD completed, he first accepted an academic position at the University of Connecticut and later at Florida State University. Disappointed with faculty politics and wanting to provide direct patient care, he remembered what he had heard about KP. In 1971 he met with psychiatrist Daniel Wesche in Florida and was recruited to Permanente. The following year psychiatric social worker Herbert Biskar[3] replaced Thomas Goff, and psychiatrist Barbara Radmore, fresh from residency training, joined the department.

In 1959, the year that BK opened, Kaiser Foundation Health Plan purchased a large, white residence—the former home of a local judge—to accommodate surgical and medical residents. In 1967 the judge's former home, with its impressive architecture and commanding views of Portland and the Willamette River, became headquarters for the mental health department. Early members of the department hold warm memories of their years in the comfortable old home. Gregory used the generously proportioned rooms to promote an esprit de corps within the department. The kitchen became a lunchtime meeting place, where colleagues could gather informally. Nordstrom enjoyed his office in the sunroom, that is, until the rains came and he discovered that the roof leaked. Biskar savored his spacious, second-floor bedroom office with its view of the Willamette River, the city, and the northwest hills. The large living room provided a friendly environment for patients, as well as a meeting space for staffers.

GROWING PAINS: CONFLICT,
NEW LEADERSHIP, INNOVATION

In 1972 Gregory was diagnosed with a cardiac condition and stepped down as Department Chief. Wesche replaced him. Abrams continued in his role as Assistant Chief. Like Gregory, Wesche was happy to delegate much of the administrative work to Abrams. Wesche was quiet, reflective, and described as a "sweet guy." A gifted therapist, he seemed able to reach patients with whom other therapists had failed. But he was no enforcer; he left that job to the more assertive Abrams.

Within a decade, by 1974, Health Plan membership had swelled to 150,000, resulting in a need to expand mental health services. Portland native and social worker Dennis Florendo joined the department. He would assert himself as an ally to Abrams in the coming department conflicts. Therapist Nicholas Kreofsky completed the roster of new hires.

In 1974 psychiatrist Barbara Radmore resigned from the department because of illness. Her departure created an opening for another woman therapist, particularly one who could address the problems of abused women. Therapist Jean Monihan who had a Master of Arts in communication replaced Radmore. Skilled in small-group dynamics, Monihan quickly became indispensable. In 1975 Gregory took a year-long sabbatical leave, and psychiatrist Katherine "Kitty" Evers took his place. She was assigned to provide hospital care at Woodland Park Hospital, where Monihan was to assist her.

By now the "judge's house," as it continued to be called, was straining at the seams from the influx of new department members, and they relocated to a one-story structure in a mixed-use area off NE Sandy Boulevard. The new building, more commodious than the now-cramped quarters at the judge's house, was less desirable in other ways. The rooms were small, dark and uninspiring. Evers occupied a basement office, reached by a narrow passageway. One day a bear of a man with a wild look and disheveled appearance confronted her at the doorway of her office. Recognizing Evers, he announced, "I know you. You committed me." Preparing for the worst, Evers remembers asking, "Did we get along?" "Oh, yes, you were very nice to me," the man affirmed. Together, Evers and the patient would go on to resume a productive therapeutic relationship.

As Kaiser Foundation Health Plan and the Mental Health Department grew, the nonphysician therapists grew increasingly restive. One of their grievances was that, given the ambiguity of the reporting structure, they were unable to effectively negotiate salary increases or benefits. (In 1968 Abrams and Fuller's request to The Permanente Clinic Executive Committee for affiliation had been denied.) Non-physician therapists continued to report to the Medical

Group but were salaried under Health Plan. In 1975 Florendo consulted an attorney for the International Longshoremen Workers Union who counseled the aggrieved therapists to unionize. Ironically, Abrams, the lead advocate for increased negotiating power, was ineligible for union membership because he was an administrator.[4] The group petitioned the local chapter of the National Labor Relations Board and won approval to affiliate with the ILWU. Not surprisingly, Health Plan administrators appealed the decision to the NLRB and prevailed in a three-two vote, arguing that the group was too small and that it should include others, i.e. nurse practitioners, physician assistants, optometrists. Discouraged at its failure to organize, the group retreated. It would make no further move to organize until 1983. (The Region's affiliated clinicians would eventually unionize in 2002.)

Other fissures within the department increased tensions. Therapists who favored the analytical approach and talk therapy found frustrating their limited time with patients. In addition, those who wanted the freedom to accept private-practice patients, separate and apart from their jobs at Kaiser Permanente Northwest, were told they could not do so. Still others within the department thought work assignments were inequitably distributed. Tensions mounted between the administrative team and department dissidents. Inevitably turf battles erupted, resulting in some heated verbal exchanges. One acrimonious confrontation, between Gregory and Wesche, required Area Medical Director Bob Senft to rush to the mental health clinic to intervene.

Department Chair Wesche finally relinquished his position in 1976, perhaps recognizing the need for a stronger administrative hand. Ron Potts, Assistant Area Medical Director, concluded that Evers had the relevant experience and collaborative skills to bring the department together. Regional Medical Director Marvin Goldberg appointed Evers Chief in 1976, the start of her 14-year tenure as Department Chief and of an era characterized by steady leadership, innovation, and growth.

Both her mother and her father were physicians, so Evers says that she was destined to become a physician. Very early in her education, even before her internship, she showed a bent for psychiatry. She earned her MD at University of Maryland in Baltimore and received her psychiatry training at Fort Logan Mental Health Center in Denver, Colorado. Moving west, she discovered and fell in love with the Pacific Northwest and took a position at Mental Health and Family Service Center in Vancouver, Washington.

In 1975 Evers joined Permanente, coincident with the release of the movie *One Flew Over the Cuckoo's Nest*—a harsh depiction of the brutality of society's institutional treatment of the mentally ill. The movie was based on Ken Kesey's

1962 novel and portrayed ECT as a punitive procedure for a rebellious inmate played by Jack Nicholson. Shock therapy shown to be effective for severe depression, and sometimes used for other conditions, became unpopular. Health Plan patients thought to need shock therapy were referred for treatment to non-Permanente physicians at Holladay Park Hospital.

Evers confronted several thorny problems as she assumed the job of Department Chief. One source of trouble was the individuality that characterized the practice. Evers wanted the department to function as an organized team, so she reassigned duties and rotated call among the three MDs and the five PsyDs. She allocated office assignments and other perks on the basis of seniority, rather than academic degree and sought opinions from each member of the department before making difficult decisions.

At this time mentally ill patients were often hospitalized for months. The department launched an effort to decrease hospitalization days for patients and began to limit hospitalizations to one-to-two weeks. Therapists used inpatient time for diagnosing, medicating, stabilizing, and planning for discharge. Patients were discharged to their homes for continued treatment.

Evers wanted to move mental health practitioners from their isolated facility and to integrate them within the Region's medical offices. The 1981 expansion of the East Interstate Medical Office, later to be renamed Health Center East, included spacious offices to accommodate mental health patients and their family members.

Psychiatrist Stuart Oken joined Permanente and the Department of Mental Health in 1978. His training at Johns Hopkins University had included a fellowship in community psychiatry. Like Evers, he advocated integrating mental health services into regular medical facilities. When the department relocated to East Interstate Medical Office, Oken moved his practice to the Kaiser Sunnyside Medical Center campus in Clackamas County. For a time, Oken worried that the progress toward integration might be thwarted; a plan was then in the works to locate a mental health clinic at a separate building on the KSMC campus, away from other medical services. Oken's objections created such controversy that an addition to the Mt. Scott Medical Office was built to accommodate the Mental Health Department. (Ironically, Oken was soon thereafter recalled to Health Center East in the BK area.)

Mental health offices eventually moved into other medical offices, including those in Salem, Beaverton, and at Division. The 1987 opening of the Sunset Medical Office would mark the first time that mental health practitioners and primary care clinicians would share a common module. The new togetherness offered both disciplines a familiarity with the other's activities and blurred the lines of loyalties so common within departments. Integration was a plus for patients too, who could now be managed in a regular medical office environment.

Managing acute psychiatric emergencies had long posed a seemingly intractable problem. Emergency room physicians had no satisfactory system to manage and hospitalize disruptive patients. Their only recourse was a call system whereby physicians and doctorate-level therapists made themselves available by pager to offer telephone advice or to go in person to the emergency room. Never a satisfactory arrangement, the chronic problem begged for a solution. After observing the psychiatric emergency service at KP Southern California in San Diego, Evers organized a 24-hour unit in the BK emergency room to be staffed by a designated group of nurse practitioners and masters-level therapists. In 1996 when BK closed, the service transferred to KSMC.

The department also introduced short-term, problem-specific group therapy and a more responsive call system whereby a patient could speak directly to a therapist by phone, be evaluated, and be directed to appropriate short-term counseling. The goal was to return the patient within five to ten sessions to satisfactory functioning.

In 1989, after 14 years as Department Chief, Evers relinquished her role. Breaking with the traditional process whereby the Medical Director appointed a Department Chief, the department held an election. Oken prevailed over Larry Cooper to lead the department for the next four years. Oken was eager to effect efficiencies, elevate the department's image, and demonstrate how an HMO could effectively provide psychiatric care. His push to adopt a managed-care model, when vestiges of a private-practice model still remained, was unpopular with some.

Oken drew up an ambitious reorganization plan, targeting 48 outpatient and inpatient clinical programs and projects, administrative functions, and educational and research programs. Then he assigned responsibilities among clinicians. Oken was determined to improve integration and teamwork. To increase access to the Mental Health Department by other disciplines, he introduced a telephone service, "the mind phone," whereby any Permanente physician could obtain direct access to a psychiatric consultant.[5] Oken also called for an extensive study to evaluate costs and effectiveness of inpatient mental health services provided elsewhere in the community. When a comparison of Oregon Health and Science University and Providence St. Vincent Hospital revealed longer hospitalization days and higher readmission rates at OHSU, Health Plan transferred its members' care exclusively to St. Vincent.

When Oken's four-year term as Department Chief ended in 1993, psychiatrists Lauretta Young and Mark Leveaux shared the role of Chief for another four years.

Young, Assistant Chief under Oken, was a natural choice. A graduate from Oregon State University, she had obtained both her medical education and residency training at OHSU, where she worked with attending Permanente psychiatrists Per Sweetman and Cooper. Like Oken she was attracted to a practice in a managed-care setting. On joining Permanente in 1983, Young was assigned to cover Health Plan patients hospitalized at the OHSU psychiatric unit and to consult at BK and KSMC. Thereafter she worked primarily in the outpatient department and she implemented a residency program at East Interstate Medical Office for fourth-year OHSU psychiatric residents. The first of its kind for an HMO, the program was lauded by health-care writer James Sabin in his 1993 book about managed care: *No Margin No Mission: Health Care Organizations and the Quest for Ethical Excellence.*

In 1997 Leveaux resigned from Permanente to become Director of Mental Health Services at Group Health Cooperative in Seattle and Young became Department Chief.

In 2008 for the first time in its history the Mental Health Department at KPNW obtained its own residential treatment beds for patients with substance abuse and non-acute mental illness. Located at Brookside Center near KSMC, the unit opened in June 2008. Today, the Mental Health Department has outpatient locations at 9 sites throughout the service area; its staff comprises 36 physicians, 6 PhDs, and 50 other therapists. It maintains a 24-hour crisis team at KSMC and a teaching program for 20 to 30 graduate students and interns.

ATP, ADRS, KPRR, AND ACHP

In 1974 KP's Health Services Research Center,[6] under administrator Theodore Columbo, began a demonstration and research project, the Ethanolism Program, to determine whether treatment for alcoholics could reduce their use of other medical services. The program's first location was a small residence at the north end of the BK parking lot. There, a small staff comprising an evaluator, an administrative assistant, and a research technician triaged patients to appropriate services in the community, as well as to Permanente physicians.

One year later, Area Medical Director Arnold Hurtado asked Mental Health Department Chief Evers to develop a protocol for treating both alcohol and other substance abuse. The Alcohol Treatment Program (ATP) provided detoxification in an outpatient setting and Antabuse to sustain sobriety. The program encouraged participants to attend Alcoholics Anonymous (AA) as an adjunct to treatment. At the time, most insurance plans, including Kaiser Foundation Health Plan, did not cover hospitalization for these dependencies. Most patients could not have afforded hospitalization.

When the treatment program became a separate entity, mental health practitioners continued to provide weekly group therapy to participants. Counselors attached to the treatment program worked with individuals. Regional Medical Director Marvin Goldberg appointed family practitioner Ray Noel, former consultant to the ethanolism research program, to lead the new department. Noel had previous experience in the field of addiction medicine, having served seven years in the U.S. Navy providing therapy to drug-addicted Marines at Camp Pendleton Marine Corps Base.

Results of both the research project and the treatment program showed that a combination of outpatient treatments, Antabuse and AA attendance, resulted in decreased unnecessary use of medical services and corresponding cost savings. Researchers submitted a proposal to extend benefits to those enrolled in the ATP. The two senior leaders, Permanente's Goldberg and Health Plan's Dan Wagster, accepted the proposal and authorized the program.

By 1981 the ATP had grown sufficiently to justify a full-time Department Chief. Noel wished to devote more of his time to family practice and less to addiction medicine.[7] His decision provided an opening for Robert Senft, who had stepped down as BK Area Medical Director. Permanente has historically offered physicians who take administrative positions, thereby losing some clinical skills, a choice of returning to clinical medicine after brushing up on skills or pursuing other avenues within the program.

As Northwest Permanente adopted a broader range of treatment options for chemical dependency, the program expanded to become Alcohol and Drug Recovery Services (ADRS). To increase his knowledge in the area of chemical dependency and treatment, Senft spent time at the Lloyd and Mabel Johnson Foundation in Minneapolis and at the Haight Ashbury Free Clinic in San Francisco. He returned with plans to further develop the service, extending its coverage to 24 hours and expanding its capability to oversee detoxification. Both Senft and Noel earned board certification in addiction medicine.

Next, department leaders convinced Health Plan to provide coverage for limited residential therapy at Cedar Hills Hospital, Medical Center Hospital, and the Hooper Center. An experiment to prescribe methadone was discontinued in 1988 after results were found to be inconclusive. At about the same time the program changed its name to KP Recovery Resources (KPRR).

The decade of the 1980s saw a spike in adolescent chemical dependency throughout the country. KPNW responded by developing an Adolescent Chemical Health Program (ACHP), led by Rick Boehm and Judi Brenes, RN. Boehm's expertise was drug dependency treatment; Brenes' was health education. Together, the two established an outpatient clinic, first in the Overlook building near the Health Center West Medical Office, then in a rented facility in North Portland. In 1986 they leased the Madeleine Convent for residential treatment.

Once again, a research demonstration project would be the seed for a unique program. Jointly funded by KPNW and the National Institute of Mental Health, the new program drew encouragement from BK Area Medical Director David Lawrence and from Health Plan administrators Michael Leahy and Timothy Carpenter. Boehm and Brenes developed a broad-based program with educational features, including individual and family treatment, as well as consultation services within Portland and Vancouver schools. The adolescent chemical health program grew to include seven outpatient counselors, seven residential counselors and ten assistant counselors. A nurse practitioner gave physical examinations to incoming patients and cared for them throughout their stay.

The Madeleine Convent, with its contemporary architecture, sits across the street from St. Mary Magdalene Catholic Church in a quiet northeast Portland residential area. There may have been some who questioned the practicality, let alone the propriety, of housing an alcohol and drug treatment center within the walls of a convent. But the Madeleine Convent proved an ideal facility. Group meetings and classes took place in the small chapel. Boys in treatment were housed on the basement level; girls were assigned quarters on the second floor. Problems between the sexes were negligible. Some on the staff swore that the spirit of the nuns who had previously inhabited the rooms instilled virtuous behaviors in program participants.

In 1987 Emergency Department physician Robert Miller assumed leadership of the Recovery Resources Program, replacing Senft. Miller continued to support the innovative work begun by Boehm and Brenes. He encouraged educational conferences, some of which registered as many as 250 attendants. In 1992 the adolescent program received the James A. Vohs Award for Quality, which "recognizes and honors projects that advance quality of care, showcase innovative techniques and knowledge that can be transferred throughout the program and underscore the value of multidisciplinary teamwork." The Madeleine facility closed, but the Department of Addiction Medicine continued to grow under the direction of Bradley Anderson, a former family practitioner trained in addiction medicine. Today the department thrives. Its staff of 50 provides services at ten facilities.

EARLY PHYSICAL THERAPY

In 1942 Alton Rogers found work as an ambulance driver in the Vancouver Kaiser Shipyard. The following year the Northern Permanente Foundation Hospital hired him as a cast man and orthopedic technician. His interests eventually led him to physical therapy and a new career. In 1959, by then manager of the Physical Therapy Department, he transferred to the new BK. Inpatient and outpatient services included whirlpool baths, hot paraffin treatments, ultraviolet light therapy, ultrasound, and Medcolater modalities. In addition, the department enjoyed a well-equipped exercise room. By 1971 daily patient visits numbered about 80. The department employed seven full-time and two part-time physical therapists.

PHYSIATRY

It wasn't until 1971 that Permanente hired its first physiatrist, John Gerhardt. Given Henry Kaiser's respect for the power of physical medicine and rehabilitation and given his determination to act on his beliefs, one wonders why a physiatry presence in the Northwest Region took 25 years.[8]

Gerhardt's life before his arrival in Portland had been one of serendipity, luck, and kismet. Austrian born and educated at the II State Gymnasium in Poland, he enrolled in an engineering school in Lwow in eastern Poland, rooming with a medical student with whom he studied anatomy. With the German invasion of Poland, massive bombing forced Gerhardt and his family to flee to the countryside. Hitler and the Russians had agreed to an equitable partition of Poland. Russian troops moved into eastern Poland and began to execute young Polish men. Gerhardt was saved from this fate because he was Austrian, rather than Polish. Fearful nonetheless and suspicious of Russian intentions, he tried to escape to German-occupied Poland, only to be stopped at the river border, not once but twice. On his third attempt he managed the river crossing over the ice. He found work in a railroad factory. Then, in December 1940 his luck ran out: all males between the ages of 18 and 25 were drafted into the German army.

Gerhardt became a motorcycle courier with a tank company. Then when Germany attacked Russia in June 1941, he was ordered to active duty on the Russian front. The following year, while visiting division headquarters, he read a bulletin seeking applicants for medical school in Berlin. He submitted his application, listing (falsely, to be sure) some medical school experience. In the admissions interview, he had no trouble providing accurate answers to questions on anatomy. Accepted at a military medical academy affiliated with the Kaiser Wilhelm University, he flew to Berlin where he saw for the first time the devastation to the city by allied bombing.

After attending classes during the day, medical students were responsible for guarding military stables at night and for manning watchtowers to locate fires. One classmate assigned to watchtower duty and fearful of heights traded duties with Gerhardt, who had been assigned to guard the stables. From his watchtower post Gerhardt watched in horror as allied bombs struck the stables below. Horses and men were instantly engulfed in flames.

Shortly before the German surrender, Gerhardt and 30 orderlies and nurses fled the advancing Russian army toward the American zone in Frankfurt. At war's end he was discharged from the German army but helped transport wounded soldiers to Munich. From Munich he made his way to Austria. He received his MD from the Karl Franzens University Medical School in Graz, Austria in 1948. For another eight years he served various residencies in trauma, orthopedics, obstetrics, and surgery. In 1956 now certified as a specialist in orthopedics, he emigrated to the U.S., where he secured and maintained a private general practice in rural Illinois for 13 years. There he met Wilhelm Jawurek[9] a physician refugee from Czechoslovakia who was practicing nearby. The two became friends. Jawurek's wife was a former Oregonian, and she often waxed poetic about the beauties of her home state. Largely because of her, Gerhardt applied for a two-year residency at the Portland Veterans Administration Hospital in physical medicine and rehabilitation—the only residency available in the specialty at the time. In 1971 he answered an ad for work at The Permanente Clinic, was hired and assigned a 6-x-6 foot office in the basement of BK. His tenure within those cramped quarters was short-lived; the new Interstate Clinic, later renamed Health Center West, opened within months. The gleaming facility included a well-designed Physical Medicine Department.

Gerhardt remained passionate about physical medicine and, when he was asked to accept a half-time orthopedics practice, he refused, insisting his energies be devoted to physiatry. Innovative and unorthodox, he introduced the controversial treatment prolotherapy[10] and advocated a multidisciplinary approach to complex arthritis and orthopedic problems. A prolific writer, he authored several textbooks. During the planning of KSMC, he convinced administrators to include a 50-x-25 foot therapy pool for the Physical Therapy Department, a standard feature in Austrian hospitals but rarely seen in the U.S.

Kadavil Satyanarayas—Satyan, as he is known to his colleagues—grew up in South India, the son of a judge. He remembers reading as a child a novel about a heroic general practitioner in England and telling his father that he wanted to become a doctor. Despite disability from polio contracted when he was two-and-a-half years old, he went on to fulfill his boyhood dream—not as the country physician he had envisioned but as a physiatrist. Skillful, gentlemanly, and kind, he enjoyed a 30-year career with Permanente.

Serendipity led Satyan to physiatry and rehabilitation. After obtaining his MD from Kasturba Medical College in Manipal in South India, he had a chance meeting with a paraplegic woman physician who had trained in the U.S. at New York University and now oversaw a modern, well-equipped rehabilitation center at Christian Medical College Hospital in Vellore, India. She persuaded him to work for her to fulfill the three-year service requirement of the Indian government. He obtained extensive experience—with the first electromyography (EMG) machine in India, with nerve conduction velocity (NCV) research for leprosy patients, and with spinal cord injuries.

India had no rehabilitation training center at the time, so he enrolled at the Rusk Institute of Rehabilitation Medicine at New York University Medical Center. His seatmate on the transcontinental flight from India was a woman who, seeing his short-sleeved shirt and learning his destination, advised him to purchase a coat without delay. During the layover in Beirut, Satyan bought the heaviest jacket he could find. He arrived in New York on a cold December day, grateful for the advice of a stranger and his new winter apparel.

Satyan followed his Rusk training with a year-long fellowship in spinal cord injury. In 1976 he and his wife flew to Montana, rented a car, and drove to San Diego. From San Diego, they turned north and drove up the West Coast to Portland where they stopped. The city's appeal was immediate and they determined to stay. Satyan wrote to the only Portland physiatrist of his acquaintance, who forwarded the letter to Permanente's Gerhardt. Gerhardt interviewed Satyan, hired him, and set about teaching him outpatient physiatry, at the time a specialty dominated by muscular skeletal disorders—a far cry from Satyan's training in rehabilitation medicine. A year or so after the opening of KSMC, Gerhardt transferred to the new hospital; Satyan remained at Health Center West. From then on, Satyan and Gerhardt ran separate departments, though each routinely provided cross coverage for the other.

The Physiatry Department made up for its slow start during the next two decades, hiring Mayo Clinic-trained Paul Raether in 1984; Northwestern University-trained Robert Young in 1988; and Oregonian Lane Barton in 1989. In 1987 after 13 years as an internist and an intensivist, Paul Jacobs wanted a change.

Influenced by Gerhardt, he had become interested in local injection therapy for musculoskeletal disorders. So, in 1984, with a newborn, a toddler, and a double stroller, Jacobs and his wife Karen took a sabbatical leave in Australia and New Zealand to visit rehabilitation centers, physiatrists, physiotherapists, chiropractors, and pain centers. On his return, he found the life of an internist with its night work unsustainable. He arranged for a three-year residency in physiatry at the University of Colorado Medical Center in Denver. Completing the residency, he rejoined Permanente, working part time in occupational medicine until a full-time position opened in physiatry. Eventually, he became Department Chief and was a recipient of a NWP Distinguished Physician Award.

In 2006 the Medical Society of Metropolitan Portland directory listed 43 physiatrists; of those, 14 were Permanente physiatrists.

—⚏—

PART V:
ADDITIONAL
PERMANENTE
PERSUASIONS

—⚏—

CHAPTER 16:
SOCIAL CONSCIENCE OF
PERMANENTE HEALTH CARE

By Kitty Evers, MD

At some alchemical point, leadership and opportunity combine to produce change. In the story of Permanente, the Great Depression of the 1930s and World War II brought about enormous disruptions, including fissures in the existing medical culture. Wartime necessity allowed Henry Kaiser and his health care program for shipyard workers to gain a foothold in the established fee-for-service world and, after some tenuous years of struggle, to flourish.

The elements of the Permanente health care model fuse social responsibility with pragmatism; they include an integrated group practice, prepayment by subscribers at affordable prices, and high-quality medical care. And these elements are generally accepted as the DNA of the Kaiser Permanente health care model. Henry Kaiser's earliest endeavors, however, fell far short of that ideal. In 1927 Kaiser was awarded a contract to build and pave a 200-mile highway across Cuba, then an area with minimal infrastructure to support the necessary labor force, which comprised expatriates, many of whom arrived with dependants, and an indigenous population of laborers. Five years later Kaiser was brought before the U.S. Congress to account for safety and health care conditions at the Hoover Dam worksite. One can speculate that this experience made him determined to provide health care for his workers on future projects. We have already pointed to his enlightened treatment of workers at the Grand Coulee Dam and at his wartime shipyards.

This attitude, or social conscience, permeated KP workplaces: in the organization's advocacy and support for its physician group; in an ever-increasing recruitment of women physicians and clinicians; in its commitment to research and development; and in instilling the volunteer spirit.

PHYSICIAN ADVOCACY AND SUPPORT
Physicians who joined Permanente were attracted by the promise that they could concentrate on the practice of medicine without the distraction of running

a business. Permanente guaranteed an interesting practice; autonomy within the exam room; the opportunity to practice evidence-based medicine and preventive care; an integrated system with no financial barriers to referral; a salary, educational leave; a liberal medical and dental benefit package (including partner health benefits for both gay and straight); and sound retirement benefits. It also provided sabbatical leaves: for some, the opportunity to obtain additional training, and for others, the time to provide medical care in underserved areas, both in the U.S. and abroad.

The size of Northwest Permanente offered physicians the opportunity to grow through their careers. Almost all administrative positions have been filled from within, often with the help of on-the-job training. The organization's Department of Continuing Education provided additional support. Still another attractive feature allowed those contemplating retirement, especially those who might feel ambivalent about the decision, to return to Permanente in a part-time or locum tenens role. An Emeritus Staff program, begun in 1981, fostered connections not only between NWP and retirees, but among the retirees themselves.

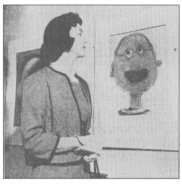

Virginia Saward, Portland artist whose painting of Mrs. Bess Kaiser hangs in the new Kaiser Hospital, examines one of 25 works by children in Saturday classes at The Portland Art Museum, which are part of the décor in lounges and wards of pediatrics division.
Courtesy of The Oregonian.

As Permanente matured, it developed other policies to support physicians. In 1970 pediatricians Jacob and Betty Reiss successfully petitioned to share a pediatric practice, setting a precedent. Working part time was certainly not the norm. Rather, from Permanente's beginnings, physicians were expected to choose between family and profession. When, in 1981, three mental health therapists were pregnant at the same time, Permanente offered each of the three a part-time practice so that they might balance their child-rearing responsibilities with their professional work. By 2007 about half of those in the Departments of Pediatrics, Family Practice, Internal Medicine, and Obstetrics and Gynecology worked part time. And though these departments attract a higher proportion of women, men too have opted, albeit in much smaller numbers, to work part time.

NWP has evolved, too, in its sensitivity to the problems of its physicians. In the early 1990s the Region's Board of Directors designated a standing advisory committee, the Physicians Health Committee, to address health issues affecting its physicians. Internist Richard Bills was appointed the committee's first chairperson. The committee encouraged each physician to seek a primary care physician, to participate personally in prevention guidelines, to adopt ergonomic changes to prevent injury at work, and to disclose through confidential surveys their satisfaction or lack thereof with their work life.

Boards of medical examiners in each state mandate reporting drug and alcohol abuse by a physician. In most states the abuse of alcohol or prescription or illegal drugs has been grounds for termination of the medical license. Oregon and Washington have slightly differing approaches, but both emphasize advocacy that entails reporting, monitoring, and treating substance abuse. Washington State monitors and treats specific mental health conditions as well. Oregon began reporting disabling mental health conditions in 2009.

In 1985 NWP established a hospital staff committee to help impaired physicians. Volunteer committee members included recovering physicians who counseled physicians seeking help. In its 7 years of existence, the committee saw 17 physicians among a mean population of 426. One might have interpreted that the relatively small number indicated few emotional or substance-abuse problems. But a 1991 physician survey of the group indicated that a significant number of physicians were struggling with symptoms of early, mid, or late burnout. The Biblical reference: "Physician, heal thyself " (St. Luke 4:23) may be an ideal, but self-care has its limits. The growing recognition in Permanente's leadership of stresses within its physician group prompted the creation in 1993 of a confidential counseling program by and for physicians and their families.

HEALING ARTS IN THE WORKPLACE

From its beginnings as a health care Region, KP Northwest incorporated the concept that the surrounding environment has a healing effect on both patients and staff. Consequently, its leaders saw art and architecture as worthy investments and set aside a fixed percentage of each building's costs for art and craft. Virginia Saward and others had the foresight to collect a sizable inventory of works by Northwest artists. Judith Poxson Fawkes' memorable tapestry, *View of Portland with Bess Kaiser Hospital*, brought the outdoors to the hospital interior. On display at the entrance to Bess Kaiser Hospital, its four woven panels reflected a bird's eye view of the Willamette River, the hospital and the city. Herself an accomplished artist, Virginia Saward began by collecting works by local artists. At first she rented works from the Portland Art Museum. Those that received favorable comment by visitors and staff, she purchased. Today the Saward collection comprises 80 works, permanently displayed at the Center for Health Research.

KP buildings, both medical offices and hospitals, combine beauty with utility, and several have won architectural awards for design. Tualatin Medical Office consciously interacts with the community and its wetlands environment. Its roof collects rainwater, which cascades in front of two-story windows outside the ground floor waiting room. The building and its landscape are featured in the City of Tualatin Art Walk. The thoughtfully designed campus of Kaiser Sunnyside Medical Center features a labyrinth, an intricate walking path leading to the center. A conscious allusion to a medieval tradition, the labyrinth at KSMC encourages a quiet walking meditation—a temporary respite from stress—for both patients and staff.

The year 1975 saw a shift in focus and a new direction for the Region's art and architecture. The Department of External Affairs determined that art should be accessible, even touchable. "Arts and crafts are especially effective [in enhancing the healing process] primarily because works of the hand are basic to all human activity and have universal appeal." Thereafter, for a time the Region purchased only craft pieces: ceramics, textiles, enamel, glass, and wood.

In the following years the Region's collection suffered some erosion of its former curatorial discipline; some facilities, for example, began to acquire framed posters that represented neither the local environment nor Northwest artists. In 1994 the Region renewed the discussion to establish criteria for collecting art. A group of leaders—controller Bill Cooper; Center for Health Research Director Mitch Greenlick; facilities services' Robert McDowell; and NWP's Harvey Klevit—articulated a general vision that included key elements: "Surroundings and the environment can aid the healing process; responsible corporations should support local artists and thus encourage an active art community; good art is timeless and therefore cost effective." In recent years photography has been featured in facilities. Sunnybrook Medical Office, for example, showcases original photographs of Northwest nature. Cascade Park Medical Office also features original photographs, though it still retains Henk Pander's watercolor *Farm in Friesland* and John Ricken's large bronze sculpture *Running Horse*.

PERMANENTE WOMEN

From ancient times women have played an active role as healers, herbalists, and midwives. In both Elizabethan England and colonial America women practiced traditional midwifery and healing. But the formation of a surgeons' guild in England in 1540, with its fierce protectionism from competition, set the cause of women back for centuries. Its provisions dictated "... no carpenters, smiths, weavers or women shall practice medicine." In America, the hugely influential Puritan minister Cotton Mather[1] further damaged the cause of women in *Angelic Conjunction* by decreeing that women were to be excluded from practicing medicine.

Change was slow to come, but in 1847, nearly a century after the death of Mather, Elizabeth Blackwell won acceptance to medical school at Geneva Medical College in upstate New York. She became the first woman to graduate from a medical school in the U.S. There followed a brief flourishing of medical schools for women students. Philanthropist Elizabeth Garrett endowed $500,000 to open Johns Hopkins University School of Medicine. Its two provisions included one that required admission to women students. Consequently, in the first class 3 of the 12 students were women. Still, old attitudes are wondrously slow to change. Even that faculty sage William Osler later lamented the experiment of admitting women to medical school as a failure, though he acknowledged ruefully that the "die was cast."

After the 1910 Flexner Report exposed sham medical schools, forcing more than half to close their doors, those that remained, including Johns Hopkins, chose to accept only a few women. And that august institution Harvard Medical School did not open its doors to women until 1945. The Woman's Medical College of Pennsylvania, founded in 1850, was the only women's medical college to survive the Flexner Report.

Four women physicians made up the Permanente medical staff of 40 in Vancouver during World War II. They were pediatricians Katherine Van Leeuwen, Cire Scheer, and Margaret Ingram. Lucille (Lucy) Hacker was not only the rare woman pathologist, she was the Region's *only* pathologist. Moreover, her male colleagues are said to have respected her skill in her specialty.

Following the war years, only one woman, pediatrician Virginia Gilliland, joined the Medical Group. Hired in 1948, she remained the only Northern Permanente woman physician for the next 20 years. Apparently unconcerned by her gender isolation, she seemed to thrive within the small Medical Group. A touch of the flamboyant characterized her persona. She piloted helicopters and drove a Mercedes SL convertible, more often than not accompanied by her Great Dane who sat imperiously beside her in the passenger seat.

In the late 1960s and early 1970s several additional women joined the Medical Group: anesthesiologist Pauline Grodsky in 1967; obstetrician Barbara Manildi in 1968; Emergency Department physician Josephine (Sunny) Colbach and internist Leonora Dantes, both in 1970. Recruitment slowed for a time in the early 1970s but picked up again mid-decade. Permanente hired pediatrician Virginia Feldman in 1975 (together with her internist husband George); pathologist Shusma Chawla in 1978; otolaryngologist Sharon Higgins in 1979; and ophthalmologist Christina West in 1981. Beginning in the

1980s women began to join Permanente in greater numbers. Table 1 shows the dramatic increase in the ratio of women physicians by department specialty in a 30-year period between 1977 and 2007. The percentage increases in internal medicine, from 2% to 36%; in pediatrics, from 3% to 61%; and in obstetrics, 13% to 63% are particularly striking.

Table 1. Permanente Women Physicians in the Northwest 1977 and 2007				
	1997		2007	
Department	Women	Total	Women	Total
Emergency	1	11	6	32
Pathology	1	5	6	12
Internal Medicine	1	54	37	103
Family Practice	1	7	28	102
Pediatrics	1	27	49	80
Obstetrics	3	23	31	49
Psychiatry	1	3	11	31
Anesthesia	2	7	10	29

As the ranks of women physicians grew throughout the country and within Permanente, the numbers of women in leadership roles grew as well. In 1981 pathologist Kathleen Holahan broke through barriers as the first woman to be elected to the NWP Board of Directors. Others followed Holahan's example, among them family practitioner Margaret Vandenbark, hospitalist Donna Strain, internist Jane Drummond, and family practitioner Carolyn Hokanson. Women also assumed other leadership positions. Psychiatrist Kitty Evers (author of this chapter) was appointed Chief of the Psychiatry Department in 1976—at the time the lone woman in male-dominated, sometimes rancorous, chief meetings. Besides the administrative assistant who took meeting minutes, she was usually the only woman in the room. Evers may have been the first woman in the role of Department Chief, but she was followed by others: pediatrician Virginia Feldman, family practitioner Margaret Vandenbark, internist Carrie Ware, psychiatrist Lauretta Young, dermatologist Mary Lyons, internist Marcia Dunham, pediatrician Joyce Liu, and medical geneticists Lessa Linck and Dana Kostiner. Radiologist Kathleen Meunier was appointed Chief of Legal Medicine in 1994 and was succeeded by Maureen Wright, who was recruited to Permanente as a hospitalist. Now Associate Medical Director of quality systems, Wright explained her reasons for joining NWP: "… they offered an innovative program that involved internal medicine physicians doing only hospital work. I came primarily because of that innovation."

Current NWP Executive Medical Director Sharon Higgins was one of only 60 women among 6,000 otolaryngologists practicing in the U.S. when she graduated from her residency. She joined the Medical Group in 1979; was Department Chief from 1985 to 1999; and assumed the top leadership position, Executive Medical Director, in 2007. In remembering her training, Higgins recalled, "As a surgical intern at the Veteran's Administration Hospital in Oklahoma City, I had a flock of six medical students, two of whom were women; our chief resident was a woman as well. In the medical school hierarchy, the patient is first seen by the medical student, then by the intern, and finally by the chief resident. The female medical student had presented [during medical rounds] a routine hernia case; the patient was a grizzled Vet. As I examined the patient he asked, 'Where are the guys?' When I explained that the chief resident was also a woman, he said, 'The VA ain't what it used to be.'"

Not all the women who played significant roles in the development of Permanente were physicians. In *The Story of Dr. Sidney R. Garfield: The Visionary who turned Sick Care into Health Care,* Tom Debley describes how Betty Runyen, the attractive and dedicated nurse at Contractors General Hospital near Desert Center, California, worked without pay for seven months before the prepayment system proved successful. As one of only two nurses at the hospital, she took on numerous challenging tasks during Garfield's frequent absences. Another nurse, Millie Cutting, Cecil Cutting's wife, together with Edgar Kaiser's wife Sue, organized a free well-baby clinic in a local church and solicited funds from local businesses, including known houses of prostitution on Grand Coulee's B Street. Historian Steve Gilford describes how Dr. Cutting himself escorted his wife to solicit a donation from one of these houses. Welcomed inside by a gracious madam, the Cuttings received a generous donation. During the course of a pleasant exchange, the host shared her family picture album with the two visitors. The madams were said to be generous contributors; the church provided the space, the madams the money.

As has already been noted, Bernice Oswald played a crucial role in the Northwest when women executives were a rarity. Controller for both Health Plan and the Medical Group from 1945 until her retirement in 1970, Oswald described to an interviewer how she became interested in accounting during her youth when, at age 13, she kept the books for a neighbor's business. She learned accounting through a correspondence course.

Other women have served long and illustrious careers within Permanente. Marci Clark[2] joined KP in 1975, hired for a nonmanagerial position. She ended her 34-year career as leader of professional resources. Over the years she recruited over 700 Permanente physicians. Deborah Hedges came to KP in 1980, having previously traveled and worked in a head-spinning number of countries. Her colorful and impressive itinerary includes travel through England, Scotland, Germany, Italy, the former Yugoslavia, the Greek Islands, Turkey, Afghanistan, and Nepal. When her companion accepted locum tenens work at the Kunde Hospital on the Mount Everest slope in Nepal, Hedges opened a restaurant in Kathmandu. In her 24 years with Permanente, Hedges has served the Medical Group in numerous demanding positions (though to be sure, none so exotic as running a restaurant in Kathmandu). She currently serves as Permanente Director of Human Resources.

Ann Stenzel responded to a 1978 advertisement by NWP seeking someone with experience with ERISA.[3] She joined the Pension and Benefits Department, working under Business Manager Jack Freis and his associate Phil Papworth. She later became Director of that department. Others with long tenures include Kathy Bailey, professional compensation; Lori Byers, Bonnie Johnson, Joyce Lavoie, pension and benefits; Patsy Lindsay, government relations and compliance; Judy Parmenter, human resources; Helena Purcell, executive administrative assistant; and Susan Gardner, senior administrative analyst.

THE CENTER FOR HEALTH RESEARCH

Both Henry Kaiser and Garfield understood the social mission of KP to include independent research. In 1943 Garfield sought and obtained $50,000 for clinical research to treat syphilis. Soon thereafter he discovered that the shipyards offered limitless potential for epidemiological studies. In 1958 the Kaiser Foundation established a research institute in Richmond, California. Grants came from both external and internal sources. Often Permanente physicians were chosen as members of the research team, sometimes as primary investigators. The institute undertook projects in cardiovascular disease, psychosomatic illness, cancer, diabetes, and allergies.

Ernest Saward saw in the prepaid group practice a social experiment for Permanente in the Northwest. For Saward, a Portland-based Center for Health Research was a natural outgrowth of this mission, fulfilling an intrinsic social obligation to the local community. After laying the groundwork for the center together with Arnold Hurtado, in 1964 he offered the position of director to Mitch Greenlick whose training at the University of Michigan was in research and in medical care organization.

Though he was sponsored by Saward, Greenlick was officially responsible to Kaiser Foundation Hospitals. Nevertheless, he was to have a close relationship to the Permanente physicians and to have a significant effect on their practice of medicine. A pharmacist by training, Greenlick was an unusual candidate to lead a pioneering research center. An indifferent student, he was also a self-described troublemaker and spent much of his time managing a grocery store. With his low grade-point average, his counselor refused to recommend him for pharmacy school. Disregarding his counselor's dismissal, he took the entrance examinations at Wayne State University and placed second in a field of 3,000. And the reason he decided to become a pharmacist? He admired the father of a friend, a pharmacist whose shirt and tie identified him as a professional, a rarity in Greenlick's Detroit neighborhood. (Ironically, in the course of Greenlick's long KP career, no one recalls ever having seen him wear a tie.)

It didn't take long for Greenlick to become disillusioned at pharmacy school. His initial performance was every bit as poor as his high school one had been. But before long, he began to distinguish himself: as editor of the pharmacy magazine, President of the pharmacy professional fraternity, and president of the campus leadership society. After graduation he sought a master's degree, then went to Michigan where his PhD work included research on health services. He met with Saward who was looking for a Director for his research center. KP with its stable population of patients and its centralized medical records was ideal for health care research. Saward offered Greenlick the position, and he took the job.

Under Greenlick's leadership, the Center identified four areas of concentration: the effects of: 1) health care services to an existing populations in an established health care system; 2) new health care services to new population within a health care system; 3) new methods and new personnel to provide existing services in a health care system; and 4) theoretical and conceptual issues. Funding came from Kaiser Foundation Hospitals and from federal and philanthropic grants. Greenlick's investigators mined medical records from KP's huge population base (the oldest and most complete in the U.S.) to abstract indispensable data on population-based care, both inside and outside KP.

Saward gave unwavering support to Greenlick's innovations. Through the years, the Center for Health Research participated in or led numerous clinical studies, but its central mission remained studying the impact of health services on social development. A decades-long KP icon, Greenlick retired from KPNW in 1990. He currently represents District 33 in the House of Representatives of the Oregon State Legislature where he is a health policy leader.

VOLUNTEERING IN THE COMMUNITY AND IN THE WORLD

The desire to help, to make a difference, calls many young men and women to the practice of medicine. After they attain their medical degrees that call to service remains, even when they feel fatigued or their days are long. For many NWP physicians the urge to give back to the community goes well beyond the office and the surgery suite.

Carolyn Polansky who joined Permanente in 1982 and worked for many years in urgency care is an example. As a fourth-year medical student at the Woman's Medical College of Pennsylvania in Philadelphia, Polansky served two months on the hospital ship SS Hope stationed in Natal, Brazil. She assisted in surgery on the ship and helped the public health staff at neighborhood well-baby clinics. She walked door to door to promote immunization and TB testing. She was one of an eye-care team that evaluated patients at a leper colony. Years later, as a Permanente physician, she served with a mobile health clinic sponsored by Northwest Medical Teams International based at Kuchavelli, Sri Lanka after the tsunami that devastated that Region. During the tsunami, the government and rebels had agreed to a cease fire. Polansky was still in the country when the cease fire ended and violence resumed, requiring the team to withdraw from the area. Polanksy's volunteerism continued into retirement. She volunteered with the Center for Personal Restoration in Arequipa, Peru, providing medical care to adults and children and, in Fiji, providing preventive health care to women.

Several mental health physicians have incorporated volunteer activities into their private time. Psychiatrist Larry Cooper worked at the mental health service of the free Portland Neighborhood Health Clinic from 1982 to 2003. He worked, not with the chronically mentally ill, but with the working poor who lacked employer-paid insurance. These patients made too much money to qualify for the Oregon Health Plan but could not afford to buy their own insurance. Psychiatrist Stuart Oken, in addition to his clinical and administrative responsibilities, worked with the organization's Care Management Institute as Director of the project on health literacy. The program targets the illiterate, a surprising 30% of the population, as well as the functionally illiterate (15%). In addition, Oken has served for 15 years on the board of Folk Time, an organization whose mission is to build community for those chronically mentally ill who otherwise remain socially isolated and disenfranchised from the community.

Otolaryngologist Jeffrey Israel developed the KPNW Cleft Palate Team and Clinic in 1985. In addition to working with patients in the Northwest, the team helped bring physicians from other countries to Oregon to learn the team's surgical techniques. His work has taken him to China, Costa Rica, Honduras, Mexico, Peru, the Philippines, and Siberia. Israel and Thomas Albert, a professor of oral and maxillofacial surgery at OHSU are co-founders of the Foundation for the Advancement of Cleft Education and Services (FACES Foundation), a foundation that provides surgical treatment for children with facial deformities.

Hematologist Stephen Chandler served with Northwest Medical Teams beginning in the 1990s. He completed 15 mission trips, most to Latin America, but also to Sri Lanka after the 2004 Indian Ocean tsunami. Now retired from NWP,

Chandler has, for six years, contributed as an adjunct faculty member at OHSU, teaching a course called "The Healer's Art." In a recent interview Chandler talked about his enjoyment in helping "these young students maintain their heart and soul and love of service throughout medical school and into practice."

Pediatrician Virginia Feldman and her husband internist George Feldman began volunteering in India during their 1984 sabbatical year. Since that first trip, they have returned to India again and again, sometimes remaining for months at a time. The two have volunteered in four different programs in various locations. For one of these, Virginia Feldman oversaw the opening of a clinic and training of community health workers. She then began work with 500 prostituted women in the area, studying their health histories and those of their children. Thirty of the 100 women with whom she worked were able to free themselves from sex work. Throughout her Permanente career, Feldman has devoted enormous amounts of her time to various local health clinics.

Jill Ginsberg, who joined the Family Practice Department in 1994 and now is lead physician for KPNW's Community Care Department, has a long history of helping the less privileged. During the course of her resident training in San Francisco, she visited pregnant women in homeless shelters. She has worked for the Indian Health Service on the Washington Olympic Peninsula at Port Angeles, Callam Bay, and Neah Bay and started free clinics for Spanish-speaking migrant workers in Forks, Washington.

Ginsberg helped relocate to Portland several families from New Orleans who were left homeless by Hurricane Katrina in 2006. In November 2005 she worked with Pastor Mary Overstreet to open a free health clinic, North by Northeast Health Center on Martin Luther King Boulevard in North Portland. Since August 2006, volunteer medical advisors have treated more than 3,000 patients. Ginsberg continues to serve the clinic as its Medical Director.

Those physicians singled out here for their volunteer work represent heroic examples of the idealism that permeates NWP. They are, however, by no means unique. Through its 70-year history Permanente physicians in the Northwest have contributed their time and expertise to volunteer in the community and throughout the world.

PART VI: THE RECENT DECADES

CHAPTER 17:
THE SEVENTIES

EXIT: THE ICON DEPARTS

In 1969, without warning, Ernest Saward announced his intention to take a two-to-three-year leave of absence. He planned to return to Permanente, he said, and thereafter divide his time between clinical practice and research. He had recently returned from a five-week trip to New Zealand and Australia, fully expecting the Region to have concluded a planned acquisition of property for a second medical center and hospital. Although he did not say so at the time, he was dismayed to learn that no action had taken place. Privately he decided that his leave-taking would force the Medical Group to develop new leadership and to eliminate its dependency on him.

His announcement naming surgeon Lewis Hughes to replace him stunned the Medical Group. Although Hughes was respected for his surgical skills and generally well liked, he lacked substantive administrative experience and, in the Medical Group's view, leadership strengths. Soft spoken, tall and slender, he was unassuming in manner and dress, usually wearing a gray suit and sometimes mismatched socks. Many believed the rightful heir-apparent to Saward should have been internist Arnold Hurtado, who had administrative interest and skills. But in a 1982 interview with John Smillie, Saward explained the rationale for his decision: Hurtado was unacceptable to the surgeons; Paul Lairson,[1] Sawards's deputy, had only been with the group three years; and neither Norman Frink nor Roger George, the two with most experience, had any interest in the position.

Some physicians were delighted that the "old tyrant" was leaving, though they were suspicious of

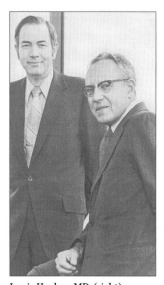

Lewis Hughes, MD, (right) Medical Director of The Permanente Clinic, 1970 – 1975. Scott Fleming, Kaiser Foundation Health Plan Senior Vice President and Regional Manager, 1973 – 1975. *Courtesy of Kaiser Permanente Heritage Resources.*

Saward's motives, especially when they learned that he planned to retain his position on the Executive Committee, thereby ensuring his ability to exert his influence behind the scenes. Others, however, were saddened, some even devastated, at the prospect of losing his strong leadership. Those in Oakland's central administrative office were perplexed, unable to understand his motivation. Saward moved swiftly, largely ignoring the upheaval swirling around his decision, and obtained a position at Yale as professor in public health. This move was to be followed by another, to his alma mater University of Rochester, as associate dean of extramural affairs and professor of social medicine. There he would launch a new career in teaching and in directing health care policy.

Not surprisingly, Saward's departure left a leadership vacuum and coincided with other events that were to have a profound effect on the organization of the Medical Group and on its relationship with Health Plan. Among the challenges of the decade would be Permanente leadership changes, a deteriorating financial picture, a long road to attain an optimal retirement plan, the opening of a second hospital, and the introduction of family practitioners, as well as of physician assistants and nurse practitioners to the organization.

As the new Medical Director, Hughes was to have a difficult time, for the physicians of the 1970s were not about to accept the working conditions tolerated by the physicians of the previous decade. For one thing, the physician-patient ratio was 1/1600. (By contrast, The Permanente Medical Group in California enjoyed a ratio of 1/1000.) In addition, the schedule required internists to take overnight call three times a month, which necessitated a grueling 31-hour work shift: 8 hours in clinic, followed by 15 hours overnight in the hospital, followed by another 8 hours in clinic. General surgeons' 24-hour call was even more frequent and required covering the hospital and the emergency room and performing emergency surgeries. Obstetrics was understaffed and overworked, and the resignation of a popular gynecologist who performed oncologic surgeries had a demoralizing effect. Pediatricians were required to take overnight call about every sixth day. Add to these working conditions the fact that physicians' incomes were not competitive with those in the community and that the Region suffered from a reputation for poor service, it's little wonder that recruiting new physicians was a difficult assignment.

Still, in spite of its problems, the Northwest was still the most productive per capita Kaiser Permanente Region. It had significant cash reserves, and it owned property for expansion—several acres in Washington County for a Beaverton medical office and 26 acres in Clackamas, Oregon for a planned medical center. What's more, the Region seemed to view its myriad challenges with an optimism that was characteristic of Henry Kaiser.

Hughes tried to appease as many of his colleagues as possible; as a result special interests influenced the Executive Committee to make decisions that a stronger leader would have opposed. These included hiring more physicians to care for surgical patients in the emergency room; hiring medical school residents as moonlighters to cover hospitalized surgical patients; increasing vacation time; and approving extra time for inpatient consultation and administrative tasks. In addition, the committee increased income scales for hard-to-recruit surgical subspecialties such as ENT and orthopedics. At the same time it authorized pay increases for primary care specialties at 15 and 20 years of tenure. Finally, the committee relaxed its policy on vacation requests and began to approve vacations on short notice, a change that inevitably created operating room inefficiencies.

Bernice Oswald, long-time auditor and supervisor for financial affairs for both Kaiser Foundation Health Plan and Hospitals and for The Permanente Clinic, retired in 1970, and named Robert Scott, previously with the Medical Group in Los Angeles, as her successor. Scott continued Oswald's dual role with the physicians and with Health Plan. Three years later, Sam Hufford, Health Plan's Regional Manager, took early retirement, to be succeeded by Health Plan veteran Scott Fleming.[2] When Fleming first joined the Health Plan Legal Department in 1955, Henry Kaiser and the Permanente Medical Groups were engaged in conflict over contractual and organizational issues. It was Fleming who successfully resolved them. But because of Fleming's paid position with Health Plan, the physicians were at first wary of him. Their misgivings gave way to respect soon enough, as they came to trust Fleming's candor, diligence, and integrity.

Despite Hughes' efforts to placate the Medical Group, physicians remained querulous under his leadership, complaining of delayed decisions, inadequate delegation, and poor communication. In late 1974 many members of the group expressed a desire for their own controller or business manager. Both Fleming and Scott supported the idea, and at the end of 1975 the Medical Group hired Jack Fries. A New Yorker with a Harvard MBA, Fries was a sophisticated business analyst. His style, direct and straightforward, took some getting used to by the Medical Group but soon won over the physicians. He would prove a good match for the next Medical Director.

In 1974 Health Plan finances deteriorated and in 1975 the financial picture darkened. Membership satisfaction hit an all-time low, and the dues structure made marketing difficult. A low point came when Health Plan asked physicians to consider reductions in their salaries. An emergency Joint Task Force on Cost Effectiveness met on March 10 with Associate Medical Director Fred Nomura as Chair.[3] On March 20 the task force submitted its first interim report with 37 recommendations.

In his "Reflections of a Lame Duck" (Appendix 4) address to his Permanente colleagues at the September 1975 Falstaff[4] conference, shortly before his term as Medical Director ended, Hughes candidly assessed his leadership shortcomings.

But he faulted the Medical Group too for placing all the blame for the Region's troubles on Health Plan rather than acknowledging any responsibility for ensuring cost control and membership satisfaction. That month a committee chaired by Perry Sloop undertook the search for a Medical Director—a new experience for the 30-year-old Medical Group. The search committee settled on Marvin Goldberg from Southern California Permanente Medical Group. More will be said about Goldberg and his influence later in this and the following chapter.

RETIREMENT PLANS

In addition to leadership challenges, the 1970s saw an almost decade-long effort by Permanente physicians to secure their retirement plan. Other Permanente Medical Groups had adopted retirement plans, beginning with the SCPMG in 1957. As laid out in the Tahoe Agreement, the Medical Service Agreement called for Health Plan to contribute 12 cents per month per member to a trust fund administered by Aetna with individual physician accounts. As a partnership the physicians were ineligible for an IRS-qualified plan with its accompanying tax advantages. (The group had first considered incorporating but ultimately decided on a non-qualified plan based on deferred earnings to be taxed after retirement.) TPMG had developed a similar plan in 1959, and the physicians of The Permanente Clinic had followed with a plan of their own in 1961.

In 1962 the Northern California regional IRS ruled that funds allocated to individual physicians were taxable as current income and that physicians were liable for back taxes. (The Southern California IRS had previously made a reverse ruling.) TPMG paid the back taxes and then sued the IRS for refunds. The first case was U.S. vs. Basye (James Basye, whose name became synonymous with the dispute, was merely first named on the alphabetical list.) The U.S. District Court ruled in favor of TPMG in 1968, but the IRS won on appeal in 1971. The case then went to the Supreme Court where TPMG lost. (In anticipation of an unfavorable decision, TPMG had already established the Common Plan in 1965 so as to comply with IRS regulations and provide a defined benefit plan for all Regions with retirement income based on years of service and peak income. But the Common Plan had limitations: fewer tax advantages, a limit on contributions, a Social Security offset, and no security against creditors.)

VERVLOET AND INCORPORATION

It was pulmonologist Albert Vervloet who almost single-handedly championed the cause of Northwest Permanente physicians in obtaining a superior pension plan. Seen by some as a polemicist, Vervloet must nevertheless be credited with an unwavering dedication to improving the status of physicians who, in his view, were treated as mere employees by Health Plan and given little say in directing their future. In pursuit of his goal, he largely ignored those in positions of authority, alienating the Medical Director, the Associate Medical Director, the Chief of Medicine, hospital administrators, and the Director of the Research Center. Both Saward (no longer Medical Director but still a member of the Executive Committee) and Kaiser Health Plan President and CEO Clifford Keene cautioned Vervloet to temper his aggressive style with more restraint. Vervloet ignored them both.

Vervloet's story is the stuff of fiction. Born in 1932 in Surabaya, Java, the grandson of a prosperous Dutch immigrant whose wealth derived from a family-owned sugar factory, Vervloet grew up in luxurious surroundings. His privileged world ended abruptly, however, with the Japanese occupation in 1941. The invaders immediately imprisoned Vervloet's engineer father who had enlisted with the Dutch army to oversee construction of concrete bunkers. Vervloet would not see his father again until after the war. The Japanese seized the family's property and transported the nine-year-old Albert, together with his two siblings and his mother, by horse cart to a holding area at a railroad station. Detained for the better part of the following morning under a relentless sun and given neither water nor a place to relieve themselves, they were herded aboard trains to an internment camp. There Albert was assigned to a youth camp, his older brother to adult quarters. Out of necessity, Albert became an expert marksman with a slingshot. When he could, he brought down birds to supplement his meager food ration.

Chronically hungry, he surreptitiously began to trade for food with local Indonesians at night under the camp fence until he learned that the punishment for this offense, at least for adults, was death by shooting. Youths received a lashing while tied to a post in the Javanese sun. When liberation came, he reunited with his family, who, together with other Dutch citizens, found protection from rampaging Indonesian insurgents within a Gurkha unit of the British Army. The family emigrated to Holland in 1946 and Vervloet received his medical degree from Leiden University in 1960. In 1964 he and his wife came to Portland where he had obtained a fellowship in pulmonary diseases with Miles Edwards[5] at the University of Oregon Medical School. After finishing his training, he entertained offers from both the Veterans Administration and The Portland Clinic. Then Charles Pinney, who attended the weekly chest conferences at the medical school, persuaded Vervloet to consider The Permanente Clinic. Attracted by its retirement program, he joined the Medical Group in 1968 devoting half his time to Permanente and half to research at the medical school.

Soon after joining The Permanente Clinic, Vervloet began to ask questions about the physicians' financial relationship with Health Plan and discovered that details of the pension plan left many questions unanswered. Winning election to the

Executive Committee, he quickly immersed himself in the business affairs of the Medical Group and began his tireless crusade to bring about incorporation.

Although Vervloet never lost his determination in pursuit of his objective, other issues periodically distracted him. One of these was the disbursal of community service funds[6] to the research center—a percentage far greater than that allocated by other Regions. In Northern California, for example, 62% went to professional library services, education, and intern and residency services, with only 14% allocated to research. But the Northwest Region allocated a much smaller percentage to physician education and training, and a hefty 62% to research. Vervloet also challenged the method by which Health Plan revised and negotiated the Medical Service Agreement, and insisted on an independent legal review of its terms and full disclosure to the partnership of its content.

At the July 27, 1970 meeting of the Executive Committee, Arnold Hurtado recommended "that an ad-hoc committee study the merits of incorporation versus the partnership." The result was the formation of a retirement plan pension committee with Vervloet as chairman. During the next four years he presided over innumerable meetings and presentations by attorneys and others regarding incorporation. The committee's objectives were twofold: one, to secure the Common Plan resources—

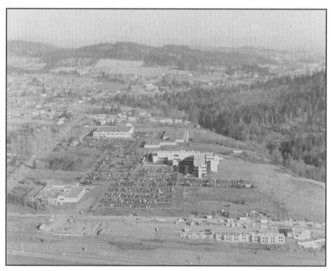

Kaiser Sunnyside Medical Center campus with the hospital in the center; Mt Scott clinic on the left; and the Regional Supply Center and Clinical Laboratories the upper building, circa 1979.
Courtesy of Kaiser Permanente Heritage Resources.

at risk to Health Plan creditors if Health Plan were to fail—and two, to obtain the favorable tax advantage of benefits through incorporation.

Earlier, controller Bernice Oswald had gathered information that seemed to argue against incorporation. Local Health Plan attorneys (Davies, Biggs, Strayer, Stoel and Boley) warned of a "two-state problem"; Oregon law required that Oregon corporations be registered in Oregon. Although Washington state law was not clear, an opinion from the Washington Attorney General implied that an Oregon professional corporation could not qualify to practice in the state of Washington.

At an early 1971 Executive Committee meeting dedicated to discussing incorporation attorney, Tom Dearing laid out both the pros and cons of incorporation. Health Plan attorney Jerry Phelan argued the merits of the Common Plan. Attorney Morton Zalutsky, retained by Permanente's pension committee, advocated incorporation. Each made presentations to the Executive Committee. Zalutsky, unable to obtain complete information about the Common Plan, learned only later that Phelan, regarding Zalutsky as an adversary, had withheld some pertinent details. Delay followed delay, but in 1972 the pension committee conducted a plebiscite that revealed that 92% of the Medical Group favored incorporation. The Executive Committee then held an official balloting confirming the result. In July the committee tabled a motion to begin action to incorporate until Saward could attend. The Executive Committee retained Zalutsky to write the Articles of Incorporation. Zalutsky remained confident that the interstate commerce law would supersede the Washington Attorney General's opinion and in 1973 he argued the case, resolving the two-state problem to the Attorney General's satisfaction.

The next hurdle was Health Plan's desire to treat all Regions' retirement plans with reasonable uniformity. At the time neither TPMG nor SCPMG had voiced an interest in incorporating. As for Colorado and Ohio Regions, neither had a retirement plan; Colorado had incorporated for reasons pertaining to state laws on fee splitting but was considering a change to a partnership. Only the Hawaii Permanente Medical Group had incorporated and remained satisfied with its decision. In May 1974 at a summit meeting in Denver, regional leaders met to hear Colorado leaders discuss

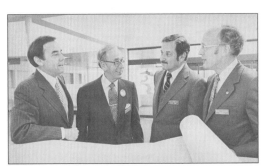

Visit at new Montana Clinic in 1978. (left to right) James A. Vohs, President Kaiser Foundation Health Plan; Edgar Kaiser, Chairman of the Board; Marvin Goldberg, Oregon Regional Medical Director; and Daniel Wagster, Vice President and Oregon Regional Manager.
Courtesy of Kaiser Permanente Heritage Resources.

their experience regarding incorporation and to review opinions and actions to date. Attendees included Hughes, Fleming, Deering, Zalutsky, Phelan, and members of the pension committee. The meeting was a disappointment. Much of the information covered already familiar ground. No decisions emerged.

Toward the end of 1974 an unexpected event diverted Vervloet's energies from his goal of incorporation. A dispute arose within the pulmonary function laboratory at Bess Kaiser Hospital where Vervloet was Medical Director. Although the quality of the laboratory was never in question, Chief of Medicine Arnold Hurtado had received reports of alleged administrative dysfunction. At Hurtado's request, two outside Seattle pulmonologists investigated the charges, evaluated the department, and recommended changes in management. Stung by the criticism, Vervloet resigned as Director in 1975. Then, during his campaign for reelection to the Executive Committee, Vervloet charged that its members had maligned him and he called for an investigation. In March he withdrew his efforts to bring about incorporation through the pension committee, leaving further activity in the hands of the Executive Committee. Hughes, who after the plebiscite had given lukewarm support to incorporation, now wavered and called for further evaluation.

Perhaps because of criticisms leveled at him about his management of the Pulmonary Department, Vervloet resigned from the partnership in September 1975, without having achieved his desired goal of incorporation. Hughes stepped down that year as Medical Director. On December 30, Marvin Goldberg from the San Diego Area accepted the position of Medical Director. But it would be another four years before the Medical Group would attain the status of a professional corporation. A new generation of NWP physicians who may take their pension plan for granted are indebted, whether they know it or not, to the tenacious Vervloet and his quest more than 30 years ago to achieve incorporation.

SUNNYSIDE UP

In 1968 KP purchased 60 acres in Clackamas, Oregon near the proposed I-205 freeway, with the idea of building a second hospital. The 1960s had seen tremendous membership growth for the organization, from 55,000 in 1962 to 125,000 by 1969. Not surprisingly, BK was hard-pressed to accommodate all its members who required beds. On some mornings the staff resorted to placing patients admitted the previous evening in hallways until a bed could be secured.

A solution seemed to present itself when, in 1970 Dwyer Memorial Hospital, financed and built by the Dwyer lumber family just two years earlier, went up for sale. KP began negotiating the purchase but, just when an agreement seemed imminent, 30 local physicians and a group of community leaders swooped in to purchase the facility and turned it into a nonprofit community hospital—the North Clackamas

Community Hospital (later to be purchased by Sisters of Providence and renamed Providence Milwaukie Hospital). Thus, the promising solution to KP's hospital bed shortage vanished. Now building a second hospital became an urgent priority. In the interim, KP had no choice but to rent hospital beds in local hospitals.

Conditional permits for Kaiser Sunnyside Medical Center had already been obtained for 161 beds and 30 medical offices, but obtaining final permits required a series of hearings. In July 1972 the Oregon Comprehensive Planning Authority granted the Certificate of Need by a narrow margin of 11 to 9, over the objections from the Clackamas County Medical Association, the Physicians Association of Clackamas County (PACC), and two local hospitals, that unsuccessfully appealed the decision.

Construction began in the spring of 1973. Designed by the Zimmer, Gunsul, Frasca Architects, KSMC would be the last KP Hospital to follow Garfield's signature design feature, the encircling outside corridor. Ken Myers was named hospital administrator, Arnold Hurtado, President of the medical staff, and Barbara Robertson, Director of Nursing. The official opening on September 5, 1975 was attended by various county and state officials, as well as by Kaiser Foundation Health Plan President and CEO James Vohs and the venerable Ernest Saward, now associate dean on extramural affairs at the University of Rochester School of Medicine.

The new hospital could not offer emergency services for a full year after its opening, posing a serious problem. Patients routinely arrived at the hospital seeking urgent treatment, reasoning that every hospital has an emergency room. One evening, before the hospital's official opening, an injured man arrived at the brightly lit main entrance where a reception for union officials was taking place in the new lobby. Fortunately, nursing personnel were present to provide interim treatment and to call for ambulance transport to another hospital.

With its pastoral location along two-lane Sunnyside Road, where it nestled in the shadow of heavily wooded Mt. Talbert, KSMC occupied an enviable site. BK loyalists referred to the new hospital as the "country club," suggesting some complicated mix of scorn and envy. Certainly the new hospital seemed worlds apart from its inner-city sister hospital. Its campus was a refuge for wildlife; deer regularly grazed on the grounds, and rabbits, keeping a wary eye for foraging coyotes, scampered about in the grass in the evening. Surgeon Ivan Altman brought his own tractor to plow plots set aside for employees who wished to plant gardens. Lunch-time joggers ran past grazing farm animals; others used the lunch hour to hit golf balls at nearby Top O'Scott Golf Course.

The opening of the Emergency Room coincided with the addition of more medical office construction and with commercial development along Sunnyside Road. In 1978 the 36,000-square foot Mt. Scott office, with offices for 22 physicians, opened on the Sunnyside medical center campus.

Meanwhile commercial development along Sunnyside Road gobbled up large tracts of farmland. In 1981 Clackamas Town Center, a shopping mall that included both a theater and an ice-skating rink, opened across the Interstate-205 freeway. And as freeway traffic and commercial development encroached, KSMC inevitably lost its cachet as the country club.

CALIFORNIA IMPORT

Marvin Goldberg, recruited from San Diego to be Medical Director in 1976, was an unusual appointment. Medical Directors have almost always come from within their own partnership. But The Permanente Clinic took this step because no one within its ranks appeared sufficiently qualified to fill the important leadership position.

Born in Brooklyn and raised in New York City, Goldberg attended Yale University for both undergraduate and medical degrees. Following a pediatric residency at Mt. Sinai Hospital, he enlisted in the Army for a two-year fulfillment of his deferral responsibility. Goldberg investigated the Permanente medical program, remembering that his chief resident had joined SCPMG. Impressed by what he learned, he joined KP's North Hollywood offices where he became Chief of Pediatrics. He then won a three-year appointment as area Medical Director in San Diego.

Goldberg had no illusions that change would be easy in Portland. As he described it, ghosts from the past still hovered. One of these was Saward, still on the Executive Committee though not in attendance at meetings. Goldberg's arrival had an impact from the beginning. Confident and charismatic, Goldberg exuded warmth and charm. He was, everyone agreed, uncanny in his ability to remember names.

At the administrative office at Crown Plaza, near what is now Keller Auditorium, Goldberg quickly obtained a corner office, rejecting the Spartan cubicle formerly occupied by Hughes. Goldberg enjoyed the status of his position but he did not neglect his clinical skills. He wore a standard-issue physician's white coat even in his administrative office and worked a half day each week in the pediatric clinic. As an administrator, he entrusted individuals to perform without close oversight. He eliminated numerous committees and replaced the unpopular centralized appointment center with appointment centers at each of the various clinics.

In 1977 Goldberg asked the still-absent Saward to resign from the Executive Committee to make way for an active committee member-partner. Awaiting a formal response and getting none, he sent his request again—this time in writing. Saward, displeased, sent Goldberg a curt reply in which he chastised the upstart for his "chutzpah." Finally, on March 18, 1977 the Executive Committee terminated

Saward as a partner. Thereafter, though Saward returned to Portland often to visit his beloved research center, he never again returned to The Permanente Clinic.

In 1978 the elusive quest to incorporate was at last achieved; The Permanente Clinic became Northwest Permanente, P.C. Goldberg and Business Manager Jack Fries had learned a great deal from Bill Dung the Medical Director of the Hawaii Permanente Medical Group. Thus, building on the previous work of Vervloet and Zalutsky and on the experience of the HPMG, they prepared their proposal. This time Goldberg met with no resistance from Health Plan to secure pension funds. Goldberg restructured the Medical Group to a more businesslike model and obtained additional benefits for physicians.[7]

It was Goldberg's belief that membership growth was essential to the organization's financial success. And it was he who would oversee the expansion to Salem and Longview-Kelso in the 1980s, and who, together with regional Health Plan Manager Daniel Wagster, would purchase property near the Tanasbourne Mall in Hillsboro for a proposed third hospital complex, to include offices for 50 physicians.

Goldberg was influential, too, in urging Permanente physicians toward active involvement in the local medical community and he himself served on local and state health planning groups. In addition, he sought out Senator Robert Packwood, chairman of the Senate Finance Committee. When the Senator made his monthly visits to Oregon, Goldberg met with him over breakfast where the two discussed health care issues. The relationship would prove advantageous; in 1987, the federal Health Care Financing Administration announced Medicare reimbursement rates for the following year. National reimbursement rates were to increase 13.5%, while those for Oregon were to drop. A subsequent review of calculations requested by Packwood revealed errors, and Oregon received an additional $5.3 million in Medicare payments.

HELP FOR PRIMARY CARE

Family Practitioners: In 1950 Ray Kay, Medical Director of SCPMG, integrated family practice into the multispecialty group in Fontana, California. Neither TPMG in Northern California nor The Permanente Clinic in the Northwest would take this step for more than two decades.

At an Executive Committee meeting in January 1973, pediatrician Peter Hurst suggested the formation of a family practice service. He believed the new department should at first be under the auspices of an already established department. Reaction to Hurst's informal proposal was muted, but representatives from primary care departments—internist John Emery, Chief of Medicine Arnold Hurtado and pediatrician James Powell—established an exploratory family practice committee. Group Health Cooperative in Seattle had begun integrating family practitioners as early as the 1950s. Seeking to learn more about how best to integrate family practice at Permanente, in 1973 the three made a site visit to Group Health, where they saw the significant role played by its family practitioners. In contrast to The Permanente Clinic, which relied exclusively on internists, pediatricians, and obstetricians, Group Health employed 70 family practitioners in primary care.

The committee decided to introduce a family practice program within Permanente, and Jack Emery became Administrative Director. In July 1974, Permanente hired its first family practitioner, Greg Swift, and assigned him to the Beaverton Medical Office.

Like others before him, Swift was attracted to the Northwest after hearing accounts of the Region's beauty. Raised in Michigan, he obtained his MD from Northwestern University, decided on a career in family practice, and became chief resident at Deaconess Hospital in Buffalo, New York. It was there that his interest in the Northwest was piqued by a fellow resident in training, a native Oregonian. But it was more than the beauty of the country that attracted Swift to the West Coast. He was interested in an organized delivery system that included prepayment, and no such program existed in his area. Thus, he applied to both Group Health and to Permanente—two very different programs. Group Health offered a well-established department. Permanente, on the other hand, was dominated by specialists. Swift chose Permanente and, in July 1974 he joined the Beaverton Medical Office. Later that year a second family practitioner, Noel Meyn, joined Swift at Beaverton. Authorization to hire three additional family practitioners followed and, in 1976 Medical Director Goldberg appointed Swift Chair of the new Department of Family Practice.

Family practitioner training includes both adult and pediatric medicine. Most family practitioners expect to see obstetrical patients as well. In 1977 Permanente's Obstetrical and Pediatric Departments declared that family practitioners were not to see patients already established with the two specialty departments. Family practice was free to develop separate pediatric and gynecological practices, but they were to be excluded from obstetrics.

In 1977 Permanente hired family practitioners Donald Herring and Jon Blackman, who were slated to establish a family practice presence at the Division Medical Office in the Sunnyside area. This initial foray into new territory was short-lived, however. A consensus voiced a preference for consolidating the department within the BK area, rather than spreading themselves too thinly at KSMC-area outposts. Thus, in 1978 both Herring and Blackman retreated to the Beaverton Medical Office. Three years later the Region would develop a more defined scope of practice for family practitioners. The continuing story of family practice is discussed in Chapter 18: The Eighties.

Physician Assistants (PAs): There is irony in the fact that graduates of PA programs, designed in the mid-1960s to provide health care in rural communities, would gravitate instead to urban areas. Well intentioned though they were, creators of PA programs might have recognized that graduates would be attracted to urban areas where most medical centers, Medical Group practices, and HMOs are located. By 1986 75% of PAs would work in managed health care systems.

The year was 1961. In response to the shortage of physicians in rural areas, Charles Hudson, President of the National Board of Medical Examiners, proposed assigning experienced military corpsmen as assistants to physicians, thus bolstering the number of health care clinicians in underserved areas. Although the American Medical Association did not act on this suggestion, in 1965 Duke University offered the first PA training program, graduating its first class in 1967. In 1970, Ben Berger, a former Naval hospital corpsman with the Marines in Vietnam, was drawn by an article in *Life Magazine* about the Duke program. He was among those who graduated from the third PA class at Duke in 1970. He was the first to join an HMO when he took a job at Permanente's Vancouver Clinic. Berger was a good fit for his new role with Permanente. The clinic had no on-site surgeon, and Berger's Vietnam experience had given him the skills to suture small wounds and provide care for minor trauma. Impressed, the Medical Group asked Berger to help recruit more PAs. Three others from the Duke program joined Berger: Ron Bean, Charles Dubay, and Michael Fitch.

By 1986, fifteen years after hiring its first PA, NWP relied on the skills of 32 PAs, the majority of whom were assigned to primary care. Others would specialize in orthopedics, minor trauma, rheumatology, diabetic care and gastroenterology. In 2007 more than 80 PAs were employed in 16 departments and subspecialties, the majority working in family practice and in urgency care.

Nurse Practitioners (NPs): Permanente pediatricians trained and began using NPs as early as 1973, but internists did not incorporate these clinicians into their practice until 1975. In the 1970s internists complained that as many as seven appointments each day were given over to physical examinations. To streamline the efficiency of conducting physical exams and thereby relieve internists from these routine, time-intensive tests, Permanente introduced evening clinics at BK where nurses administered various screening tests, measured height and weight, tested vision and hearing, measured blood pressure, and administered a health questionnaire. It was thought that these preliminary tests would provide essential information and thus streamline a patient's annual exam. Unfortunately, physicians reported that these steps did not reduce appointment time.

Chief of Medicine Arnold Hurtado was familiar with a multiphasic program already adopted by other KP Regions, in which a nurse, rather than a physician, performed physical examinations.

The Internal Medicine Department, in cooperation with University of Oregon Medical School, trained six nurses to evaluate and manage patients. In 1975 a small clinic on SE 52nd avenue, previously used by Permanente internists, opened as the Health Appraisal Center. Here NPs conducted the multiphasic testing and the physical examination, making necessary referrals to the physician. The program also evaluated and managed patients for hypertension, diabetes, and obesity. The program was extremely popular with members; they were impressed by the various tests to assess their health and by the time allocated to them with the NP. As the program expanded, the Health Appraisal Center hired more NPs, many from out of state. As NPs came to be seen as more and more indispensable, they matriculated to the primary care medical offices. Today primary care NPs are as numerous in the organization as are PAs.

CHAPTER 18:
THE EIGHTIES:
NEW DIRECTIONS

—⚋—

SOUTH TO SALEM

As early as 1975, Kaiser Permanente members living in Salem, including State employees and union groups, began lobbying for medical services closer to home. KP was slow to act, as initial marketing studies suggested an insufficient pool from which to draw potential Salem-area members. Four years later, in 1979, another feasibility study conducted by family practitioner Greg Swift and administrator Tim Carpenter, was more encouraging. Moreover, leaders calculated political advantages to locating in the state's capital city. Consequently, in January 1980 the organization opened rented offices on Center Street, adjacent to the Salem General Hospital, and established a Salem-area office. Family practitioners Swift and recently trained Peter Jernigan, together with Physician Assistant Carlos Giralt, began seeing patients. Janet Neuburg joined the core group five months later, to be followed by four others during the next two years. Cramped quarters meant sharing office space, two physicians to each office. The pharmacy occupied a closet, and the small laboratory and x-ray rooms were within steps of the patient exam rooms. Giralt remembers that when all clinicians were present some patients in the crowded waiting room were obliged to stand.

KP's entry into the Salem market galvanized the local medical community to form an Independent Provider Association (IPA)[1] called Capital Health Care. This action followed a familiar pattern wherever KP expanded into new territory. Thirty years earlier in 1954, the first IPA was formed by the Medical Society of San Joaquin Valley to compete with the anticipated entry of KP into the Society's area. On the arrival of KP in Salem, Capital Health Care quickly exerted pressure on local specialists to refuse care to KP members. Soon thereafter, local ENT and urology physicians withdrew from a previous contract agreement to attend KP members. In this hostile environment two emergency cases (one ENT, the other urology) required transfer to the Kaiser Sunnyside Medical Center, some 40 miles north, for treatment.

Only when KP complained to the Salem Hospital Board, the Marion-Polk County Medical Society and the Oregon Board of Medical Examiners did local ENT and urology specialists reluctantly agree to provide emergency care for KP members. Then in December, Salem ophthalmologists announced their refusal to see non-emergent KP patients. Local general surgeons followed suit. Northwest Permanente now had no choice but to ask its own urologists, otolaryngologists, and ophthalmologists to make the 40-mile trip to Salem to provide consultations for KP members. Patients requiring surgery had to travel to either Bess Kaiser Hospital or KSMC. Permanente responded to these setbacks as it had always done—by making adjustments and persevering. Permanente surgeon Paul Smith transferred to Salem to care for area members. Thereafter, until additional NWP physicians could be hired in Salem, a core of Portland-based Permanente surgeons provided coverage during Smith's absences and on weekends, relying on overnight quarters in Salem motels. Permanente surgeon David Moiel remembers stays at the Chumaree Inn, sometimes in the presidential suite. His children learned to swim one summer in the motel swimming pool.

Permanente surgeons still remember attacks against them by local area surgeons. At one staff meeting, Moiel was accused of unethical practice for engaging in "itinerant" surgery. One surgeon went so far as to recommend sanction by the American College of Surgeons (no matter that Moiel was not affiliated with that professional group). During this period of relentless attacks, one local surgeon accused his colleagues of hypocrisy, pointing out that they performed itinerant surgery when they worked at the hospital in nearby Silverton. Despite the hostility that surrounded and threatened to swamp the Permanente physicians in Salem, Smith remained remarkably resolute. Not only did he endure, he appeared to enjoy his Salem practice.

In 1980 KP purchased 8 acres in northeast Salem, the site for the first phase of its own medical office in the area. North Lancaster Medical Office opened in 1982 with 14 physician and 2 optometry offices, optical facilities, and the requisite laboratory and pharmacy. The building was unique, featuring a circular design and exterior cladding of 6-by-6 foot Alaska yellow cedar panels. Architects commissioned artist LeRoy Setziol, noted for his carvings at Salishan Resort on the Oregon Coast at Gleneden Beach, to provide the distinctive woodcarving on the panels.

KP continued to attract Salem members: by November 1982 membership had grown to 15,500—a number too substantial to be administered as a satellite from far away KSMC. Greg Swift was appointed the Salem office leader and named physician-in-charge. He reported, not to Sunnyside leaders, but directly to Regional Medical Director Marvin Goldberg.

Throughout 1984 Capital Health Care campaigned actively against KP. One local newspaper quoted the Capital Health Care President: "Kaiser is a super organization ... [but] why cooperate with them? You are just cutting your own throat."

One Salem anesthesiologist went further, warning that KP was like a cancer. "It's very powerful and will eat into the community." Others outside the medical community differed. The Director of the State of Oregon Public Employees Benefit Board rhapsodized, "[Kaiser] is so wonderful ... [and] can manage complete hospital and doctor care for any employee. They have probably done more for cost containment than any other group." For a time, Capital Health Care considered excluding physicians who treated KP patients, backing down only when legal counsel advised that such an action would violate antitrust statutes.

Some local non-Permanente otolaryngologists, ophthalmologists, and orthopedists from nearby Dallas and Albany contracted to see KP patients at the North Lancaster Medical Office but performed surgeries at West Valley Community Hospital 15 miles west in Dallas. Permanente family practitioners incorporated routine obstetrics in their practice, for while some local physicians had finally begun to cooperate with KP, Salem-area obstetricians remained obdurate, treating only those patients at highest risk. Finally, in 1995 NWP hired its first obstetrician, Michael Lewis, for the West Salem Medical Office. Lewis later won a NWP Distinguished Physician Award for patient care.

In 1985, as Salem membership continued to grow, KP completed a second phase of construction at the North Lancaster Medical Office. Michael Krall was appointed Chief for primary care, encompassing family practice, internal medicine and pediatrics. By 1988, 36,000 Health Plan members relied on the North Lancaster Medical Office for their medical care; overcrowding was the inevitable result. Several obstetricians and surgeons relocated to a leased building on Oak Street, within walking distance of Salem Hospital and near the city's center. And that year KP purchased property on the outskirts of suburban Salem, 12 miles southwest of the North Lancaster Medical Office. Two years later, in 1990, the Skyline Medical Office, the southernmost KP facility in Oregon, opened its doors.

WILLIAM DE'AK AND FAMILY PRACTICE

Family practitioner William De'ak figures hugely in two NWP developments in the early part of the 1980s: he better defined the role of family practitioners within primary care, and he led the expansion of NWP into the Longview-Kelso area in southwest Washington. Trained as a pediatrician, De'ak gained adult medicine experience when, working for the National Health Services Corp. in Alaska, he placed physician assistants in remote Alaskan villages. It was during this time that he met David Lawrence, then Director of the MEDEX program at University of Washington. In 1978, preparing to leave Alaska, he contacted Lawrence, now Director of Multnomah County Health Department. Lawrence referred De'ak to Permanente's Regional Medical Director Goldberg. Permanente had no open positions at the time for a pediatrician but did have an opening in its Family Practice Department. So pediatrician-turned-family practitioner De'ak came to Permanente in 1978 and started work at the Vancouver Medical Office.

When in 1980 Greg Swift relocated to the Salem Medical Office, De'ak, a relative newcomer to the organization and to family practice, took over as Department Chief. In his four-year tenure as department leader he would change the role of family practitioners and elevate their status. Nicholas DeMorgan, who joined the department in 1978, remembers competing for resources with internal medicine and struggling to "find a place rather than that of a poor relative." De'ak steered family practitioners toward the outpatient arena, that is, medical office visits, and to urgent care. He recommended that internists with their adult medicine expertise attend the bulk of hospitalized patients. To this end, he changed protocols so that patients seen in urgent care who required hospitalization but who had no designated primary care physician would be assigned to internists. Family practitioners continued to follow their own hospitalized patients.

The second achievement (some would say debacle) for which De'ak is remembered is his responsibility for rolling out the Longview-Kelso program. To understand De'ak's predicament in carrying out his assignment requires a fuller discussion of the Longview-Kelso expansion.

NORTH TO LONGVIEW-KELSO

For some time KP leaders had contemplated moving into the Longview-Kelso area in Washington State, a 40-minute drive from Portland. Health Plan's Regional Manager Daniel Wagster, a graduate of Kelso High School, was familiar with the industries and labor unions in the area and he believed that KP would attract members from that segment. In addition, expansion was the hallmark of the 1980s and there were fears that Group Health might move into the Longview-Kelso area. In 1984 the likely entry of KP into Longview-Kelso spawned considerable interest and enthusiasm. The reaction by the local medical community, however, was predictably negative. One newspaper article recounted the experiences of Salem community physicians after KP entered the Salem market. One Longview physician interpreted the move as another attempt by major employers to control medicine in Longview. Another recalled his grandfather's negative experience some 50 years earlier when Longview Memorial Hospital had provided a prepaid health plan with salaried physicians.

Others, however, eagerly awaited the arrival of KP. One union member, angered by his employer's cuts to his health care benefit, said "Kaiser may be a godsend if … [it] can provide coverage at a good equitable level." And a union official harshly criticized local physicians who boycotted the Monticello Medical Center in Longview, WA, when its leaders met with KP administrators. In general, local industries, including Longview Fiber, Weyerhaeuser and Crown Zellerbach, welcomed KP's entry into Longview-Kelso. At a May 24 news conference in Longview, Area Medical Director Lawrence announced plans to open a medical office staffed by a small cadre of family practitioners. The next day, Blue Cross Cowlitz Medical Service reacted. It announced a Preferred Provider Organization (PPO)[2] called Community Choice Care. And one day later, amid rumors that KP planned to purchase the financially struggling Monticello Community Hospital, the parent company of St. John's Medical Center in Longview announced its intention to buy Monticello. In this atmosphere of rumors and escalating tensions, Lawrence appeared on *Liveline*, a Sunday morning radio program, where he took calls from community residents and tried to dispel rumors.

In 1984 as the organization readied for the expansion into Longview-Kelso, De'ak was appointed physician-in-charge for the northern outpost. He and Ray Dockery, administrator for Health Center East Medical Office, traveled to Longview-Kelso in June of that year to secure the necessary physicians and support staff. De'ak soon found himself in a near-impossible position. He had received assurance from Goldberg of full support from Portland and assumed that some of the physicians would, if necessary, rotate at Longview. The promised support did not materialize. Permanente's Portland Clinical Departments did not believe they could deprive their departments of resources for the Longview expansion. Desperate, De'ak met personally with every physician in Longview with no success. Dockery remembers that by the end of July they were still empty-handed: no physicians, no medical offices. Yet contracts to provide care were set to begin in November, and that date crept inexorably closer.

Under mounting pressure, Dockery supervised the gutting and renovation of the one-story Bell Telephone Company building. At last De'ak negotiated generous (critics would say lavish) contracts with three established local family practitioners and provided in-service education to them about the intricacies of prepaid group medicine. One of these, William Nelson, a private practitioner for ten years, joined saying that he couldn't turn down the offer of a higher income, generous pension and health care plans, and the option to continue to see his existing patients on a fee-for-service basis. (Most of Nelson's patients would, however, decide to join KP.) As was the case in Salem, specialty care from community physicians was difficult to obtain. But whereas Permanente physicians in Salem covered routine obstetrics, NWP obtained an exclusive contract with outside obstetricians in Longview-Kelso. As well, the organization contracted with general surgical, orthopedic, ENT, internal medicine, pediatric, anesthesiology, and radiology groups. Many of these contracts still exist.

KP opened its doors to Longview members in November 1984, having turned the former office building on Ninth Avenue into a serviceable medical office. By the end of that month, clinicians there had provided care to nearly 90 patients. By the time Permanente hired family practitioner Frank Eigner in 1985, Longview already had a busy department of six other family practitioners and a nurse practitioner. Family practitioner David Westrup joined the department the following year. KP had not foreseen its rapid membership growth in the Longview-Kelso area having projected a five-year growth of only 9,500. Instead, after just two years, membership was 14,000, nearly 50% over projections and straining the capacity of its single medical office. The organization quickly leased another building on Delaware Avenue near St. John's Medical Center for physical therapy, optometry, optical care and mental health services. Four-year Air Force Veteran Joseph Davis joined Permanente in 1986, and the following year he took over the struggling work-injury medical program. By visiting local sawmills, paper mills and other work places, Davis began to build effective relationships with local industries, and the program steadily expanded.

The year 1986 saw NWP's Longview program over budget by $3 million—the amount that Permanente was paying to contracted non-Permanente physicians. A delicate renegotiating process took place in which NWP secured more favorable contract terms with local physicians and assured them of its interest in maintaining long-term relationships. At the same time, Permanente decided to internalize Departments of Ophthalmology and Allergy.

Some in the organization blamed De'ak for his part in the budget problems of Longview-Kelso. By his own account, he increasingly felt himself a pariah by his Permanente peers. He later resigned from Permanente—and for a time from medicine—and moved to Hawaii to start a bed and breakfast. (In 1992 De'ak resumed his Permanente career, but far from the Northwest, as Area Medical Director for the Carolina Permanente Medical Group in North Carolina.) Davis replaced De'ak and he was immediately drawn into planning for a new medical office. In 1989, a 43,000 square-foot medical office opened on 20 acres 1 mile east of the interstate freeway. The modular structure was designed to incorporate expansion. Member growth in Longview continued to race ahead of projections, requiring additions to the medical center in 1994, 1996, and 1997.

FAMILY PRACTICE DEVELOPMENTS

The Department of Family Practice, well established in the BK area, was slow to gain acceptance in the KSMC area. Family practitioners Donald Herring and Jon Blackman set up practice for just one year at Division Medical Office before returning to the BK area and to a consolidated department. Then, in 1980, Arnold Hurtado, Area Medical Director at KSMC, asked Blackman to help plan the future Rockwood Medical Office in east Portland. In addition, he asked Blackman to develop a family practice model, both for Rockwood and for the Sunnyside area, and to become Chief of the new department. In Blackman's experience, the KSMC area, with its reliance on internists, was not receptive to family practitioners. Despite this reservation, he put forth his proposal to the Department Chiefs. Gratified when, in 1981, the KSMC Chiefs accepted the proposal, Blackman took a prolonged vacation. On his return, he was dismayed to learn that plans for the Rockwood Medical Office had been cancelled because of budget problems. The cancellation meant that the family practice presence in the Sunnyside area had been scuttled as well. Blackman recalls that he sought answers to his questions about the status of Rockwood, as well as assurances regarding his professional future. Despite his best efforts, he got no satisfactory answers. Discouraged, Blackman resigned from Permanente and established a private practice in Beaverton.

In the BK area, Thomas Syltebo succeeded De'ak as Department Chief in 1984 and held the position until his promotion in 1989 to Area Medical Director. During this time family practice was asked to accept more adult medicine patients and to decrease its pediatric role. Permanente saw as advantageous the flexibility of family practice to handle minor injuries, a role with which internists had minimal experience. In 1989 the organization opened the Cascade Park Medical Office in suburban Vancouver; family practice versatility would be a major factor in the success of the facility.

That year KSMC hired its first family practitioner since the departures of Blackman and Herring. William Nyone took up a solitary post at the Rockwood Medical Office and began building a panel of patients. Nyone says that though he regretted that his scope of practice would not include obstetrics, he didn't hesitate to accept the job offer. And for the next six years he remained the sole family practitioner in the KSMC area. Then when the Rockwood Urgency Care Clinic disbanded, those physicians joined Nyone in the Family Practice Department. Today the Region's 105 family practitioners outnumber internists, and they have a strong voice, exerting influence on the Board of Directors and in various administrative posts throughout the organization.

FRIENDS TO THE NORTH

The physicians at Seattle's Group Health were in some ways like cousins, though their staff model differed from Permanente's group model. Permanente's John Thompson, whose brother Robert headed Group Health's Preventive Care Program, said, "When my brother and I compare notes, it is like putting on a comfortable shoe. I consider ... Group Health ... a sister organization." And just as the decade of the 80s ushered in an era of change and expansion for Permanente, so it did for Group Health.

Group Health had hired Don Brennan, its first non-physician Executive Director, in 1976. During his tenure, Brennan asserted himself more forcefully than his predecessor had in dealing with both the Medical Group and its administrative staff—a role that some on the board of trustees resented. Under Brennan's leadership, co-op membership dwindled to just 29% of the total health plan membership. To counteract the trend of increasing non co-op members in 1978, the board adopted a three-year, slow-growth policy restricting annual enrollment to 10,000.[3]

After Brennan's retirement in 1980, the Group Health Board waited nearly a year to name his replacement, Gail Warden, former Vice President and CEO at Rush Presbyterian St. Luke Medical Center in Chicago. In agreeing to accept the Group Health job, Warden asked for and got the title CEO and President. He was also given authority to hire and dismiss administrative personnel. Warden warned of two particularly ominous perils to Group Health. First, national and local recessions threatened government payrolls. Second, an aging population, heavy users of medical services, posed a significant drain on resources. Accordingly he proposed to the Board a strategic plan to deal with these externals. And soon thereafter he made several difficult business decisions, mandating a change to the dues structure to include experience, rather than community rating,[4] as well as co-payments for drugs and office visits. In these and other changes, Warden was proceeding down the path toward a corporate business model and away from Group Health's social mission. That year the administrative personnel moved to spacious quarters in an office complex overlooking Elliott Bay, thus geographically distancing themselves from clinicians and health care staff.

In 1982 Group Health physicians were unable to agree on a Medical Director from within their ranks. (Part of the difficulty lay in the decentralization of the Medical Group. During the previous 5 years a restructuring of the 300-member Medical Group had resulted in 3 separate service areas, each with its own Executive Committee and Chief of staff.) At last they selected an outsider, Turner Bledsoe, formerly Associate Dean at Johns Hopkins University and Vice President for health affairs at the Maine Medical Center. That year Warden appointed Phil Nudelman Chief Operating Officer. NWP would hear from Nudelman in 1990.

In 1982 the Insurance Companies of North America, renamed CIGNA later that year, offered for sale their 20,000-member HMO in Spokane, Washington. At first Group Health showed little interest but in January 1983, despite the fact that the Spokane-based HMO lacked a hospital and specialists, Group Health made the purchase, renaming it Group Health of Spokane. Unlike its parent, Group Health of Spokane was not organized as a consumer cooperative, but rather as a nonprofit corporation owned by Group Health. The Seattle-based parent company did, however, allow consumer participation by its Spokane subsidiary. In 1986, a new branch, Group Health of Washington, formed to provide service to Yakima and the tri-cities areas. Trouble arose almost immediately when activities by some of its members. The Nuclear Awareness Group (NAG) began to interfere with marketing and enrollment in the tri-cities, which included employees of the Hanford nuclear complex. NAG placed antinuclear literature in all Group Health facilities including those in Richland, Washington, which angered residents, many of whom depended on their jobs in nuclear weapons research and production. After a heated membership meeting, the Board suspended the privileges of NAG.

Under Warden's leadership, despite turbulence in the health care marketplace and distractions by the Board on social issues, Group Health extended its geographical coverage and added new facilities. Among these were the new Rainier Medical Center in a South Seattle neighborhood, The Silverado Medical Center on Kitsap Peninsula, a medical center in South Tacoma, and another on Bainbridge Island. In Bellingham, 80 miles north of Seattle, local physicians contracted to care for Group Health members.

In 1987 a disgruntled Board rejected Warden's operations budget, and the physicians declared their lack of confidence in Bledsoe. The previous year had been a difficult one, marked by a hiring freeze, an increased patient load for physicians and difficulties negotiating the 1987 contract with Group Health. The physicians refused to renew Bledsoe's contract and, in October, Warden resigned.

It was time for Group Health to return to its cultural roots as a cooperative. The administrative office moved to the former *Seattle Post-Intelligencer* building, where the traditional cooperative culture reclaimed Warden's corporate one. Group Health veteran Aubrey Davis[5] was tapped to be the new President and CEO.

NUCLEAR MAGNETIC RESONANCE TOMOGRAPHY

The 1980s saw a rush by Portland radiologists to acquire Magnetic Resonance Imaging (MRI) units. In December 1984 alone, the state received six applications for MRIs; in addition three MRI units were already under construction. Radiologist Ben Brown presented a request to the Executive Committee for an MRI unit, calculating its cost recovery to be no more than three years. Still, KP took no immediate action to acquire an MRI, content for the time being to rely on community services. At first KP routinely referred patients to one of two sites, usually based on the distance from the patient's home to the test site. When one of these, Northwest Magnetic Imaging, was found to be superior in quality and service, KP relied almost exclusively on that service, where it developed an excellent working relationship with its Director, radiologist O.D. Haugen.[6] Haugen welcomed Permanente radiologists to regularly attend their patients during exams at his imaging facility.

Despite this satisfactory working arrangement at an outside facility, it was just a matter of time before KP purchased its own MRI unit. And in 1989 the first MRI unit was installed at KSMC. Almost immediately, scheduled MRIs jammed the appointment schedule, weekdays from 8:00am to 5:00pm. High demand soon led to expanded evening hours and then to weekends. Even so, organization leaders saw that a single MRI unit was woefully inadequate to meet demand. A second unit was followed by a third. A fourth MRI installed in 2005 at the Salmon Creek Medical Office has a unique open design to accommodate severely obese and claustrophobic patients. In recent years, two additional MRIs have been installed: a mobile unit based at KSMC and another based in Salem.

ALLERGY AND AIDS

The decade of the 1980s is associated, especially for immunologists, with the acquired immune deficiency syndrome epidemic. Allergist Robert Lawrence, who had trained in pediatrics, allergy, and immunology, joined Permanente one year before the first reported cases of the unusual syndrome that was affecting homosexual men. Little did Lawrence realize that these and a growing number of other cases would dramatically affect his career or that he would play a prominent role in managing the frightening scourge, later discovered to be of infectious origin.

NWP's first allergist was Donald Tatum, hired in 1967. Until that year, pediatricians and internists had overseen care for patients with allergies. Tatum received his allergy and immunology training at the National Jewish Medical and Research Center in Denver, Colorado, and practiced in Fairbanks, Alaska, and in Portland before coming to Permanente. Registered Nurse Darlene Fortuny was assigned to assist him. Together they organized an allergy service. Their quarters were in the basement of the 35-year-old Weidler House next to the Broadway Clinic in Northeast Portland. They were rewarded for their work in this inauspicious setting when they were included in the planning for an allergy suite at the new Health Center West Medical Office. Opening in 1971, the allergy suite was equipped with injection rooms and equipment to mix solutions. Its effective operation suffered a blow however, when Tatum, vacationing at Lake Tahoe in 1972, collapsed and died of a heart attack. He was just 49.

Fortunately, Permanente got help from local allergist Michael Noonan who was building a private practice at the Metropolitan Clinic in Northeast Portland. Noonan provided both part-time and full-time service to Permanente's Allergy Department for the ensuing four years. Permanente pediatrician Earl Pierce and pulmonologist Charles Pinney trained with The Permanente Medical Group in San Francisco under Ben Feingold, and returned to staff the Portland-area allergy clinic. Microbiologist Arthur Fritsch from the Oregon Medical School helped out on a part-time basis.

In 1977 Permanente hired two allergists: Kuo Chang[7] and Raymond Brady, and the Allergy Department again moved, this time to the vacated Broadway Clinic. Brady grew restless and left after a short time but then, in 1980, Lawrence joined the small department. Again the Allergy Department moved—this time to the newly constructed Health Center East Medical Office, where it settled into permanent quarters. Chang provided consultations in Salem until pediatric allergist Jean Carney joined the Salem staff.

In 1981 the first U.S. cases of opportunistic infections in homosexual men were reported together with cases of an unusual skin malignancy called Kaposi's sarcoma. These cases associated with an unidentified wasting disease and characterized by a lack of T helper cells in the blood, qualified the disease as an immune deficiency disorder. In 1982 the disorder was given a name: acquired immune deficiency syndrome (AIDS). Physicians across the nation observed with alarm the increasing numbers of case reports. Lawrence, recently trained as an immunologist, sent a memo to his Area Medical Director suggesting some early planning to deal with the growing number of cases, not only in homosexuals, but in heterosexuals, hemophiliacs, recipients of blood transfusions, and IV-drug users. The first case of AIDS in Oregon appeared in 1982. One year later KP Northwest identified its first case, though it is likely that there were earlier, undiagnosed cases.

The public reaction to what some called a "gay plague" was fear and rejection of those afflicted, both adults and children. Even health care professionals expressed reluctance to work with these patients. Lawrence reacted by co-chairing, together with administrator Marna Flaherty-Robb, a regional AIDS multidisciplinary task force of 40 representing nursing, pharmacy, social services, mental health, laboratory services and hospital infection control. Under the leadership of Judi Brenes, an AIDS Education and Prevention Subcommittee educated staff and Health Plan members on how the disease was spread and how to minimize risk. Mental health therapist Jeanne Monahan and social worker Phyllis Heims devoted much of their time to afflicted patients.

In 1986 an immune deficiency clinic opened at Health Center East with Lawrence as Director. Lawrence found his life becoming consumed by an unforgiving work schedule, centered mostly on AIDS cases. In addition to his clinic practice, he lectured across the nation and served on both an interregional and an Oregon AIDS task force. Infectious disease specialist Keith Riley joined Lawrence in 1989, and they shared the clinical workload, each devoting half time to AIDS. Diana Antoniskis joined the two in 1991. The daily occurrence of death and dying might have taken a heavier toll on staff had it not been for the camaraderie and frequent group meetings within the department from which all members derived support.

The discovery of effective drugs helped turn AIDS into a chronic disorder and the toll of daily deaths subsided. In 2005 Lawrence returned to a full-time practice in allergy and immunology; he no longer sees AIDS patients. And 27 years after the appearance of AIDS, 5 infectious disease specialists and internists, together with a staff of 20 including nurses, pharmacists, and social workers, attend the immune deficiency clinic at East Interstate Medical Office.

KSMC OBSTETRICAL DEPARTMENT CONFLICTS

When, in 1975, the Ob/Gyn Department established offices at the new KSMC, Area Medical Director Hurtado appointed Milton Lee as Chief of Gynecology for the KSMC area. Lee was popular and had a strong personality. Although he was ostensibly to report to Regional Chief Sheldon Spielman, he quickly asserted his independence, scheduling KSMC department meetings at the same time as regional department meetings. No longer willing to ignore Lee's behavior, Spielman restricted his responsibilities. Disinclined to accept this apparent rebuke, Lee resigned from the Medical Group.

Department Chief Spielman continued to argue that all obstetrics services should be centralized in the BK area. Richard Wong succeeded Lee as Area Department Chief and, ignoring Spielman's arguments, began to work closely with Area Medical Director Bowne to plan OB services at KSMC. (Bowne had by then replaced Arnold Hurtado as Area Medical Director.) By 1980 planning was well under way for a second hospital wing to include a labor, delivery, and nursery unit. KSMC obstetricians, although supportive of an obstetric service at the hospital, believed they had not been fully brought into the decision-making and planning process. John Linman was appointed to replace Wong. Linman worked with pediatrician Klevit and RN Lynn Didlick to oversee the 1984 opening of the KSMC obstetrical and neonatal service. The physical space included six birthing rooms, two labor rooms, three delivery suites, and a four-bed recovery room.

When BK closed its doors in 1999, KP contracted with Providence St. Vincent Hospital and, for a time, Legacy Emanuel Hospital to provide obstetric services for BK members. KSMC continued its robust obstetrical service for area residents.

LEADERSHIP CHANGES

In 1981, after five years as Area Medical Director at BK, Robert Senft was ready to step down. His replacement was David Lawrence, whose hiring can be traced to a dinner party and a serendipitous encounter some years earlier. At that gathering hosted by family practitioner De'ak, the Goldbergs and the Lawrences met. Seated beside Lawrence, Sarah Goldberg disclosed that, nearing completion of an MBA, she was eager to find a job. At the time Lawrence oversaw the Multnomah County Health Department, and he offered her an administrative post. Subsequently, the Goldbergs and Lawrences became close friends. It was this earlier connection between the two men that led Goldberg to select Lawrence as Senft's replacement. And it was at another dinner—this time at Goldberg's Black Butte home, that Goldberg offered the Permanente position to Lawrence.

Lawrence's previous experience had been heavily weighted toward administrative rather than clinical roles. He had joined the public health service after his medical internship and had had Peace Corps assignments in the Dominican Republic, Washington, DC, and Chile. Obtaining a Master of Public Health at University of Washington, he went on to head the MEDEX physician assistant program for five more years. Returning to Portland, he was hired as Medical Director of the Multnomah County Health Department before heading the Department of Human Resources in Multnomah County.

Given Lawrence's administrative background, and the fact that he came from outside KP, no one should have been surprised that Lawrence was to find the position of Area Medical Director challenging. From the first, he experienced conflict with physicians, most notably with the Obstetrics Department. He did, however, enjoy the support of two primary care chiefs: James Brodhacker, in internal medicine and Fred Nomura, in pediatrics. And he had an amicable relationship with his fellow Area Medical Director at KSMC, Hurtado.

In 1982, Goldberg made additional changes to his administrative team, deposing 25-year Permanente veteran Hurtado from his post as KSMC Medical Director. This time Goldberg would appoint someone from within the ranks of Permanente and, in fact, he had already determined on his choice to succeed Hurtado: Bowne from the SCPMG. Bowne had been Chief of Surgery at San Diego and physician-in-charge at the Kaiser Foundation Hospital in El Cajon. Goldberg's decision to devise a means to recruit Bowne with a more generous salary inducement almost certainly contributed to his undoing at NWP and his 1985 resignation. In 1985 the Colorado Region underwent administrative changes with the appointment of a new Medical Director and a search for a new Health Plan manager. CEO and President of Kaiser Foundation Health Plan James Vohs surprised Lawrence by offering him the position, and in March 1985 Lawrence moved to Denver. Now on the Health Plan administrative team, his long suit, he flourished; before long he was given the position of Regional Manager for KP's huge Northern California Region. In 1992 he would become Chairman and CEO of the programwide Kaiser Foundation Health Plan.

With Lawrence's departure in 1985 from the Northwest Region, Potts succeeded him as Medical Director for the BK area. His confirmation by the Board of Directors in March started a chain of events that sparked a controversy, one with dramatic consequences. It began with some on the Board who objected to the process by which Potts had been appointed. They asked for a review of the by-laws and, at a special Board meeting on April 15, some members called into question Goldberg's leadership. Another meeting followed three days later at the Salishan Resort on the Oregon Coast, this time with a facilitator. When Pott's salary was disclosed, the Board learned for the first time that the administrative team received physician base pay for the four-and-a half-day work week plus 11% more for the additional half day of an administrator's five-day week. They discovered as well that administrators awarded themselves compensatory time off for work after hours, often in cash. In the ensuing two months Goldberg received considerable criticism from Board members, but he continued to enjoy support, even popularity, among some physicians. In the end, Goldberg said he could not remain in his leadership post without unanimous support from the Board. He submitted his resignation July 18, 1985 to take effect August 23rd.

THE QUIET PEDIATRICIAN

Goldberg's announcement to resign as Regional Medical Director in the middle of his term posed a problem for the Permanente Board of Directors: any interim stand-in, Board members reasoned, would receive an unfair advantage over others who might seek the leadership position. The two Area Medical Directors, Potts and Bowne, were asked to share the role until a permanent leader could be

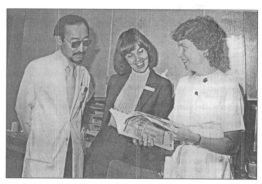

Fred Nomura (left) and Barbe West (center) at the Beaverton Clinic, 1984. Nomura was the Northwest Permanente Director, 1985-1992; West was the Kaiser Permanente Regional President, 1997-2001.
Courtesy of Kaiser Permanente Heritage Resources.

chosen. But another problem lay beneath the surface. Permanente leaders, both locally and in Oakland, lacked confidence in Bowne, who clearly coveted the position. Quietly, the Board sounded out Nomura about his willingness to stand for the position. Nomura was reticent, lacking the enthusiasm to become a career administrator. Nevertheless, he reluctantly agreed to finish Goldberg's term, but he made clear his intention to serve only a single three-year term thereafter and then return to his pediatric practice.

Nomura's personal story is that of thousands of other Japanese Americans living on the West Coast who were viewed with suspicion after the Japanese attack on December 7, 1941. Nomura was just four years old when, in April 1941, President Roosevelt signed Executive Order 9066, decreeing that 110,000 Japanese

Americans were to pack what belongings they could carry and leave their homes within two days. Nomura, his parents, and three brothers were bussed from their Seattle home to a holding facility at the state fairgrounds in Puyallup, 30 miles south of Seattle. The hastily arranged shelters were horse barns whose stalls were converted to bunks. After three months the Nomura family endured another forced move, this time by train to a newly constructed relocation camp at Minidoka in the Idaho desert, 18 miles from Twin Falls.

Nomura recalls that despite the traumatic displacement of his family, his young age offered a kind of protection against the psychological scarring that others suffered as a result of internment. Rather, he remembers far more acutely the temperature extremes, the bitter cold of the winters, the intense heat of the summers, and the inadequate thin plank walls of the barracks, the outdoor plumbing, the communal mess halls, and the ever-present barbed wire.

Released after two and a half years, Nomura's family eventually returned to Seattle. Scholarships enabled Nomura to attain higher education. He graduated from the University of Washington Medical School and served a pediatric residency at Tripler Army Medical Center in Honolulu, Hawaii. One cannot escape the irony that the man once classified as an enemy alien by the U.S. was now assigned to a U.S. military base and at the very site of a Japanese attack just two decades earlier.

In 1968, Nomura joined Permanente. Quiet, soft spoken, reserved, and focused, Nomura proved to be politically adroit. When, in 1973, Hurst stepped down as pediatric Chief, Nomura prevailed over Klevit to replace Hurst. Then, after a three-year term as Chief, he served another eight years, from 1976 to 1984, as physician-in-charge at the Beaverton Medical Office where he and his Health Plan counterpart Barbe West created a partnership that was described as a model of cooperative management.

In his first year as Regional Medical Director, Nomura faced the inevitable problems, both internal and external. His two priorities were to reorganize the administrative team and to solidify the partnership with Health Plan. In addition to replacing Permanente Business Manager Mark Knudsen with Mary Liberator, he created the new positions of Assistant Regional Medical Director and appointed James Brodhacker and Klevit to those posts. He retained both Bowne and Potts as Area Medical Directors. But Bowne, who believed himself to be the appropriate heir to Goldberg, had been stung by his rejection from the Medical Group. He began to interfere with Nomura's agenda. When finally Nomura removed him as Area Medical Director, Bowne refused to step down as a Board member and stubbornly continued to attend Board meetings.

Added to these internal vexations, Nomura confronted a tough financial year in

1986; both membership growth and revenue fell below forecast, and the region faced a troubling increase in expense. Unexpected accruals for 1985 had to be paid in 1986, and Longview-Kelso expenses were out of control. And as if these headaches weren't sufficient, Permanente was finding physician recruitment difficult. Predictably, access to services suffered, forcing the organization to rely on costly outside referrals and adding still further to unanticipated costs.

Inevitably, financial reversals led to a crisis. NWP and Health Plan each faced a deficit of $3.5 million. Under the risk-sharing agreement between Health Plan and Permanente, Health Plan assumed most of Permanente's deficit. But the organization still faced a net loss of $1.1 million without sufficient reserves to pay it. Nomura and Katcher developed a plan to deal with the dilemma. Health Plan was to give Permanente additional funds to reduce its deficit, a portion of which was to be made up in 1987 by reducing physician salaries. In turn, Permanente would help Health Plan reach its financial goals and, if they were met, the salary reductions were to be returned to the physicians in 1988. Happily, 1987 was a remarkable financial success. Service improved, and the Region recruited physicians. That year, Health Plan reached its highest enrollment since 1945, gaining 19,383 new subscribers. It also reported its highest-to-date earnings, with income of $12 million. But the success of 1987 was the calm before the storm.

THE NURSES' STRIKE

On July 6, 1988, the Oregon Nurses Association (ONA), the Oregon Federation of Nurses (OFN) and the union Local 49, representing medical assistants and other support staff, went on strike. This unprecedented work stoppage by KP nurses would last two months and create bitterness never before seen in the organization. The major issue was over health care benefits. Health Plan requested that part-time workers pay a portion of their health care benefits as well as co-payments for office visits and laboratory tests. (Six months earlier Health Plan had reached an agreement with 180 radiology clerks and technicians that called for part-time workers to pay a higher service fee.) Though Permanente and Health Plan had braced for a nursing strike, no one anticipated the stand-off to last more than one month.

The NWP administrative team supported Health Plan leaders, but members of the Permanente Board, as well as members of the rank and file in the physician group, were divided in their sympathies. Dissenters openly criticized management and some physicians went so far as to join the picket lines in support of their nursing colleagues. KSMC was forced to close its inpatient nursing units but continued to staff outpatient and Urgent Care Departments. BK continued to staff 30 inpatient beds, its labor and delivery service, and the Emergency Department. Nursing supervisors assumed the work of staff nurses, shouldering 12-hour shifts. KP

Regions in other states as well as Group Health sent experienced nursing supervisors who crossed the picket line under the protection of security guards. Most local hospitals agreed to accept KP patients. The exception was Southwest Washington Medical Center in Vancouver. Its refusal to open its doors to KP physicians and patients created a cool relationship that lingers even today.

The two Area Medical Directors were relatively new to their leadership roles. Allan Weiland had recently replaced Potts at BK when Potts left to become Medical Director in Ohio, and Seth Garber had succeeded Bowne at KSMC. The two nevertheless coordinated physician assignments at outside hospitals. Surgical specialists received staff privileges at six Portland hospitals. Internists at BK followed members at Providence Good Samaritan and Providence St. Vincent hospitals; those at KSMC attended patients at Portland Adventist and Woodland Park hospitals, which also accepted overflow obstetrics patients. High-risk obstetrical patients were admitted to Oregon Health and Science University. Administrators implemented an emergency operations group that met every day at 7:30 am to debrief and plan. Staff physicians, however, were not nearly so well informed. Those who remember the time recall knowing little about the progress toward a settlement. Like the general public, they depended for their news on the daily news reports in *The Oregonian*.

Permanente physicians reported that throughout the nursing strike, community hospitals were cooperative and sympathetic, and they were given a respect sometimes lacking at their home hospitals. And while the strike took an emotional toll on nurses, the economic impact was not so significant as it might have been for, because of a general nursing shortage in Portland and the surrounding metro area, KP nurses easily found temporary work in community hospitals, sometimes, ironically, caring for KP patients. The conclusion of the strike saw nurses agreeing to some minor rollbacks. No clear winners emerged from the bruising, exhausting experience. On the other hand, there was no reported instance of poor care to patients.

Although Nomura intended to resign at the end of his term in December 1988, the Board entreated him to remain for another term. The Region had been through a traumatic experience, and the organization's leaders recognized the imperative to address the conflicts that had led to the strike and to begin a healing process. Nomura pursued a discretionary course, working quietly with Health Plan managers and nurses to address issues and resolve conflicts, determined that the Region would never again find itself on the brink of a strike.

In the first post-strike year, 1989, Nomura oversaw several significant changes. After Permanente Business Manager Mary Liberator resigned, Harry Stathos replaced her and continues in that position in 2010. Nomura increased physician benefits, adding an extra week of vacation after 12 years of service. Two years later, he implemented another benefit: the Rule of 80, a provision of the Permanente

Physicians Retirement Plan. The Rule of 80 allows a participant to retire at an age younger than 60 and, if at retirement age plus service equal or exceed 80, receive an unreduced benefit by deferring payment to age 60. Nomura and Katcher continued their successful partnership through the end of Nomura's term as the Region's Medical Director.

COMPETITION

The 1980s saw numerous relatively new and struggling health plans in the area merge and affiliate.[8] One of these organizations however was not new, having originated a half century earlier. In 1988 Physicians Association of Clackamas County (PACC) adopted a more corporate model under its assertive new CEO, Lawrence Filosa.[9] Not all physicians welcomed the new model, resulting in a split between those who supported and those who opposed the change. The Clackamas County Medical Society distanced itself from PACC and no longer used its office facilities. Other changes followed including expansion by PACC to Multnomah, Washington, and Clark counties. In 1994 a proposed merger with Medford-based Health Future to cover 16 Oregon communities came to nothing. That same year Filosa was replaced by Martin Preizler from Wisconsin, who inherited a situation whereby more capital was needed for PACC to upgrade its information system and expand its product line or be overtaken by larger and better-financed competitors. In 1995 responding to growing physician complaints, retired Permanente pediatrician Klevit, then Medical Director for the Oregon Board of Medical Examiners, became PACC Vice President for Medical Affairs.[10] Then in 1997 PACC was bought out by the parent company of QualMed, signaling the demise of PACC. The pioneering physician-sponsored plan was lost forever, its profits to be applied to fund the nonprofit Northwest Health Foundation whose stated mission was to "advance support and provide for the health of the people of Oregon and Southwest Washington." (In 2004 the KP Community Fund[11] contributed $26 million to support the Northwest Health Foundation.)

CHAPTER 19:
THE NINETIES

—ᶆ—

By Allan J. Weiland, MD

BECOMING THE DEVIL

In the early 1990s health care costs posed one of the top problems for American industry, emerging as a major issue in the 1992 presidential campaign. With its 45-year history, Kaiser Permanente was by then well established as an integrated delivery system, providing cost-effective care for its members. Its Medical Group comprised salaried physicians—one of the only capitated Medical Groups in the area. Because of its renegade roots and its slow acceptance by the community, the Kaiser Permanente Northwest program remained within the walls of its two hospitals—Bess Kaiser Hospital and Kaiser Sunnyside Medical Center—except for small outposts in Longview, Washington, and Salem, Oregon. In those communities, KP had established medical offices but contracted with local community hospitals for inpatient care.

Fred Nomura, approaching the end of his second full term as Regional Medical Director, decided not to seek reelection. The Board began a search for Nomura's successor in June 1992, its focus on the two Area Medical Directors: Seth Garber at KSMC and Allan Weiland (the author of this chapter) at BK. Weiland won the October election and assumed his new position as Regional Medical Director in January 1993. Garber resigned as Medical Director of KSMC in March to become Regional Medical Director of the Texas Region. Thus, a turnover of the Medical Group leadership took place almost simultaneously.

In the late fall of 1993, newly elected President Bill Clinton with his wife Hillary introduced a sweeping proposal

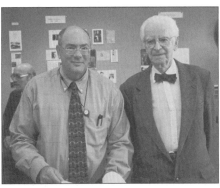

Allan Weiland and Charles Grossman, 2004. Weiland was Northwest Permanente Medical Director, 1993-2004; Grossman was an original Permanente Clinic partner in 1949. *From the author's collection.*

to overhaul America's health care system. Embracing Alain Enthoven's "managed competition" philosophy, the proposal—an enormous, unreadable tome—was put forth without collaboration with industry stakeholders, a fatal miscalculation by its proponents. Weiland and Phillip Nudelman from Group Health Coopera- tive in Seattle attended the formal unveiling of the plan on the south lawn of the White House.

Though never adopted, the Clinton health care plan nevertheless called the na- tion's attention to the financing of health care and endorsed a managed care model as the answer to rising costs. Consequently, during the next several years, existing health plans, as well as a number of newcomers, underwent swift transformations to "managed care." Portland was no exception. Area Health Maintenance Organi- zations proliferated almost overnight. The local Blue Cross plan converted its tradi- tional indemnity business to a managed-care model, instantly becoming the largest HMO in the area. Suddenly the entire nature of competition changed. KP, previ- ously viewed as just different from (and inherently inferior to) plans that offered unlimited physician choice, was suddenly cast as the old way to provide managed care. Almost every Medical Group became capitated, at least to some extent. Sev- eral affiliated with national practice management companies such as PhyCor and MedPartners and signed long-term management leases to acquire capital. These companies then swiftly introduced new managed-care practices to control costs. Primary care physicians became gatekeepers and were given strict limitations on referrals to specialists. Draconian programs required pre-authorization for every treatment, including emergency hospitalization, and for every test. Most insurers installed 1-800 numbers, requiring physicians to phone call-center staff for per- mission to order tests, medications, and referrals. Some plans implemented gag rules, prohibiting physicians from disclosing financial arrangements they had with a payer. Health plans aggregated claims information to determine which physicians were most prolific in generating billings. Those found lagging were dropped from the network. This practice—called economic credentialing—was at first crude, in that it failed to adjust for severity of illness within a practice.

These cost-cutting practices did reduce the upward trending costs of health care in the mid-1990s, but not by truly managing care more effectively. Instead, cost savings were more often the result of frequent denials of appropriate care, significant delays in treatment, and substantial underpayment for physician services. So prevalent were the stories about cost-cutting by HMOs that they became a staple in the anecdotes of late-night talk-show hosts and other venues of popular culture. The movie *As Good As It Gets* lambasted "damn HMOs," drawing spontaneous cheers and whistles from those in the audiences and capturing the public's mood against managed care.

With its long history as an HMO, KP was a highly visible presence. And although it never engaged in the egregious measures of other insurance companies, it was nevertheless tarred by the same brush, predictably becoming the target of bad press. The organization's leaders, recognizing the now pejorative connotation of "managed care," considered describing the program a new way. In the end, however, no one could think of a better term to characterize the KP mission.

But, whereas KP was far different from the newcomer HMOs, some of its bad press was deserved. Its level of service and access to care, for example, fell short of the community standard, which offered open access to specialists. Not surprisingly, given its service and access reputation, KPNW saw no membership growth between 1990 and 1993.

Meanwhile, KP at the national level was undergoing a series of changes under David Lawrence, MD, CEO of Kaiser Foundation Health and Hospitals since 1991. Although Lawrence had initially enjoyed the support of the 12 Medical Directors, within a short time he grew frustrated with their unwillingness to relinquish autonomy and their reluctance to embrace strategic change. In response, Lawrence disbanded the KaiPerm Committee, a national forum where Medical Directors regularly met with Regional Managers and Program Office leaders to discuss organizational issues. Furthermore, he stopped including regional leaders at Health Plan Board meetings. Lawrence asserted that the program would have to double in size to compete with the largest health plans in a rapidly consolidating marketplace. He questioned whether Health Plan's exclusive relationship with each of the Permanente Medical Groups could support the required growth.

To lead a strategic expansion initiative, Lawrence brought in outside expert James Williams and engaged management consultants McKinsey and Company to help redesign the organization. Each Region was charged with preparing a strategic assessment as well as a plan to achieve substantial growth in its marketplace. A team from McKinsey duly descended on Portland in late 1993 and began the assessment process, examining the marketplace, the organization's cost structure, its reputation, and its results. This comprehensive assessment set the stage for a number of dramatic decisions, some local, some national, that would have a huge impact on the Northwest Region and its physicians for years to come.

In addition to his emphasis on membership growth, Lawrence complained to the regional Executive Medical Directors that they had failed to take responsibility for improving quality of care. This accusation caused outrage at the time, but on reflection, many of the Medical Directors agreed with Lawrence's assessment. The group commissioned a team to develop standards for quality review within the organization. Ron Potts, then the Ohio Region's Medical Director, together with Weiland, the newly elected Regional Medical Director in the Northwest Region, participated with experts in quality from the other Permanente Medical Groups to develop standards. A new quality review process became the basis for two new committees—the Medical Directors' Quality Committee (MDQC) and the Medical Directors' Quality Review (MDQR)—both of which proved instrumental in seeing the various Regions achieve and then maintain the highest accreditation status from national regulatory review bodies.

EMERGING FROM FORTRESS PERMANENTE

The McKinsey team, as part of a Strategic Positioning Assessment (SPA), evaluated the competitive position of KPNW, using a framework of strengths, weaknesses, threats, and opportunities. The evaluation included interviews of members, staff, patients, and competitors. Over the course of a year the team gathered significant information about the local health care environment to determine how the Region was positioned to succeed over time. In a nutshell, the team found that the Region was among the higher-priced health plans, that it provided mediocre service and access, that hospital facilities, particularly BK, were not positioned in rapid growth areas and that both hospitals suffered from a poor reputation when surveyed against other Portland-area hospitals. As the team leader dryly stated, "You won't grow if you have high price and poor service."

These messages, painful to hear, were nevertheless a wake-up call. Membership growth in the Northwest Region had been stagnant for four years. An aging BK needed $60 million in capital investments to meet community and seismic standards. (Geotechnical engineers had discovered that the 34-year-old hospital sat on a potentially unstable hill, along a seismic fault, and doubted that the hospital could be reinforced to meet new seismic standards.) In addition, the hospital location was in a section of Portland where growth was stagnant. Moreover, suburban populations in rapidly growing Washington County to the west and Clark County, Washington to the north, were not likely to bypass excellent local facilities to travel to an inner city hospital. Although KP had high name recognition (99%) only 11% of nonmembers said they would consider enrolling in the program.

The McKinsey group presented the sobering findings to the senior leaders in a series of meetings, together with an analysis of nine potential options for future hospital services. Together, Medical Director Weiland, Regional Manager Michael Katcher, and other leaders reviewed the options in the coming days. Given the slim chance for approval by Oakland for a major capital investment in the aging hospital, the two reluctantly concluded that Bess Kaiser Hospital, beloved to a generation of physicians and staff, would have to close, relocating its services to more strategically placed hospitals to the west and the north. Their decision was met with disbelief and outrage, primarily by staff physicians at BK. Skeptics questioned how the Region could duplicate the services offered at BK in outlying areas, which would surely require building two small suburban hospitals. Where was the capital for such an investment to come from? The alternative would mean contracting with existing community facilities, but this alternative offered only a limited number of options: Providence St. Vincent in rapidly growing Beaverton to the west, was one; Providence Portland another. Legacy Health System was less attractive, as its two major hospitals, Emanuel and Good Samaritan, were both located in the city's stagnant core. A third small Legacy hospital, Meridian Park, was, however, located to the south of the city in Tualatin, Oregon. But neither the Sisters of Providence nor Legacy offered a presence in Southwest Washington's Clark County to the north of Portland. There Southwest Washington Medical Center zealously guarded its position against intruders, an unfriendly monopoly in the city of Vancouver.

In its previous dealings with community hospitals, Northwest Permanente had found Providence a better business partner than Legacy. In fact, NWP had sued Legacy over breach of contract a mere two years before when Legacy announced its radiation therapy services would double the agreed-on cost.[1] So Weiland and Health Plan's Katcher determined to try to form an alliance with Providence Health System. They appointed Skip McGinty, Director of Contracting, to begin negotiations with Providence. John Bakke, a former Chief of Internal Medicine, was to work with McGinty. A team led by Permanente's Deborah Hedges with numerous primary and specialty care physicians formulated a service delivery plan. Tom Syltebo, Area Medical Director at BK, teamed with his Health Plan partner, KSMC administrator Barbe West, to oversee the process.

As plans developed, the team shared them with the Permanente Board of Directors in a series of evening meetings. The atmosphere at these discussions was tense. Confronting the idea of losing the flagship hospital and of working in non-Kaiser hospitals where NWP physicians would be a minority among a likely hostile medical staff was traumatic. Discussions became sufficiently heated, the atmosphere increasingly tense between Board members and Medical Director Weiland that he decided to step down from his position and not seek reelection in 1995. In time, with the help of facilitator Bob McCarthy, discussions resumed, becoming more businesslike and less emotional, and Board members asked Weiland to run for a second term as Medical Director.

As planning progressed, the Region's leaders shared them with North Portland community leaders, primarily the North/Northeast Portland Neighborhood Association. Area residents, especially African Americans, expressed great concern about the loss of neighborhood health care services; BK was one of just two hospitals in the area serving low-income residents. Mayor Vera Katz summoned Katcher and Weiland to a meeting; she was fully prepared, she said, to use her mayoral clout to ban KP from enrolling City employees in its Health Plan unless it would maintain some hospital services within the city. Increasing the pressure, the North/Northeast Portland Neighborhood Association contacted Jesse Jackson who sent a letter threatening a boycott and a march. With tensions high, program leaders held a series of meetings with community leaders, finally agreeing to maintain some services in the community.

North Portland residents were adamant that obstetrics services remain in the neighborhood. "You are not taking our babies out of the community!" KP spokespersons tried to argue that St. Vincent Hospital was a beautiful facility, and they promised to transport KP patients free of charge to that hospital, but to no avail. So KP acquiesced, agreeing to provide obstetrics services at Legacy Emanuel[2] and at Portland Providence. These programs would be costly to the Northwest Region, as they meant major inefficiency of call schedules and the necessity of providing additional staff to cover more hospitals.

Nevertheless, the relative ease with which KP assimilated into the Providence system can be traced to a 20-year history of collaboration between Permanente cardiologists and the cardiac surgeons of Providence St. Vincent Medical Center. Beginning with cardiac angiographer Phil Au's integration into the cardiac team at St. Vincent in the early 1990s, KP's cath lab had achieved preeminence. Au himself, the busiest angioplaster in the Northwest, performed 350 angioplasties a year, always achieving superior results. His reputation, as well as that of the three other cardiologists who joined him later, almost certainly explains the mostly neutral attitude with which Providence physicians accepted in their midst 250 Permanente physicians at St. Vincent and another 75 at Portland Providence Hospital. Even so, KP had to overcome very different hospital cultures, as well as resentment by physicians in the contracting hospitals. In planning for the move to Providence St. Vincent, for example, two obstacles became apparent immediately. The first was integrating high-risk maternity services, a staple at BK, to St. Vincent, with its carriage-trade, low-risk obstetric service. There, patients labored, delivered, and received after-delivery care in the same room. Whereas this model worked well for the majority of St. Vincent's typically healthy maternity patients, it was inadequate for the BK patient population with its high rate of illness and premature delivery. Martin Schwartz, Kathleen Kennedy, David Weil, and others worked to create training programs for St. Vincent nurses to familiarize them with KP protocols and procedures. Perhaps not surprisingly, their efforts were met with resistance by St. Vincent administrators and staff, who viewed KP as second rate. It would take another year and several near-tragic care incidents to convince the staff and the administration that Permanente physicians knew what they were talking about.

Once on site at Providence hospitals, Permanente physicians began to look at hospital processes, both to suit their practice styles and to effect greater efficiencies.

Since Permanente worked with national purchasing standards, its surgeons had their lists of agreed-upon instruments and equipment, which they presented to the St. Vincent administration. Because so much had been standardized, they had little trouble in getting all the equipment they requested. This astounded the St. Vincent staff physicians, who were routinely turned down for their individual and idiosyncratic equipment requests. Cries of favoritism went up. In fact, the seeming preferential treatment was instead a matter of cost savings for the administration through KP's standardized, organized practices.

Permanente physicians made other changes as well; they introduced aggressive discharge planning; created a hospitalist service to decrease utilization; introduced an antibiotic-review program; and provided 24-hour in-house obstetrical coverage. Observing that operating room turnover at St. Vincent was twice as long as at BK, they requested and got dedicated operating rooms, brought in their own highly skilled certified nurse anesthetists and operating room nurses, and promptly reduced turnover time by half. Providence administrators were sufficiently impressed that they asked NWP to perform OB anesthesia at all Providence hospitals, including Providence Milwaukie Hospital, a small facility where KP did not practice at all. This outside community contract, the first for NWP in 50 years—required explicit permission from its Health Plan partner, with whom Permanente shared an exclusive service clause. Health Plan's Katcher agreed to the contract, authorizing an outside entity to pay NWP directly to care for non-KP patients.

BettyLou Koffel, Permanente's Westside Anesthesiology Chief, endorsed the expanded program, and once the Region resolved how to provide gain sharing for staff affected by the new contract, NWP suddenly became one of the largest community providers of obstetrical anesthesia services. In doing so, it served notice to some old-line community physicians known to have denigrated Permanente as inferior that KP's quality could compete with all others. Today, primarily because of KP's presence, Providence St. Vincent maintains the busiest OB service in the state of Oregon. With obstetrics service hallways stretching a quarter of a mile, some staff have joked that roller skates would improve timely access to patient rooms.

If the move to the Providence hospitals was reasonably accomplished, the transition across the river to Vancouver's Southwest Washington Medical Center, the monopoly Clark County hospital, was not so easy. Unlike the collaborative history between KP and St. Vincent, the history of relations between Southwest Washington's medical staff and Permanente was a troubled one. To cite one example, Southwest Washington was the only hospital in the metropolitan area not to come to the aid of KP during its 1988 eight-week nursing strike. In addition, Southwest Washington physicians had long accused KP of shirking its responsibility to care for the indigent in Clark County and to share the city call burden. Though hospital

CEO Jeff Selberg saw the advantages of collaborating with Permanente and personally adopted a welcoming attitude, the medical staff was anything but. Particularly egregious were the openly hostile attitudes of surgeons in the specialties of orthopedics, neurosurgery, and ENT. All were threatened by the prospect of the Permanente physicians joining them en masse and instantly becoming one of the largest groups on the medical staff.

Clark County physicians and Southwest Washington Medical Center formed a physician-hospital organization called Clark United Providers (CUP) to contract services; its leaders offered Katcher a reduction in the hospital rates if he would contract with the community physicians of CUP. This proposal was clearly an attempted end-run around Permanente. Had Katcher accepted the offer, he would have endangered the mutually exclusive agreement between Health Plan and the physicians of NWP. As it was, Katcher considered the offer but ultimately decided against the arrangement. Not long thereafter the physician component of CUP collapsed. Negotiations resumed, and the two medical centers agreed to move KP services to Southwest Washington in April 1997. To accommodate the additional volume of patients, the medical center first needed to enlarge its Emergency and its Labor and Delivery Departments.

Now the planning entered a more intense phase. Unlike the arrangement at St. Vincent where KP maintained a full cadre of its own specialty services and enjoyed dedicated office space, Southwest Washington provided neither office space nor OR time to Permanente staff on its campus. Even as it built a large new medical office building for community physicians attached to the hospital, it reserved no quarters for its new contract partner.

The plan called for housing internal medicine, family practice, obstetrics, and general surgery at the hospital and for contracting orthopedics, neurosurgery, ENT, and urology with local Clark County physicians. But this plan, too, derailed. Most community physicians in these specialties, led by neurosurgeon Jay Miller, were hostile to a contract with NWP. In an early 1997 meeting between senior Permanente leaders and Southwest Washington orthopedists and neurosurgeons, community physicians restated their old complaint that Permanente physicians didn't do their fair share in caring for the indigent at Southwest Washington—where Permanente had as yet no medical staff presence. Permanente's Vice President of Operations James Brodhacker remained calm, pointing out that both parties were merely doing their jobs. The orthopedic group then agreed to contract with Permanente for coverage, but only at six times the usual and customary charges. Not surprisingly, Permanente rejected the orthopedists' terms. Left with few options, KP had to rethink its strategy. To offer full service in Clark County the organization would have to provide its own subspecialists. But where to house them? Southwest Washington had already made clear that it could offer no office space; to exacerbate the situation, a local building moratorium prohibited new construction in the area near the hospital. Finally, specialty space became available across the street from KP's Cascade Park Medical Office. The renovated facility named Mill Plain One,would house Permanente specialists. And, in April 1997, NWP physicians began practicing at Southwest Washington Medical Center, its inhospitable ally.

From the start, the medical staff at Southwest Washington welcomed Permanente internists and obstetricians, happy to have help with 24-hour coverage. And, as it had done at Providence hospitals, Permanente quickly demonstrated its efficiencies and innovations, installing a hospitalist service, taking over hospital epidemiology and antibiotic review functions, and supervising family practice residents. KP staff participated in quality improvements and helped prepare for Joint Commission accreditation. Permanente's Weiland was asked to join the Southwest Washington Medical Center Board of Trustees. Still, despite the considerable and obvious contributions by Permanente, hostilities lingered. Hot-button issues centered around city call coverage, OR time, and the transfer of KP patients from the Emergency Department at Southwest Washington to KSMC for inpatient care.

Led by Jay Miller, the Executive Committee of the medical staff tried to amend the by-laws to change the formula by which city call was distributed. Instead of apportioning call based on number of physicians, Miller wanted to tie coverage to the percentage of KP patients. In response to this proposal, Weiland threatened the hospital with legal action for discriminatory practices. Miller, Chief Medical Officer of Southwest Washington Medical Center Gilbert Rodriguez, and Executive Committee leaders tried four times to amend the by-laws and thus, discriminate against Permanente physicians. Each time these efforts were met with vigorous opposition by Permanente physicians including the threat of legal action. And though the three-year campaign by Southwest Washington's medical staff to single out Permanente physicians for additional call rotations failed, the effort poisoned the atmosphere still further.

One long-held KP policy—stabilizing members seen in outside hospital emergency rooms and transferring them to KP hospitals—also contributed to hard feelings. Southwest Washington Medical Center wanted these patients admitted there, where its Emergency Department physicians received reimbursement for admissions through the Emergency Room. Several ugly confrontations occurred when Emergency Department physicians and Rodriguez accused KP of violating federal anti-patient "dumping" legislation. The medical staff went so far as to censure several Permanente orthopedic surgeons for trying to transfer KP members to KSMC.

Another source of conflict was the continued practice by Southwest Washington's old-line medical staff to assign Permanente the least desirable OR times. Time and again, they reserved the desirable morning blocks for themselves, relegating Permanente surgeons and staff to late afternoon hours. Worse, Permanente's Ob/Gyn physicians on staff at Southwest Washington were assigned no OR time at all; they were obliged to travel to KSMC for all but emergency cases. Permanente's Medical Director for Specialty Services Sharon Higgins worked hard to problem-solve collaboratively with a stubbornly obdurate Southwest Washington medical staff. Rodriguez helped resolve some issues, but the dispute about transfers from the Emergency Department ultimately required legal intervention.

After two years Permanente was one of the two largest Medical Groups on the medical staff at Southwest Washington Medical Center. Business from Permanente brought an average annual revenue of $25 million. Yet despite the obvious benefits of the collaboration, the new hospital administrator Jeff Lang remained cool to the presence of KP staff. When Legacy Health System decided to build a hospital in Clark County, thereby ending the monopolistic hold of Southwest Washington, KP supported Legacy's plan, angering Lang, who was waging a battle to oppose Legacy's certificate-of-need application. Subsequently, Weiland resigned from Southwest Washington Medical Center's Board of Trustees, a position he had held for four years.

After Lang's sudden retirement from Southwest Washington Medical Center, new hospital administrator Joe Kortum continued his predecessor's refusal to acknowledge contributions of the Permanente staff. During his first two years as administrator, he visited each of the major Medical Groups on the staff but pointedly ignored Permanente—the only large Medical Group in Clark County with an exclusive affiliation with Southwest Washington. Still, in spite of its troubled relationship with its contracted partner, KP resolved to remain at Southwest Washington rather than to contract with Legacy. The rationale for this decision was twofold: first, providing services at two hospitals would be too costly; second, members now familiar with Southwest Washington would find unsettling a change to a new hospital.

By the end of the 1990s, Permanente had emerged from its fortress and had integrated into several large community institutions successfully, for the most part. Even in the hostile environment of Southwest Washington Medical Center, Permanente physicians became heads of medical staff committees, including the quality and credentialing committees. One, Permanente general surgeon Alden Roberts, became Chief of the Medical Staff and head of the Executive Committee. In every community institution that it joined, Permanente assumed leadership positions of clinical departments, including those of family practice, internal medicine, and Ob/Gyn. At meeting after meeting the same question was likely to arise: "How does Permanente do this?"

LEADING THE ELECTRONIC REVOLUTION

One of the ways that Permanente clinicians distinguished themselves on quality and cost effectiveness was to implement an electronic medical record. The planning that led to the Northwest Region's installation of the largest nongovernmental electronic medical record system took place gradually over a period of about 15 years. As early as the 1970s, the Kaiser Foundation Health Plan Board of Directors had mandated annual visits by the quality committee to each Region. In the early 1980s Board member Mary Reres asked Weiland, then Director of Quality for the BK area, and Area Medical Director Lawrence about the timeliness of the delivery of the medical record for patient appointments. An audit found that the medical record could be counted on only 80% of the time as long as the appointment was scheduled 48 hours in advance. For an urgent appointment the results were far worse: in most cases clinicians had only a blank piece of paper with vital signs, dubbed a "white sheet" by someone with a rueful sense of humor.

Judging this response time unacceptable, Reres challenged the Region to improve medical record delivery. Weiland, together with Barbe West and Alide Chase from BK administration, led the ten-year effort to do just that. A team worked on every aspect of the record delivery process: from filing systems to procedures for pulling charts to delivery schedules. The existing system was a "unitary" record system, one medical record for each patient. When one physician or administrative department used a chart, it became unavailable to others. Fearful of relinquishing charts, some physicians were known to squirrel them away, even in the trunks of their cars! Ten years of study and work to improve the system resulted in a mere 4% improvement for prescheduled appointments, hardly the results that Reres thought acceptable.

By the beginning of 1993 medical record delivery had grown worse; the system was simply unable to keep pace with the membership growth or the growing number of medical offices throughout the service area. The basic premise, that a single copy of a medical record could fulfill all possible needs, was hopelessly flawed.

Health Plan's Katcher and Permanente's Weiland met with a group of senior leaders to discuss options. They concluded that the only permanent fix would require replacing the paper charting system with an electronic one, and they commissioned a small group, including Homer Chin, Assistant Regional Medical Director for information systems, to evaluate existing electronic systems. Chin, recently recruited from The Permanente Medical Group, and Dan Azevedo, Director of the Information Technology Department, evaluated approximately 50 existing electronic systems. Within two months they narrowed the choices to eight, and then to three. Next they visited sites to observe how the three systems performed in the work place. Ultimately the group recommended Epic Systems and its EpicCare product, installed in one Arizona clinic with 20 users. At the time, Epic was a small company of only 55 employees headquartered in Madison, Wisconsin. Its products were mostly hospital billing and scheduling systems; the small company had only recently deployed an outpatient medical record system. In its favor, it had a good reputation for delivering on time and on budget and with a high degree of integrity. Chin and Azevedo worked closely with Epic's CEO Judy Faulkner and Senior Project Manager Carl Dvorak to create a plan to demonstrate the system; they selected the Rockwood and Sunset Medical Offices and a total of 100 users. Faulkner and Dvorak knew that the Northwest Region would require a system that would eventually support 1,000 practitioners with 4,000 or more total users at more than 25 sites. A team representing both the Medical Group, Michael Krall, Lawrence Dworkin, and Thomas Stibolt and Health Plan, Peggy McClure, Nan Robertson, and Dawn Hayami, led the project.

The pilot rollout began in 1994, with EpicCare version 1.3, to test whether the system would work in the KP environment and whether users would find the system acceptable. Both Rockwood and Sunset were primary care clinics, where computer-savvy physicians were willing guinea pigs and early adopters. The pilot set stringent criteria to measure success and to regularly report progress to the NWP Board. Chin, together with Stibolt, Michael McNamara, Richard Wong, Steven Lester, Neil Blair, Steven Gordon and others, oversaw the implementation for NWP. Within several months, staff in the two clinics could maintain normal patient schedules using the electronic record exclusively. Now all lab work; physician orders; progress notes; allergy, medication and problem lists were computerized. In addition the electronic record now made readily available hospital dictations, operative reports, histories and physicals, and discharge summaries.

The pilot completed, senior leaders concluded that the system was usable. But it showed, too, that the system was not as robust as users wanted, nor as seamlessly integrated with other systems. Even more serious, the workload for physicians was going to increase. Under the old system orders could be handed off to nurses; but with EpicCare, physicians would be required to perform data entry. The electronic chart thus expanded the primary care physician's workday by 60 to 90 minutes. But the benefits! Suddenly notes were legible; orders were transmitted instantly, and the medical record was available in multiple locations simultaneously. In addition, patients now routinely received an "after-visit summary," including their diagnosis, orders, and instructions—additional information that patients loved. With EpicCare, the old problem of recurring unavailability of a patient's record was a thing of the past.

With the system's limitations and workload implications understood, Chin and his team developed a regionwide implementation plan. Primary care clinics would be the first to go online, followed by the specialty clinics. In the meantime, Chin solicited help from savvy physicians to create charting shortcuts using "dot phrases." They developed a training program, beginning with live trainers and followed with a CD-ROM-based program. Implementation spanned two years; by early 1997 all Permanente clinicians were using EpicCare as the medical record. Emergency departments, including those in contracted hospitals, adopted the new system. Now when a KP patient visited an ER at Providence Portland, Providence St. Vincent, or Southwest Washington Medical Centers, his or her medical record was instantly available, at any hour of the day or night, bringing an enormous improvement in the quality and efficiency of emergency care.

The implementation of a regionwide electronic system wasn't entirely smooth, of course, and some casualties resulted. Several respected senior clinicians chose to retire rather than to embrace the new system. Others adopted it grudgingly. But implementation proceeded. After several years, nearly all physicians agreed that they would not wish to return to a paper medical record.

The power of the electronic record was not only its instantly available, legible information, but also its ability to code encounters, to aggregate information so as to understand the natural history and prevalence of medical problems and disorders, and to track the effectiveness of interventions on populations.

"Population-based" disease management first debuted in 1988 when a small group led by endocrinologist Harry Glauber and Jonathon Brown, PhD, from the Center for Health Research developed the first disease registry: The Diabetes Project. The project's sponsors were Weiland, as the BK Area Medical Director along with Timothy Blakely, Director of Strategic Planning; Ted Carpenter, Health Plan Manager; and Mitch Greenlick, Director of the Center for Health Research. The first step was to identify diabetic patients, a daunting task at the time. Glauber and Brown, with help from IT's Dan Azevedo, had to query numerous databases, including the pharmacy for insulin prescriptions, the lab to identify abnormal glucose values, and hospital admission records. Ultimately, they identified about 9,000 diabetics. A team then worked to understand which services these members used, the costs associated with their care, the variation in care from recognized guidelines and the agreed-on outcomes to measure. They then put in place a quality improvement approach to test interventions, measure outcomes, and retest.

Over several years the project team learned that providing cost-effective care for this population would require a 500% increase in health education resources to encourage self-management. Once the team developed management protocols, provided outreach, and feedback tools for clinicians, outcomes of care began to improve rapidly. Between 1988 and 1991, for example, the annual use of glycohemoglobin assay to assess diabetic control increased from 32% to 70%, the highest rate in the country at the time. Educational interventions improved the rate at which diabetics monitored their own blood glucose from 58% to 90% in the same period. Results included improving blood pressure control, reducing cholesterol levels, and reaching greater numbers of diabetics to provide treatment. In 1993 the project won the first Annual James A. Vohs Award for Quality, KP's most prestigious quality award. While the award and recognition throughout the program were welcome, the most important result of the first population-based project was to encourage similar projects for other chronic conditions, like heart disease, asthma, and chronic lung disease, using the population-based care management approach. The success of the first project convinced leaders to call for a new Quality Management Department. As the first Director for Population-Based Care, Paul Wallace, a medical oncologist, led and supported numerous project teams, whose work ultimately reduced complications, improved quality, and lowered the cost of care for those with chronic illnesses. (In 2000 Wallace would become the second executive director of the KP Care Management Institute, a program established in 1997 to bring about care improvements throughout the program.)

Once EpicCare was in wide use, the Region dramatically improved its ability to identify patients with a particular problem, aggregate information about care, test new interventions, and provide feedback. Besides creating a legible medical record and making that record instantly available, EpicCare became a critical tool to improve patient care. Mary Reres, the Health Plan Board member who had pushed so hard to ensure the availability of the medical record at time of care, pronounced the Northwest Region's accomplishment "bodaciously awesome!"

Yet another dramatic improvement brought about by the electronic record was the Region's new ability to influence practitioner behavior using the new electronic tools. Suddenly information could be disseminated instantly, including formulary changes, alerts about product problems, and more. For example, the program changed the contract from one SSRI drug to treat depression to a more cost-effective, therapeutic equivalent. Information about the change, the new guideline, and the subsequent cost savings was distributed electronically and instantly to every clinician. As a result, clinicians began prescribing the new drug so quickly that the pharmacy sent out a plea, requesting continued prescribing of the older medication until existing inventories had been used.

When a product was recalled, the program was now able to instantly identify and notify affected patients. An example of this new ability was the recall of a new cardiac pacemaker found to be defective and the quick removal from the market of the drugs rofecoxib (Vioxx, Merck) and celecoxib (Celebrex, Pfizer). KP members were among the first to receive notification and to obtain replacement products. When new clinical information came out, like the estrogen study from the Women's Health Initiative, the clinical guideline was changed in a matter of days, and disseminated electronically. Follow-up education programs were then developed and presented throughout the community.

At the same time that KPNW was successfully implementing EpicCare, other Regions throughout the KP organization were struggling. The Colorado Region had been working with IBM to develop its own homegrown system. That project, begun at the same time as the Northwest Region's, was delivered two years late and substantially over budget. The Northern California Region was working on its own system, the Southern California Region on another. In 1995 Lawrence, Health Plan CEO, convened a meeting of his top regional leaders: David Pockell, Northern California; Hugh Jones, Southern California; and Richard Barnaby, representing Regions outside California. Lawrence included Permanente physicians: Harry Caulfield, from TPMG; Oliver Goldsmith from Southern California Permanente Medical Group; and Weiland, representing the Northwest Region.

Their mandate was to create a programwide clinical information system, one that could be used by all Regions. In the meantime, the Northwest Region would use its EpicCare system already in production; Colorado would continue work on its IBM system. California representatives expressed concerns that the EpicCare system was not sufficiently robust to work for the entire KP program; they believed it was not "scalable" to support the huge California Regions. The Colorado Region still lacked a real product, and the organization's leaders had no confidence that a programwide solution would emerge from that Region's work. Consequently, the group elected to create a third product, a national clinical information system, to be built in-house or in conjunction with a vendor larger than Epic Systems. Advocates for this decision theorized that the program would learn a lot from all three electronic medical record systems, and that the program would eventually converge on a single, programwide solution. However, whereas this decision was beneficial to the Northwest Region, allowing the Region to continue working with Epic, it turned out to be both "bodaciously" costly and traumatic for the rest of the KP program.

Throughout the next five years the national program tried unsuccessfully to build the elusive national clinical information system, spending well over $1 billion in the process, a cost that the program would ultimately have to write off. The Hawaii Region, eager to implement an electronic medical record, volunteered to be the test site for each new attempt. Each time, that Region gamely worked to make difficult or unusable systems function. Three times Hawaii tested a new system, and three times it was obliged to pull the plug on yet another failure.

Meanwhile, the Colorado Region rolled out the first version of its IBM-developed system. Though it functioned and contained some good features, the system required considerable maintenance. As costs skyrocketed for each failed national system, Lawrence and Richard Barnaby made a decision to stop further development of the Colorado Region product. In the following five years Colorado struggled with an outmoded and poorly supported system, awaiting the conversion to a product that the entire program could use.

Meanwhile, the Northwest Region continued to upgrade EpicCare two or three times a year, and its little jewel just got better and better. In November 2000 the national system experienced vast overruns and poor performance. So sponsors of the national clinical information system asked the senior leaders of EpicSystems to meet in Portland to discuss whether Epic could support the entire KP program. Its scalability was the hot topic. When the Epic staff said they could scale their product, the top information engineers representing the national clinical information system called them liars. The heated exchange nearly became a food fight. The NWP management team, particularly Homer Chin, Dan Azevedo and Weiland, were mortified at the behavior of the national KP team, and the three apologized to the Epic staff. It was only after Lawrence retired and George Halvorson became Health Plan CEO in 2002 that the failed programwide project was at last laid to rest. Finally, after a struggle of eight years, the national KP program adopted the Epic system—that sturdy, dependable local product that the Northwest Region had built and used for nearly a decade and that had been dismissed by previous planners as unworthy.

BECOMING A DIVISION AND FLIRTING
WITH A KISSING COUSIN

In the mid-1990s Lawrence announced a plan to create divisions—collections of Regions to be administered as a unit. His recommendation came as the result of his work with McKinsey Company, which concluded that Health Plan needed to expand to roughly double its current membership of eight million to compete with the consolidated giants in the industry. Lawrence also concluded that the existing regional partnership structure with the Medical Groups prevented Health Plan from growing more rapidly, and gave too much decision-making power to the Medical Groups. Subsequently, Northern and Southern California Regions were consolidated into a single division under Richard Barnaby. The two very experienced and highly regarded regional Presidents, David Pockell in Northern and Hugh Jones in Southern, were fired. Similarly, the Colorado and Kansas City Regions were combined to form the central division, and regional President for the Colorado Region, Kate Paul, took command. Ohio and Mid-Atlantic Regions merged, with both under Bernard Tyson. Georgia and North Carolina Regions were combined in the Southeast, with both reporting to Chris Binkley, regional President for Georgia. The Texas Region closed in 1997 after suffering large operating losses in a regulatory environment that Medical Director Garber described as "toxic." Although the Texas Region had never performed well in its limited territory, Dallas-Fort Worth, it was the first Region in the history of KP to shut down completely. Its demise sent a chilling message throughout the organization that no Region was safe or exempt from that fate.

Lawrence determined to expand through acquisition, and he sent James Williams, a Senior Vice President, to the East Coast to acquire some marginal health plans. He returned having purchased a Humana plan of 100,000 members in Washington, DC, that had lost money for three consecutive years. The purchase came with an unmanaged network of 5,000 community physicians, most of them specialists. Forty-six were neurosurgeons, more than the combined number employed in KP's huge California division of six million members! Williams also arranged a merger between KP Northeast Region with the Community Health Plan of Albany, New York. With that merger, the Northeast Region increased from 150,000 to 500,000 members, incorporating a vast network of community physicians, including essentially every physician in the state of Vermont.

What the program, suddenly bloated beyond recognition, quickly learned (but nevertheless learned too late) was that the business systems to manage these huge networks were nonexistent. Payment of claims in Washington, DC, came to a halt as the systems were overwhelmed. Kaiser Foundation Health Plan, long a prepaid program with a single contract with a Permanente Medical Group, had never developed the infrastructure to cope with large claims-based, fee-for-service networks. The absence of business systems, when added to the restructuring and the weakening of the partnership between Health Plan and the physicians, nearly led the entire program into bankruptcy.

And although the Northwest Region was spared the divisional restructuring, it nevertheless suffered from the effects of the new imbalance in the partnership. Lawrence systematically excluded Medical Directors from large program decisions, even from forums to share information, and he reduced almost all joint planning meetings to the division level.

Then Lawrence and Williams met with Phillip Nudelman, CEO and Chairman of the Board of Group Health in Seattle, with the idea of merging KPNW and Group Health operations into a single entity. Nudelman described these meetings as "kissing cousins getting together." Neither the Group Health Board nor the cooperative membership would agree to an acquisition or even to a merger. The two parties agreed on an affiliation structure instead, wherein both entities would share a single KP-Group Health Board. The parent Board of each entity would maintain its decision-making sovereignty. Several KP leaders negotiated the mechanics of this relationship: James Williams, Senior Vice President in Oakland; Michael Katcher,

Health Plan's Regional President in the Northwest; Kate Paul; Group Health's Nudelman and his COO Cheryl Scott. The plan called for almost all operating functions—finance, human resources, legal and strategic planning—to merge and to be administered together from Seattle headquarters. Medical operations were to be locally managed. As this plan began to be executed, KPNW Regional CFO Deborah Stokes resigned. Other key administrative managers from finance, human resources and legal departments in Portland left as well. With their departure, whole areas of planning expertise were decimated.

Meanwhile, Weiland worked with Allan Truscott, President of Group Health's Medical Group, to form a single Permanente Medical Group. This organizational change required that Group Health physicians become, like their Permanente counterparts, an independent medical corporation, no longer employees of the cooperative. Thus, Group Health physicians contracted with their cooperative in much the same way that all Permanente Medical Groups contract with Health Plan. And after a series of meetings, Permanente shareholders passed an amendment by a 90% vote to create a new entity, Pacific NWP, and a new governing Board.

But all this work to create an alliance between the two Medical Groups was placed in jeopardy when Group Health's Truscott announced his retirement as Medical Director. His successor Louise Liang from the Hawaii Straub Clinic and Hospital in Hawaii disliked the proposed alliance and rapidly moved to squelch the approval process, though more than 90% of the cooperative's physicians had approved the principle of a merger. With the collapse of the Medical Group alliance, the two parties saw little value in merely merging administrative departments, particularly in this loose affiliation. As a result, KPNW endured almost two years with no effective finance function, no financial forecasting or reporting, and no strategic planning. Eventually the whole flawed concept of an affiliation fell apart. In its place a marketing agreement allowed reciprocal benefits to members of both organizations. In addition the entities were represented jointly in the Washington State legislature. And that was the end of a grand plan for a dominant HMO in the Northwest. Weiland had to return to the NWP Medical Group and ask them to rescind the by-laws amendment they had previously passed.

After its formation the new Group Health Permanente Medical Group was welcomed into The Permanente Federation, a newly formed entity to increase the influence of the Medical Groups in negotiating with Lawrence. Thus, the decades-long working relationship between the Medical Group in Portland and the physicians at Group Health was subsumed by The Permanente Federation.

By 1997 and 1998 the performance of the divisions was so poor that the program had lost $1.5 billion and was borrowing money for operating expenses. No business infrastructures existed to manage the large networks now in place in the Northeast and Southeast Divisions. And those operations, previously financially sound, were losing vast sums. Eventually the program closed its entire Northeast Division, leaving the states of New York, Massachusetts, Connecticut, and Vermont. And by the end of 2001 the program would also close in North Carolina and Kansas City.

SURVIVING THE CAPITAL FREEZE
AND A NEAR-DEATH EXPERIENCE

With the program in deep financial trouble, in 1998 Health Plan's Board of Directors essentially froze all capital investment. Planning for all new facilities halted. The Northwest Region had started to grow again as the results of service improvements and the hospital decentralization bore fruit. Most of the credit can be attributed to efforts by Medical Directors: Thomas Syltebo and Michael Kositch in primary care; Chong Lee and Sharon Higgins in specialty care.

The Region's leaders exerted a tremendous push to control costs on all levels, including referrals to non-plan hospitals. They adopted a protocol to return all KP patients admitted to ERs in non-plan hospitals to KSMC. Inevitably the hospital and its ER began to burst with the overflow.

The Medical Group worked to control hospitalizations on all fronts. The hospitalist program expanded in every facility and began to reduce hospital stays as the coordination of care improved. Calvin Leong had led the hospitalists and utilization management at Southwest Washington Medical Center, and he took on expanded duties as Regional Director of Utilization Management. Leong organized discharge-planning rounds with the utilization management staff in each hospital, adding more case managers to help lower admission rates for those with chronic disease. Another committee, led first by Wallace and later by Richard Bills, worked with steering committees to promote population-based care tools within the electronic system to better manage major chronic illnesses. This targeted approach led to improved immunization rates; screening for breast, colon and cervical cancer; and screening and care for those with heart failure, asthma, diabetes and depression.

The program grew, and service and quality of care improved, despite the disruptive move to unfamiliar community hospitals. But lack of capital was taking a toll; the Region was unable to meet the need for new office space to handle the growth. With more crowding, both at KSMC and in the medical offices, morale began to erode. Physicians in primary care shared office space and had fewer exam rooms to practice efficiently. Chin, Assistant Medical Director for IT, had overseen a time-and-motion study that demonstrated how much more efficient the physicians could be with terminals in the exam room. But the proposal stalled; the Region could not fund the project.

In 1999 Health Plan hired Dale Crandall as President, sending a no-confidence message about Lawrence's ability to bring fiscal health to the program. Though Lawrence remained as CEO and Chairman of the Board, those positions had little operational responsibility. Barbe West was the local Regional Health Plan President, having succeeded Michael Katcher two years earlier. In the divisional restructure she first reported to Kate Paul, head of the western Regions outside California, and later to Bernard Tyson, when in still another restructuring, Paul was fired.

Crandall came from PriceWaterhouseCoopers and had an excellent business reputation, but he didn't know much about health care. Immediately he set out financial margin goals—"2-4-6"—to represent the percentage margin for each of the next three years. He asked the Regions to submit financial plans that would hit those targets and extended the capital freeze until each Region's budget met the goals.

The Northwest Region, including the Medical Group, had shown positive financial results for most years, with the exception of 1997 when it lost several million dollars because of the hospital reorganization. Despite its good financial performance, Dale Crandall asked the Region to improve service, maintain a rate advantage, reduce the cost trend, and create a margin—without spending capital to invest in equipment and facilities. How was the Region to achieve all goals simultaneously? Something had to give.

THE RISE OF THE PERMANENTE FEDERATION

Lawrence's efforts to shrink the influence of the Medical Groups, described earlier in this chapter, acted as a catalyst to bring far-flung Medical Directors together. For some years one voice, that of Martin Bauman, Medical Director in the Mid-Atlantic Region, had urged his fellow Medical Directors to join together as a single national entity. Until 1997, however, the two largest Medical Groups—from the California Regions—had opposed Bauman's plan, reasoning that such a restructuring would decrease some of their power. But the 1997 financial crisis, together with the specter of closure of some Regions, changed their thinking. Even Harry Caulfield, leader of TPMG, concluded that not even his group was big enough or strong enough to survive. His shift in thinking helped turn the tide, and a small group, led by Ian Leverton, liaison to the national program in Oakland, began putting together a plan to create a national Permanente entity. The work group included Leverton, Jay Crosson from TPMG, Irwin Goldstein from the SCPMG, and Weiland from NWP.

The group proposed a Federation, a legal association of the Medical Groups that would be headquartered in Oakland. Its Executive Director would be empowered to partner with the Health Plan and to develop a national strategy for the Medical Groups. In addition, Medical Directors of Northern and Southern California Regions would be permanent members of a five-person Executive Committee that would develop policy positions for the Federation. This stipulation ensured that the California groups would always be well represented on the decision making and would not be outvoted by other Permanente Medical Groups. At least one of the two permanent California members had to vote to pass any policy. The Medical Groups outside California would elect two representatives to the Executive Committee, each for a two-year term.

After some negotiation, the Medical Directors authorized the Federation and selected Crosson from TPMG as the first Executive Director. Oliver Goldsmith from the SCPMG was the first Chairman of the Executive Committee. Committee members included Weiland from the Northwest, Caulfield from TPMG, and Adrian Long, now Medical Director from the Mid-Atlantic Region.

Like Leverton before him, Crosson experienced difficulty in establishing a good working relationship with Lawrence. In 1998, alarmed by financial losses, and blaming much of those losses on the new divisional restructuring, the newly formed Executive Committee of the Federation requested a meeting with Kaiser Foundation Health Plan and Hospitals Board of Directors. Granted a brief hearing, they listed their concerns and volunteered to solve problems collaboratively. Health Plan Board members gave them an icy reception, and the meeting concluded without accomplishing anything.

Still, Health Plan's Lawrence realized that cooperation with Permanente Medical Groups was a necessity to overcome the program's financial straits. He listened when leaders of the Federation proposed a restructuring of the relationship between the Medical Groups and Health Plan. A group representing both entities produced a national partnership agreement—a joint governing body to develop program policy; to make major recommendations; to create special entities; to conduct research and to implement quality programs; to improve service; to provide a blueprint for closing a Region; and to determine major investments in new ventures. Both the Health Plan Board and the Federation formally adopted the national partnership agreement, which ameliorated some of the damage of the divisional restructuring. And with the newly formed joint governing body, the Medical Groups again had an equal voice in program policy and a forum for discussing strategic planning. It was no coincidence that the financial fortunes of the organization began to improve shortly thereafter.

When Dale Crandall replaced Lawrence, the working relationship between Health Plan and the Federation improved fairly quickly. Crandall made clear his willingness to let the Medical Groups and three Health Plan leaders take the lead but did not change the divisional structure.

KPNW began to make needed capital investments. It leased two floors of a five-story office building next to the Emergency Department at Providence St. Vincent, installing high-volume minor procedure rooms for a variety of services.

Fulfilling a commitment to the North and Northeast Portland community, the Region built Interstate South, a new medical office on the Interstate campus. With an imaging center, a surgicenter, and a 24-hour emergicenter, Interstate South could treat all patients except those requiring ambulance transport. The Interstate campus could now provide 80% to 90% of the services previously provided at BK. Another major investment was the $30 million dollar project to construct exterior and interior bracing systems to ensure that KSMC conform to seismic standards.

By the end of the decade the Region had undergone dramatic change. It had closed its flagship hospital and decentralized hospital services into the community as never before. It had successfully implemented the nation's most advanced private electronic medical record system with over 3,000 local users, while the rest of the national KP program continued its efforts in fits and starts and failed attempts, to create an internal system. KPNW had also substantially improved service through a period of continued growth, while keeping its rates competitive. And although it had been forced to abandon its aging BK as well as the culture that had flourished within its walls, the Region had invested in a new facility to support the inner city and had created specialty offices on the Providence St. Vincent campus. The Medical Group had grown as well, maintaining mostly positive financial results. The Region had survived the division restructuring, although its brief flirtation with Group Health had caused major disruption for the Health Plan. Health Plan, too, had shown positive financial results, though not those that Crandall had demanded in his "2-4-6" percent margin.

A RITUAL BEHEADING

After the debacle with Group Health, Health Plan regrouped under the leadership of regional President Barbe West and two trusted Operations Managers, Alide Chase and Ray Robertson. The Medical Group enjoyed stable leadership with Weiland as President. His team included James Brodhacker, Thomas Syltebo, and Sharon Higgins, operations; Homer Chin, information services; Ron Potts, quality management; Tom Janisse, Health Plan liaison; Harry Stathos, CFO; and Marci Clark, human resources; Ann Stenzel, pension and benefits; Deborah Hedges, communications and governmental affairs. In early 2000, Weiland was asked to represent the relatively new KP Partnership group to oversee a turnaround in the Mid-Atlantic Division; he agreed to relocate to Washington, DC, for six months. In his absence the Board named Brodhacker to take over day-to-day operations; Syltebo agreed to serve as interim Chairman of the Board and to oversee Board meetings. At the time, the Mid-Atlantic Division was losing $30 to $40 million dollars a year, had a huge unmanaged network of specialists, and major quality and regulatory problems. Weiland worked with the two Mid-Atlantic leaders to produce a plan for the ailing Region. He returned to the Northwest in October 2000. During his absence the Medical Group had run smoothly. One year later, after his second term, Syltebo decided to return to his clinical practice in family medicine.

Meanwhile Health Plan, though it had positive net income, had not met its aggressive financial targets—2% margin for 1999 and 4% in 2000. Several regional Presidents reviewed program office budgets and finances. Barbe West was one who expressed criticism of certain expenses. On a Friday in October 2001 Dale Crandall and Bernard Tyson scheduled a visit to West. They told her that she was no longer a good fit for the organization and fired her. She was to vacate her office over the weekend. So ended the 25-year career of the well-liked and much-respected West. One month later, Crandall and Tyson attended a meeting of the Board of Directors and explained that West had not gotten the kind of results they required. Health Plan did nothing to recognize or celebrate her accomplishments over a quarter century with the organization. It was NWP that sponsored a going-away celebration for West.

TIGHTENING UP

Throughout the 1990s NWP's Board of Directors demanded of physicians ever-more stringent requirements for joining and remaining in the Medical Group. Achieving senior physician status now required board certification. As a result, several physicians whose work was satisfactory but who could not become certified, resigned. In addition, the evaluation period lengthened from two years to three years for eligibility to senior physician status. The Board held Department Chiefs and Operations Medical Directors accountable for conducting thorough evaluations.

As requirements for remaining with the Medical Group grew more stringent, the Board invoked the disciplinary process more frequently. And although the hearing process was neither arbitrary nor capricious, the Board was tough on the individual in question. The process was effective; a number of marginal physicians, either because of quality or of service concerns, resigned after these hearings.

The new emphasis on excellence within the physician group paid dividends: the perception of the program by both members and non-members in the community improved. The physicians themselves gained recognition as they moved into leadership positions. Chapter 6 "Pariahs and Presidents" elaborates on

Permanente physicians and their leadership positions in the community. By the end of the 1990s, physicians at NWP had integrated into the fabric of the community, a dramatic change from just a decade before.

TRANSITIONS: NEW PARTNER: NEW COMPACT: AND WE'RE NUMBER ONE!

After Barbe West's sudden departure, Tyson, now President of the KP Regions outside California, began a search for a new regional President. A number of promising candidates emerged, and ultimately Cynthia Finter, the former regional President responsible for closing the Kansas City Region, earned the position. She began in February 2002 with a mandate from her boss to hit the numbers of the financial margin. Finter set out to do just that. She replaced almost all her senior leaders, a group that had a long history of working collaboratively with Permanente partners.

The atmosphere in the regional headquarters chilled. Whereas medical operations partnerships remained strong, at least for a time, other partnerships between Permanente and Health Plan cooled. Relationships in communications, government relations, legal, compliance and finance became dysfunctional.

In one instance Finter asserted her right as Health Plan President to terminate a physician. Weiland balked at Finter's unabashed encroachment into Permanente personnel matters. Dueling legal conflicts led all the way to Program Offices in Oakland. All joint management meetings stopped; communication between Health Plan and the NWP Board occurred only on matters that posed a crisis. Still, despite tension in the administrative realm, operations continued to run smoothly, with access and service steadily improving in most areas. KSMC remained busy, and plans proceeded to upgrade the facility, particularly the nursing units.

David Lawrence retired as Chairman of the Board of Kaiser Foundation Health Plan and Hospitals in 2002. George Halvorson from HealthPartners in Minnesota took over. Soon thereafter Dale Crandall left as well, and Halvorson completed the dismantling of the divisional structure. Once again the regional management teams became the local governing bodies. Strong partnerships were the norm throughout the program, except in the Northwest. Thus, the Region that for many years had embodied a powerful and functional partnership now had the most dysfunctional leadership in the entire program.

In addition to reversing the divisional structure, it was Halvorson who, together with Jay Crosson, moved to halt work on the extremely expensive and underachieving national clinical information system and to contract with Epic Systems.

In addition, the group planned various business and inpatient modules to form a single integrated suite, now called KP HealthConnect. The Northwest Region, though pleased that Epic Systems was now the program choice, lost some of its ability to introduce new features. The Region would now be part of a large national effort. Inevitably, bureaucratic processes slowed local progress significantly. On the bright side the large-scale process forced discussions for standardizing clinical definitions, vocabulary, guidelines, and tools. Ultimately, this large national clinical system, tied to business and pricing systems and an enormous national data warehouse, promised to create the most powerful clinical and decision-support system in the nation.

In 2003, *Consumer Reports* magazine ranked KPNW first in the nation for consumer satisfaction. In 2005, the magazine again recognized the Region as number one. Externally, KP was on the move and healthy. But internal relationships between the Medical Group and Health Plan continued their downward spiral. Finter's removal of 80 seasoned operations managers caused an almost instant crippling effect on planning processes throughout the Region.

Meanwhile the Permanente Board of Directors was working with a consultant to create a new compact between the corporation and the physicians. Its objective was to create a roadmap to earn Permanente recognition as the best Medical Group in the country. Though work toward this compact continued for nearly a year, it was derailed by Health Plan disruptions. When Weiland, President of the Medical Group for 12 years, announced his intention to seek reelection in 2005, a group of senior shareholders, citing his inability to create joint leadership with Health Plan's Finter, asked him to step down. Weiland acquiesced and removed his name from the ballot. Weiland's term ended on January 1, 2005. Sharon Higgins was appointed Acting Regional Medical Director during the search for a new Regional Medical Director. The search culminated with the hiring of Andrew Lum from the Colorado Permanente Medical Group. Lum officially became Regional Medical Director in April 2005, and a new chapter in NWP history opened.

AFTERWORD:
WHAT HAPPENED TO
THE PIONEERS?

—⚬—

ERNEST SAWARD

When Saward announced his leave of absence in 1970, he intended to join professor Richard Weinerman, Chairman of Public Health at Yale as Professor of Epidemiology and Public Health.[1] And, as has been stated earlier, he intended to return to clinical practice at Permanente and to continue his research interests.

In 1969, the Rochester New York Industrial Management Council (IMC) asked him to present a series of lectures at the University of Rochester Medical School to local medical societies. As well, he was asked to consult with Eastman Kodak and Xerox about containing health care costs, including the role of prepaid group practice (the term Health Maintenance Organization was not introduced until 1970). The Rochester community had innovated with health care as early as 1919, when George Eastman and other industry leaders created the IMC. In the 1930s, IMC proposed a single hospital system for the city, which the five Rochester hospitals rejected. But a newly created Hospital Council dealt with communitywide problems, leading to the 1935 formation of the Rochester Hospital Service Corporation, later to become Blue Cross.

After a visit to Rochester, Saward cancelled his Yale plans to help establish three Rochester HMOs under the auspices of Blue Cross and with support from Eastman Kodak, Xerox, and General Motors. The school of medicine in Rochester created a new position for Saward as Associate Dean for Extramural Affairs; in addition he was appointed Professor of Social Medicine. Though the three HMOs were different, they provided common benefits: Genese Valley Group Health was sponsored by Blue Cross, Health Watch Plan by the medical society, and Rochester Health Network, with support from the federal government.

David Steward, a former CEO of Blue Cross and Blue Shield in the Rochester area, described Saward's role: "Without his knowledge and leadership we never could have done what we did with HMOs. While he represented the essence of … a revolutionary philosophy of comprehensive care by salaried doctors, he fit in like an old shoe with Wenkert … as well as Blue Cross, IMC, and the medical school staff. He had a unique knack for identifying problems and prejudices and for offering solutions in a very general way."[2]

As a professor, Saward was enormously popular; students, residents, and fellows filled his courses on the social and economic aspects of medicine. Time and again, he received admiring letters from those who attended his classes. A note from one student, dated August 23, 1981 is typical: "Thank you for the time and guidance you gave me during the fellowship program. Despite demands on your time you always made time to see me."

Even before his appointment at Rochester, Saward was a familiar figure on the congressional scene. As a member of the Physicians Committee for Health for the Aged, he visited President Kennedy in 1962 and, in 1965, he attended the signing of the historic medical bill at the Truman Library. Saward served on numerous advisory committees and task forces and traveled frequently to Washington to testify before congressional committees: Ways and Means, Interstate and Foreign Commerce, Finance, Labor and Human Resources, and Government Operations. His first appearance was in 1968 before a Senate subcommittee headed by former Health Education and Welfare Secretary Senator Abraham Rubicoff, where he described the advantages of prepaid group practice. And it was as Chairman of HEW task force that he met Lady Elizabeth Gallagher, a fellow task force member, whom he was to marry in 1982. Gallagher had spent her career on Capital Hill, beginning in the Eisenhower administration, and she was a Washington insider. Together, she and Saward would collaborate on various health care issues.

Saward was a popular speaker at home and abroad. His appointments included a fellowship at Villa Scoleone in Bellagio, Italy; visiting lectureships at Salzburg, Austria; and at hospitals in London, Cambridge, and Oxford. He delivered the memorial lecture at the 360th anniversary for the University of Edinburgh Medical School. Saward was one of the original members of the Institute of Medicine; in 1987 he received the prestigious Gustav Leinhard Award for his leadership in establishing prepaid group health plans.[3]

In 1987 Saward, retired for two years, underwent a valve replacement for the heart murmur he had had from childhood. Two years later he was discovered to have inoperable lung cancer. His last visit to Portland, in April of that year, was to commemorate the 25th anniversary of the Center for Health Research, where he delivered the first Saward Lecture, an annual event that still carries his name. He died in his sleep two months later. He was 74 years old.

At his memorial service in the Senate Room of the Mayflower Hotel in Washington, DC the written program described Saward: "physician; prepaid group practice pioneer; medical director, Permanente medical group; developer of a national HMO strategy; leader in the effort for a national Medicare program; recipient of the Institute of Medicine Award for Advancement of Health Care; founder of the Health Services Research Center; educator and education administrator; chairman, National PSRO [Professional Standards Review Organization] Advisory Council; GHAA [Group Health Association of America] chairman, president, and board member; writer; friend."

WALTER NOEHREN

Walter Noehren and Saward were classmates at the University of Rochester Medical School. Both were influenced by socialist George Mackenzie, MD, at Mary Imogene Basset Hospital. Both spent time at Hanford providing care for workers. Saward followed Noehren to Permanente in Vancouver, and the two were among the few physicians who remained at Permanente after the end of World War II, when Permanente's future was very much in doubt. Always a dreamer with a vision about what health care should be, Noehren departed the program before the first partnership was established. It was Saward, ever the pragmatist, who remained and who was instrumental in the survival and the eventual success of the Northwest program.

After a failed attempt to develop a comprehensive community health center in Troutdale, Oregon, Noehren moved to nearby Sandy where he opened a conventional independent practice. But, stirred by John F. Kennedy's 1961 inaugural address and his famous words, "Ask not what your country can do for you; ask what you can do for your country," Noehren dreamed again of a comprehensive national health care system. He resurrected the program he had initiated in 1947, which he called "medical care for every man." For a time the Clackamas County Plan, as it was renamed, held some promise and was even supported by both the Oregon Medical Association and the American Medical Association. Consumed with promoting this plan, Noehren neglected his own medical practice. Then, with the passage of Medicare, his dream was shattered. Abandoning his private practice, he began to accept work in emergency rooms in Portland and in Reno, Nevada. His disappointment in failing to see his dream of universal health care realized likely contributed to a debilitating depression. In 1977 at age 63, Noehren took his own life.

CHARLES GROSSMAN

When Grossman left Permanente in 1950, he continued his research on amino acids at the University of Oregon Medical School and opened a private practice in an office building at 610 SW Alder Street in downtown Portland. At the same time, he devoted a significant amount of his time to social activism. In an April 1999 newsletter of the American College of Physicians, Grossman reported that in his early years as a physician, few physicians related to the causes that mattered to him—that is, war, poverty, and injustice.

In 1967, as part of its war-on-poverty platform, the Office of Economic Opportunity (OEO) introduced a plan to underwrite 50 neighborhood health centers throughout the U.S. Saward proposed another plan to integrate an indigent population into the Kaiser Foundation Health Plan, at the time a revolutionary idea. He cited his plan as more efficient, economical, and amenable to a research project. Grossman, representing the Albina Citizens War on Poverty Committee, challenged his old foe, objecting to Saward's proposal unless he would agree to hire an African-American physician. Saward's program proceeded. An early advocate for welfare reform, Grossman chaired two local committees to advance the cause. In 1974 he led a contingent of 40 to Salem to meet with Governor Tom McCall requesting action to deal with the welfare crisis. In a heated exchange, McCall accused Grossman of being a "professional welfare rabble rouser." Later, he softened his rhetoric, acknowledging that Grossman's concern came "from his heart and not his pocketbook."

In 1974 Grossman established contact with physicians in communist China, founding the Evans F. Carlson Friends of the People's Republic of China.[4] Throughout the next 20 years this organization arranged annual group tours of up to 50 to China to meet officials and visit institutions. As a result, Chinese scholars and others were able to visit the U.S., often as guests of those who had participated in the tours.

Grossman actively protested nuclear energy. As a founding member of the Northwest Radiation Health Alliance, he co-authored studies showing the incidence of thyroid disease, cancer, and spontaneous abortion in residents downwind from Hanford. He was the recipient of numerous awards for his work, among them Citizen of the Year, Oregon Chapter of the National Association of Social Workers, 1980; Albert Schweitzer Peace Award, International Visions for Prevention of Nuclear War, 1989; National Physicians for Social Responsibility Broad Street Pump Award for Lifetime Achievement, 2004.[5] In July 2005 he was honored at the Legacy-Emanuel medical grand rounds for his education and public service. The July 2008 issue of the *Annals of Internal Medicine* features an article by Grossman on the first civilian use of penicillin in the U.S.; the event took place at the Yale-New Haven Hospital where Grossman was a young house officer. Until 2009 Grossman continued to practice medicine in the same building where he began his practice in 1950, and he continued to advocate for social justice.

NORMAN FRINK

Norman Frink experienced difficulty during the first year of his retirement in 1977. At a retirement seminar for Permanente physicians in 1982, he described anxiety over loss of income (retirement benefits for Northwest Permanente before incorporation were not generous); loss of social identity; a sense of isolation; and

unaccustomed leisure time. Fortunately, Frink had established the Kaiser Permanente Northwest Risk Management Department late in his career and had acquired
expertise in malpractice, personal injury, and disability law. As a result, he was
able to launch a new career as a consultant and lecturer on medical-legal matters.
Among his constituents were Farmer's Insurance Group and various legal firms.
Still active at age 75, Frink died suddenly of a heart attack in 1986.

ROGER GEORGE

After delivering 17,000 babies, including the Anderson quintuplets, Roger
George retired in 1977 to his home on the Royal Oak Country Club golf course
in Vancouver, Washington, where he could enjoy his favorite recreational activity.
After his wife's death, the Andersons invited George to live with them and built an
apartment for him in the lower level of their home. In 1987 he traveled with his
adoptive family, including the now 14-year-old quints, to Peoria, Illinois to welcome the just-born Helm quintuplets. Living in the Anderson household, George
was able to watch the famous youngsters grow to near adulthood. He died in 1990.

NORBERT FELL

Norbert Fell retired in 1973 but, at the request of his department, he continued
to work part time for another year before he and his wife moved to a retirement
community in Laguna Hills, California. Periodically he attended medical luncheon
meetings at the hospital where his son-in-law, an internist, worked, becoming a familiar guest. He attended his wife as her health failed. She preceded him in death.
Fell died in his 100th year.

MORRIS AND BARNEY MALBIN

The Malbin brothers both left Permanente in 1951, establishing practices in
Portland, where they continued their close association with Grossman. Radiologist Morris worked part time in McMinnville, Oregon. In 1971 he closed his
Portland practice and worked three days a week at the McMinnville hospital. Like
Grossman, Malbin was involved in a variety of causes, including raising funds for
the Black Panthers in 1969 and protesting the Vietnam War. His FBI file was a thick
one; the file cover warned that Malbin's alias was "Moe." He named his son, born
in the Northern Permanente Hospital in Vancouver, after Canadian physician Norman Bethune, a member of the Canadian Communist Party. Bethune established
a blood transfusion service in Spain during that country's civil war, and he died
serving as a battlefield surgeon for the communist Eighth Route Army in China.
Malbin retired in 1983 and died in 1991 of complications of Alzheimer's disease.

Barney Malbin practiced internal medicine in Portland. An active member of the American College of Physicians, he published several articles in the *Annals of Internal Medicine*. Like his brother, he was a social activist. Marked for suspicion for his service with the Abraham Lincoln Brigade in the Spanish Civil War, Malbin was called to testify before the Committee on Un-American Activities. Barney Malbin died suddenly in 1959 of a heart attack at age 49.

HAROLD COHEN

After 51 years with Permanente, where he held the record for newborn deliveries, in 1996 Cohen retired and devoted an increasing amount of his time to gardening. He and his wife Charlotte traveled extensively, but when he was home he chauffeured his grandchildren to and from their various activities. As his memory began to fade, he liked to relax on his deck where he could watch the activity below on Lake Oswego. Cohen died in 2004 at age 88.

ENDNOTES

PART I: A LENGTHY PROLOGUE

CHAPTER 1: THE ROOTS

1. Henry Kaiser, himself having joined the Everett, Washington chapter of the Elks Lodge in 1916, was undoubtedly familiar with prepaid medical systems typically offered by fraternal groups.

2. The Industrial Workers of the World (IWW), or Wobblies, had formed a national labor union of Northwest timber workers as early as 1905; in 1917 and 1918 the IWW organized strikes that were marked by violence.

3. By 1978 enmity between King County Medical Society and Group Health Cooperative became a thing of the past when the Society elected Group Health physician William Spence as its President.

4. Neuberger, elected to the Senate in 1948 and in 1960, was chairman of the Senate subcommittee managing federal health benefits legislation. As a former reporter for *The Oregonian*, a member of the Permanente Foundation Health Plan and a patient of Ernest Saward, Neuberger knew the advantages of prepaid group practice and dual choice. He persuaded the committee to back a plan that would include dual choice and thus allow Kaiser Permanente to participate in the 1960 Federal Employees Health Benefits Act.

5. Alonzo B. Ordway was Vice President of the Industrial Indemnity Exchange, which serviced the Los Angeles Aqueduct Project. Hired by Kaiser in 1912 to oversee Kaiser's venture building roads in Cuba, Ordway was an advocate for the Portland-Vancouver Permanente program during the difficult post-war years when supporters were few.

6. It was not until the 20th century that man produced an atom bomb, but the idea of the atom is ancient—first attributed to the Greek philosopher Leucippus in 500 B.C. From the 17th century onward, physicists postulated the existence of atoms. H.G. Wells described an atom bomb and atomic warfare in his 1914 novel, *The World Set Free*. In December 1942, Enrico Fermi, in his laboratory beneath the football stands at the University of Chicago, produced the first self-sustaining nuclear chain reaction, providing the means to produce an atomic bomb. Fermi visited Hanford and other production sites during the war years. Later a professor at University of California at Berkeley, Fermi was a Kaiser Foundation Health Plan member.

7. In 1945 Oak Ridge supplied the uranium for the atomic bomb that destroyed Hiroshima. Hanford produced the plutonium for the bomb that ravaged Nagasaki.
8. Saward's wife, born Virginia Wagner in 1915, was raised on the family farm in Phelps Township, New York. She received a Bachelor of Fine Arts from Syracuse University College and from 1935 to 1937 was an August Hazard Fellow in European study. An accomplished artist of oil portraits and watercolor studies, she returned to painting after the couple moved to Vancouver, Washington. In the 1950s and 1960s, she became more active in the Northwest arts community, frequently exhibiting her work. A prizewinner in the 1959 Oregon Centennial Show, she was recognized as one among the group of distinguished Northwest artists, including Louis Bunce, Byron Gardner, George Johanson, and Jack McLarty.
9. Ernest H. Aebi owned the Merry Abbey, a popular Richland restaurant. After the war he opened the successful Chalet L'Abbey restaurant in Milwaukie, Oregon and became a Health Plan member. In 1972, his son, Ernest P. Aebi joined Permanente as an ophthalmologist where he practiced for 27 years before retiring in 1999.

PART II: THE EARLY DECADES
CHAPTER 2: WARTIMES 1941-1945

1. The St. Johns shipyard was near what is now the Port of Portland Terminal 4 and the site of the scrap yard for Schnitzer Steel.
2. The former site of the Vancouver shipyard is adjacent to the three-story Kaiser Shipyard Memorial Tower at Marine Park.
3. After the war, Permanente physician Charles Grossman was the Runquist brothers' physician; they paid him with their artwork.
4. Forrest Rieke, though not a Permanente physician, played a significant role in providing health care to shipyard workers. He was in charge of emergency and preventive medicine in the shipyards and was Medical Director of the day care centers. Rieke would go on to become a leader in the community for health planning and safety. In 1973, the Oregon Medical Association named him Doctor Citizen of the Year. In 1978, while traveling through Costa Rica to promote exchange programs for students and teachers, he was killed on a rural highway in a one-car accident.
5. A chipper smoothed and finished metal surfaces.
6. In 1954 the author, then a medical student at Queens University Medical School in Kingston, Ontario, discovered the *Kaiser Foundation Medical Journal* in its small library. Impressed with its simple format, green cover, and absence of advertising, he obtained a free subscription. At the time, he was more interested in the article about cat scratch disease than with the review of the

presentation by Saward and Gilbert Rogers on post-operative atelectasis at a Northern Permanente Foundation Hospital staff conference.

7. Tom Janisse, MD, an anesthesiologist, is editor-in-chief of *The Permanente Journal*. From 1996 to 2005 he was Assistant Regional Medical Director of NWP.

CHAPTER 3: HARD TIMES 1945-1950

1. Bertha Hallam was a favorite with the physcians. In 1963 she received a commendation from Multnomah County Medical Society for outstanding service. Her portrait hangs in the historical library of Oregon Health Sciences University.

2. Barney and Virginia Malbin were among the worldwide coalition of social activists who participated in the struggle against General Franco and those conservative nationalists who were determined to wrest control from Spain's newly elected coalition government of liberals and leftists. Assigned to the American Medical Bureau as Chief of Medicine in various Spanish hospitals between 1937 and 1939, Malbin fought to contain typhoid epidemics and helped repatriate wounded soldiers. Virginia, a social worker, helped refugee children and worked with wounded soldiers from fascist countries who, having fought against Franco, found themselves unwelcome in their home countries.

3. They settled on the name The Permanente Clinic for the second partnership in 1950. The first partnership was recognized by the Health Plan as The Permanente Medical Association, but they also used Roger George and Associates and The Doctors Clinic, and discussed calling it The Frink Clinic.

4. Grossman was on leave of absence, completing a one-year research fellowship with the American Cancer Society in Berkeley.

CHAPTER 4: THE FIFTIES: FIRM FOUNDATION

1. KP historian Steve Gilford recorded a 1991 conversation with the late Clifford Keene. In 1962 Keene traveled to Portland to view the new Bess Kaiser Hospital. Health Plan Administrator Sam Hufford met him at the airport. On the return trip, Hufford mentioned to Keene that a senior spokesperson at First National Bank had told him that the bank was very willing to loan money to Kaiser, recognizing an excellent potential customer. "If we ever need any money they'd be willing to talk to us." On hearing Hufford's remark, Keene snapped to attention. "Stop the car," he remembers saying. "Pull over to the side of the road. I want to talk to you about this!" Keene's interest was, well, keen. Bank of America had been KP's major financial source, albeit a reluctant one at times, as hospitals, because of their single-use, were considered a liability should they default. Keene and the surprised Hufford drove directly

to First National Bank, and the talks that day led to major loans. In retrospect, Keene said that the Portland loan set an example for other financial institutions to lend money for expansion. As he recounted that day's events, Keene said with a smile, "I never got to Bess Kaiser [Hospital] that trip."

2. After the final transfer of patients, the Vancouver facility was sold, becoming for a time a psychiatric hospital. Later, it changed hands again to become Rose Vista Nursing Home until its eventual closure in 2002. The structure was demolished in 2005 to make way for a condominium development.

PART III: PEOPLE, POLITICS, AND PARADISE

CHAPTER 5: VIENNA, VLADIVOSTOK, AND VANCOUVER: THE NORBERT FELL STORY

1. Schloss Schonbrunn, with its baroque landscaping, is the oldest zoo in the world and a UNESCO World Heritage Site.

2. The pogrom known as Kristallnacht (The Night of the Broken Glass) that took place November 9-10, 1938, was the result of Propaganda Minister Joseph Goebbels' order to avenge the shooting death of a German diplomat in Paris by a Jewish youth. Nazi sympathizers destroyed 7,550 businesses and homes, destroyed 267 synagogues, murdered 91, and rounded up 26,000 Jews for deportation to concentration camps. Nowhere was the destruction more widespread than in Vienna.

3. Internist Ekhard Ursin joined Permanente in 1960. In 1957, after completing his residency training in Madison, Wisconsin, he returned to his native Austria to work in a small hospital and spa run by a Herr Professor whose distinguished clients came to the spa for mineral waters, mud baths, hydrotherapy, and massage. Ursin's duties included taking admission histories and physicals. One morning a client presented his card with the name Duke von Hohenberg. Since 1918, when Austria became a republic, titles of nobility had been outlawed, and those who continued to trade on their former titles were generally disparaged. In the course of obtaining routine family history, Ursin inquired about the Duke's parental history including cause of death. The Duke took exception to the query, the atmosphere grew tense, and the interview ended awkwardly. The following day, Herr Professor accused Ursin of offending a key patron; Herr Hohenberg was one of the two sons of Archduke Francis Ferdinand, assassinated 43 years earlier in Sarajevo. The Hohenberg name and title had been given to the sons to reflect their mother's lineage and to annul any future claims they might make to the Hapsburg succession.

CHAPTER 6: PARIAHS AND PRESIDENTS

1. Garfield was an AMA member and a member of his local California Medical Society.

2. Proprietary schools, however, with minimal standards and little regulation, continued to flourish.

3. In 1905 the annual meeting of the AMA took place in Portland to coincide with the Lewis and Clark Exposition. Attendance was an estimated 1,700.

4. Pinney, a lieutenant colonel in the U.S. Army Medical Corps during the Korean War, was based in Pusan where he earned the Bronze Star. Pusan is remembered as a turning point in the war where the Allied forces in September 1950 halted the Communists' most significant advance.

5. Brad Davis, Executive Director of the Medical Society of Metropolitan Portland, and others had expressed concern that Aebi's presidency could erode membership. It did not, but neither did it increase membership by Permanente physicians.

6. Bernardo, the son of retired Permanente physician Augusto Bernardo, practices surgery in Salem and is the 2009 President of the Oregon Medical Association.

CHAPTER 7: ISLAND PARADISE

1. After Kaiser's death, his residence was used for various events including President Lyndon Johnson's 1968 meeting with South Korean President Chung Hee Park. Visiting press found accommodation in the air-conditioned dog kennels. But a protest there led by a local KP physician, marred the event. Willis Butler, together with two students, staged an antiwar demonstration featuring an effigy of the President outside Portloch and was promptly arrested for disregarding police orders. Found guilty, Butler was fined $500, but the judgment was reversed by the State Supreme Court in May the following year. Butler had taken previous controversial stands, one two years earlier when he announced his intention to join a group to deliver medical supplies to the North Vietnamese. At that time, amid rumors that Butler's job with KP was in jeopardy, Medical Director Chu had been obliged to issue a statement to the press denying the rumors and vouchsafing Butler's job.

2. Dodge was the first Director of the Rehabilitation Center of Hawaii; Durant, past President of the Honolulu County Medical Society. Yee was past president of the Hawaii Medical Society. Izumi was a former delegate to the AMA.

3. Excerpts from articles by the *Honolulu Star-Bulletin* reveal the heat in the dispute between Kaiser and the physician partners of Pacific Medical Associates (PMA):

August 22: "Changes in Hospital Staff Seen at Kaiser Meeting" quotes unnamed KP physicians: "There is disagreement between PMA regarding working conditions and financial arrangements." "Today's meeting is to air the problem." "If individual doctors don't like the arrangement they can quit."

August 23: "Top Five Doctors to Leave Kaiser Foundation Hospital" reports, "contracts soon to expire" and "the doctors were offered much less attractive terms for any [contract] renewal."

August 24: "Further Conflict Between Doctors and Kaiser" reports "When the doctors came out of the meeting with Kaiser Hospital officials they felt their contracts had been terminated without advance notice or a month to wind up their affairs," "... doctors hired attorney Kenneth Young and held a long meeting to try to find some settlement."

August 26: "Kaiser, Doctors Bare Hospital Row" quotes one PMA spokesperson as follows: "[PMA doctors] are remaining at the hospital and doing their best to carry out normal operations despite continued interference of officials of Kaiser Health Plan." Taking off the gloves, the unidentified official adds, "They have not and will not permit a hospital under their medical control and supervision to be operated as some might operate a cement factory." The response by a Kaiser official bristles with indignation: "The statement from PMA is completely misleading and irresponsibly reckless in every material respect."

August 26: "Kaiser Denies Doctors are Hired Help" offers an explanation by KP spokespersons about its arrangements with physicians. The article quotes PMA attorney Kenneth Young, who makes no effort to conceal his scorn and enmity toward KP: "Clifford Keene, a suitcase executive of Kaiser Health Plan who arrived from California, informed the PMA five doctors that at 12 noon their relationship with Kaiser Foundation Hospital would be terminated and that Dr. Saward, a doctor not licensed to practice medicine in Hawaii ... would be Director of Professional Services at Kaiser Foundation Hospital. Saward called a meeting of the doctor employees and solicited them to join a new Medical Group. ... Kaiser's action is an attempted control and supervision of the practice of medicine by a lay group. In brief, the doctors of PMA are tired of being pushed around by a myth of giganticism."

August 27: "I Won't Pay Doctors $60,000 Each, Angry Kaiser Declares" is followed by another headline revealing Henry Kaiser's willingness to tangle with his adversaries: "Kaiser Charges Doctors Padding."

August 28: "Kaiser Blocked by Doctors' Suit" and "Docs Slam Propaganda, Kaiser Cites Record" reveal the escalating rancor between the two sides.

August 29: "Judge Signs Restraining Order" reports "Circuit Judge William Fairbank signed a restraining order preventing Kaiser from interfering with the practice of medicine by PMA." A second headline reports, "Kaiser Fights Doctors' Restraining Order."

September 1: "Kaiser Winner in Hospital Row" reports, "PMA partners agreed not to treat Kaiser Health Plan patients and to recognize the newly formed Hawaii Permanente Medical Group. They will be allowed to remain in their [Kaiser] offices until September 20."

4. Honolulu-born Phillip Chu got his medical school education during the war years, beginning his studies in Shanghai and earning his MD in the U.S. at the Pennsylvania Medical School. For two years he served as China Regional Medical Officer for the United Nations Relief and Rehabilitation Administration (UNRRA). After his surgical residency he was senior surgeon at U.S. Public Health Service hospitals in Arizona and Detroit. He spent his last years in Honolulu. Attending business on the island of Maui in July 1970, Chu suffered a fatal heart attack and died at age 52.

5. Offered the permanent job of Regional Manager, DeLong declined the job offer and returned to the Northwest.

6. Tung Kwang Lin was Henry Kaiser's personal physician and a daily visitor to his famous patient. At one meeting Kaiser showed his new Cadillac to Lin. Asked what he thought of the purchase, Lin responded that for the price of the car he could have outfitted a cardiac catheterization unit. Two weeks later Lin had the money for the unit. Until that time, all KP medical centers had contracted with non-Kaiser facilities for cardiac catheterizations. The Hawaii Region was the first to bring the service in-house.

7. Anderson began her career with KP in 1966 as Director of Nursing at the KP Oakland Medical Center. That year she authored *Obstetrics for Nurses*. In 1972 she was hired as Assistant Hospital Administrator at the Hawaii Region's hospital. An acknowledged expert in nursing management, Anderson consulted with the Northwest Region in 1980 to help implement team nursing.

8. Dorothea Daniels joined Permanente Hospitals in 1949 as Director of Nursing at the Oakland Hospital and was the first Director of the School of Nursing for Permanente Foundation Hospitals. In 1955 she rose to become the first woman hospital administrator for KP, joining Ray Kay at KP Los Angeles Medical Center in Southern California. Later Barbara Robertson was to blaze a similar trail in the Northwest, hired as the first Nursing Director for Kaiser Sunnyside Medical Center and, in 1978, as the first woman hospital administrator in the Northwest when she took the reigns at KSMC.

PART IV: SPECIALTIES

CHAPTER 8: THE ER AND THE OR

1. The Kaiser Vancouver Shipyard first-aid station resembled today's fully equipped emergicenters. It had 14 treatment rooms—nine for surgical cases and five for medical; a four-stall exam room, an x-ray department, a cast room, a four-booth heliotherapy room, a hydrotherapy room capable of treating eight patients simultaneously, a reception area and a business office. Staff comprised five physicians, 42 nurses, 13 cast technicians, three x-ray technicians and eight nurses' aids. Twenty-one other employees provided services for the various therapies. Two substations for minor injuries or ailments were located elsewhere in the shipyard, staffed by two nurses for each of three shifts. Two ambulances stood ready at all times.

2. Barnhouse resigned from Permanente in 1974 to accept the position of Director of the Emergency Care Department at Meridian Park Hospital in Tualatin, Oregon. In 1977, he was President of the Oregon College of Emergency Physicians. He rejoined Permanente in 1986 as Chief of Urgency Care at KSMC, a post he held until his retirement in 1998.

3. Nursing technician Peg Pemberton enjoyed a long history with KP. During World War II, both her mother, Margaret Campbell Slowik, and her grandmother worked as welders in the shipyard; her father worked there as a pipe fitter. The working parents placed little Peg in the shipyard's day care center. After the war, Peg's mother found work in the nursery of the Northern Permanente Hospital. Fourteen years later, when Bess Kaiser Hospital opened, she transferred to the new hospital's emergency room. Pemberton followed in her mother's footsteps; in 1969 she too, found a position in the Bess Kaiser Hospital emergency room on the 4 p.m. to midnight shift.

4. Violence in Emergency Rooms is not uncommon. The April 2005 issue of *Massachusetts Nurse* reported that "nationally, crimes against nurses and health-care workers are as common as assault of police and correctional officers ... In 2002 more than 4,000 hospital employees were assaulted while working in the emergency centers across the state." A 1988 survey of Emergency Department Directors in 127 teaching hospitals reported that in the preceding five years 43% of those working in an ER reported a physical attack at least once each month; 57% had been threatened by a weapon. The author's own interview with ER security guards at KSMC was aborted because security personnel were called to subdue and handcuff two disruptive young men in the reception area. But according to those who work in the KSMC emergency center, violent incidents at KP Northwest have averaged just three or four a month.

5. Potts was named assistant BK Medical Director in 1980, Assistant Regional Medical Director in 1982, and BK Medical Director in 1985. In 1987 he

was appointed Associate Medical Director of the Ohio Permanente Medical Group and, the following year, Medical Director. He returned to NWP in 1994 where he served as Assistant Regional Medical Director for Quality Management until his retirement in 2005.

6. In 1980 John Johnson replaced John Smillie as physician representative for the KP Medical Care Program in Washington, DC. In that role, Johnson represented the interests of the Permanente Medical Groups to Congress and the Executive Branch agencies.

7. McFarlane completed his residency training at Portland's Good Samaritan Hospital, together with Permanente internist Eberhard Gloekler. From 1968 to 1969 he performed medical ministry work at a Presbyterian Hospital in Iran. Gloekler and McFarlane had remained in contact during McFarlane's absence, and it was Gloekler who alerted McFarlane to an opening in Permanente's Surgery Department. McFarlane applied for the position and received a transcontinental phone call from Hughes offering him the job on the basis of Gloekler's recommendation. At that time a transcontinental phone call was an extraordinary event; 35 years later the memory of that phone call is still vivid to McFarlane.

8. Physician's Assistant Josiah Hill, retired from KP after 23 years of service, died suddenly at age 61 of cardiac arrest as he sat on a bench at NE 15th Avenue and Fremont Street in Portland. The bench now bears his name. Though Hill was a relentless community activist, he was gentle and disarming, rather than confrontational. President of Physicians for Social Responsibility in 1998 and active with the Coalition for Black Men, he helped educate the community about the dangers of lead poisoning in children in low-income and minority communities. He and Rick Bayer, MD, helped establish a free clinic, now named the Josiah Hill Clinic, in Northeast Portland to screen blood levels for children. Former Governor John Kitzhaber declared the day of Hill's memorial service Josiah Hill Day. Mark Kroeker, the city's police chief at the time, recognized Hill's work as co-chairman of the Chief's Forum and as a member of the chief's blue-ribbon panel on racial profiling. The City of Portland formally declared February 21, 2001, Hill's birthday, as Josiah Hill Day.

9. The Scholl College is named for William Scholl, MD, founder in 1912 of the Illinois College of Chiropody; he achieved fame for his Scholls sandals and other foot-care products that bear his name. The terms chiropodist and podiatrist are no longer synonymous; podiatrists undergo more extensive training and have a broader scope of practice.

10. Ironically, Nag's career was cut short after just 12 years when he underwent neurosurgery for a pituitary tumor.

11. Stradley received the first Allied Health Council Award of Excellence in 1985 and again in 1994.

12. Hirohisa Ono was ten years old and less than one and a half miles from the epicenter when the U.S. dropped the atomic bomb on Nagasaki. Moments before the explosion, he was standing outside his home gazing skyward at scattered clouds. He remembers the air raid siren and the sky turning suddenly pink and purple. He remembers little else; he was thrown in the air from the blast and rendered unconscious.

13. Although there are other techniques for treating benign prostatic hypertrophy, transurethral resection of the prostate, or TURP, is considered the gold standard. Its development in the 1920s and 1930s was made possible by several other innovations: the invention of incandescent light, the cystoscope, the fenestrated tube and high-frequency electrical current for resection of tissue. The technique distinguishes urologists from other surgeons.

14. Thomas Joyce, one of the founders of The Portland Clinic and Chairman of the Department of Surgery at Oregon Medical School was puzzling to many in his contradictory stands on issues. A friend to and personal physician of Edgar Kaiser, he nevertheless prevented Kaiser from building the Permanente Foundation Hospital in Portland and restricted Permanente's Portland presence to treating workers' injuries. He persuaded fellow Mayo alumnus, anesthesiologist John Hutton, to head an anesthesia division at the medical school but then did an about-face and advocated for nurses, rather than physicians, to administer anesthesia. In any event, Joyce retained a full-time anesthesiologist, Debra Defaccio Mills, for all his surgeries at St. Vincent Hospital. Oregon Medical School graduate Marjorie Nobel, interviewed for Klein and Kenrick's *The History of Anesthesia in Oregon*, remembered Joyce as domineering and rigidly opinionated. Others, including Haugen, shared her assessment.

15. Membership in the Oregon Society of Anesthesiologists (OSA) required co-membership in the local medical society. This posed an obstacle for Permanente physicians, who, as stated earlier in this history, were excluded from membership in the Multnomah County Medical Society. Thus they were automatically barred from the OSA. Equally restrictive was the American Society of Anesthesiologists, which required as a prerequisite to membership simultaneous affiliation in both county and state societies. Edwards was one of the few Permanente physicians who managed to slip through the discriminatory roadblocks. From his pre-Permanente days he still held his membership in Multnomah County Medical Society. Two others who retained pre-existing Medical Society memberships were radiologist Henry Kavitt and opthalmologist Egon Ullman. Thus, these three, and perhaps a handful of others,

were able to retain memberships in local societies otherwise closed to Permanente physicians. It wasn't until 1963 that the Multnomah Medical Society reversed its discriminatory policy and welcomed Permanente physicians to membership. And ten years later OSA members elected Permanente anesthesiologist Rex Underwood their President.

16. Rex Underwood participated in some memorable pioneering surgeries at the Medical School, including the first cardiopulmonary bypass procedure to repair a child's congenital heart defect. Together with classmate John Roth, he administered anesthetic to conjoined twins, Underwood to one, Roth to the other, so surgeons could separate the twins' shared liver. He took part in the first transplant surgery, an unsuccessful attempt to transfer a baboon's kidney to a human. He participated in the successful kidney transplant between two identical twin girls by Nobel Prize winner Joseph Murray, who traveled from Boston to perform the surgery. Despite these opportunities and the rich training and experience he enjoyed at the Medical School, he found his salary inadequate. He noted that other disciplines, obstetricians, surgeons, and internists, were free to pursue private practices in other facilities. Anesthesiologists, on the other hand, were not allowed this means to supplement their incomes, except after 5p.m. or on weekends. Finally, he objected to a pattern of abuse of anesthesiologists by surgeons.

17. Singh, a graduate of the University of Otago Medical School Dunedin New Zealand, completed his residency at Portland Good Samaritan Hospital and at the Oregon Medical School. In 1985 Singh received the Permanente Distinguished Physician Award.

CHAPTER 9: PEDIATRICIANS, OBSTETRICIANS, AND QUINTS

1. Bradley would later become Professor of Pediatrics at the University of Maryland Medical School in Baltimore.

2. As a pediatric resident, Varga co-authored a nationally recognized book, *Handbook of Pediatric Emergencies*, published by Mosby. Later he took the book through several revisions and reprints, and it became a staple on many pediatricians' bookshelves. Two years after Varga's early death in 1980 Oregon Health and Science University established the annual Charles Varga Memorial Award to recognize the OHSU pediatric resident who best exemplified the spirit of Varga. In announcing the award, Harvey Klevit, Chief of Pediatrics at KSMC and a colleague of Varga, cited Varga's "deep regard for psychosocial, emotional, behavioral, and developmental problems of childhood and adolescence."

3. Whooping cough has reappeared in Oregon, with 187 reported cases in 2002 and 390 in 2003. The rate of pertussis has climbed from 1.81 per 100,000 in 1995 to 17.5 per 100,000 in 2005. Public health officials think the increase may reflect the growing number of exemptions from school immunizations.

4. Blair continues his full-time practice with NWP at its Beaverton Medical Office. In 1993 his son Neil joined the Department of Internal Medicine.

5. In 1984 Massengale, Eleff, and Klevit, all of whom were clinical professors at OHSU, received the school's alumni association Meritorious Achievement Award for "their outstanding contribution to the school of medicine."

6. In 1952 Arthur Roth, MD, started the first teenage medical clinic in the U.S. outside an academic medical center at the KP Oakland Medical Center. In 1960, Roth's book, *The Teenage Years*, published by Doubleday, became the first guide to managing teenage medical problems.

7. In November 1978, the 17-member Board of Directors of the Kaiser Foundation Health Plan and Hospitals met in Portland, where they toured the Region's facilities. At the dinner banquet the last night of the meeting, Vivian Terral, administrator at the Vancouver Medical Office, sat beside Board Member Henry Mead Kaiser, and they discussed the Northern Permanente Foundation Hospital in Vancouver, where Kaiser was born. The Vancouver Medical Office was about to open a new addition, and Terral spontaneously invited Kaiser to attend the opening ceremony. Only later did she discover that mere additions to buildings do not warrant official opening ceremonies. Nevertheless, in January 1980, the medical office hosted an official opening ceremony, and Kaiser and his wife toured the building and visited his birthplace.

8. At Rochester, George had attended a lecture by Allan Dafoe, famous for his 1934 delivery of the Dionne quintuplets.

9. Both Spielman and Sarda would serve long terms as department chiefs. Sarda's tenure of 17 years, from 1983 to 2000, gives him the distinction of longest-serving Chief of Obstetrics and Gynecology to date.

10. At the time of this publication, Stadter continues her work, now at the Salmon Creek Medical Office in Vancouver.

CHAPTER 10: OPHTHALMOTORHINOLARYNGOLOGY

1. Hilbourne was the first optometrist in Oregon to join a Medical Group. Both Hilbourne and Grebstad would go on to enjoy long careers with KP, Hilbourne's tenure spanning 34 years, Grebstad's 37.

2. In phacoemulsification the diseased lens is reduced to a liquid by high-frequency sound waves from a microsurgical instrument inserted through a small

3-mm incision and drained from the eye. The tiny, self-sealing incision promotes wound healing and resumption of normal activities.

3. Higgins became Executive Medical Director in 2007, the first woman within NWP to achieve that position.

4. In 1985 Jeffrey Israel founded the KP Cleft Palate Clinic and introduced a multidisciplinary approach to managing the associated problems of cleft palate. Thirteen disciplines include dentistry, speech therapy, orthodontics, facial plastic surgery, nutrition, social work, psychology, oral surgery, and audiology. Israel and Thomas Albert performed the first surgery in Oregon to correct Pierre-Rob Syndrome, which required breaking the jaw to move it forward.

5. In 2009, William Borok received a Distinguished Physician Award from NWP.

CHAPTER 11: PATHOLOGICAL NEEDS

1. In a frozen-section procedure, the surgeon gives portions of tissue to a pathologist in the operating room who then freezes tissue in a cryostat machine, cuts it with a microtome and, after staining, examines the specimen under the microscope, all within minutes.

2. In 1969 Lehman requested an increase in his monthly per capita payment, from five to eight-and-a-half cents per member per month. He also proposed that his laboratory group provide full-time in-hospital coverage at BK.

3. Holahan would distinguish herself as the first woman to be elected to the NWP Board of Directors, a position she held for six years.

4. Later an FDA audit found no wrongdoing; auditors pointed out that a review of 2,000 informed consents found irregularities in just one percent.

5. In 2000 Jones established and became both President and CEO of JMI Laboratories in North Liberty, Iowa. A multimillion-dollar-a-year operation, the laboratory is the largest of its kind in the country, providing molecular biology services and antimicrobial surveillance, as well as support for biotechnical and pharmaceutical companies in their drug discovery programs.

6. The autoanalyzer relies on a special technique called continuous flow analysis. Other machines that use the same technique include the sequential multiple analyzer (SMA) and SMA with computer (SMAC). These analyses, now automated, previously required a technician to perform them manually.

CHAPTER 12: RADIOLOGY

1. During his long career Rosenbaum held a number of leadership positions, among them Chief of Medicine and President of Holladay Park Hospital, as well as Director of the rheumatology clinic at Oregon Medical School. Though active in the medical establishment and an opponent of Medicare, he never

showed hostility toward Permanente. Indeed it was because of Rosenbaum that Henry Kavitt was able to join the Multnomah County Medical Society after his arrival in Portland. In 1938 Rosenbaum gained fame for his book, *A Taste of My Own Medicine,* wherein he described his experience as a patient with life-threatening illness. The success of his book helped him launch a new career lecturing medical students across the nation on the importance of empathy toward their patients. The 1980 movie *The Doctors,* based on Rosenbaum's book, starred actor William Hurt in the leading role.

CHAPTER 13: INTERNISTS AND MEDICAL SUBSPECIALISTS

1. The term internal medicine comes from the German "innere medizin," to describe the discipline of physicians who, in the 1800s, combined laboratory science with care of patients. American physicians who studied in Germany brought the name, together with the discipline, to the U.S.

2. The AAP continues as an elite organization of academic physicians and scientists with approximately 1,000 members. The ACP, far more inclusive, comprises 124,000 members.

3. During his career with KP, Hooker was active at the Center for Health Research; earned both an MBA and PhD in health policy; and published numerous articles on the role of PAs. He co-authored a widely used text, *Physician Assistants in American Medicine,* in 1997. In 1999 Hooker joined the faculty of the University of Texas Southwestern Medical Center at Dallas as Chief of Health Services Research and Associate Professor of PA studies.

4. In 2007 after 25 years of interviewing thousands of patients with stress-related gastrointestinal symptoms, Clarke published *They Can't Find Anything Wrong!: 7 Keys to Understanding, Treating, and Healing Stress Illness.* During his years of practice, he focused on the relationship between emotional distress and gastrointestinal symptoms, particularly in adults abused as children. He published several papers and gave numerous presentations at local, national, and international meetings; he also directed a monthly clinic for patients with stress-related illness.

5. After leaving Permanente, Blank went on to become Program Director of the Neurology Residency Program and Department Chairman at the Medical College of Pennsylvania. He then became Associate Dean for Medical Education and Affiliated Affairs at the college and continued with an expanded role when the college merged with Hahneman School of Medicine in 1977.

6. Arthur Hayward and George Feldman first met during their freshman year at Yale. It was Feldman who urged Hayward to come to Oregon and to the Oregon Medical School for residency training, and it was Feldman who influenced Hayward to join NWP and the ICU team. Their Yale classmate George W. Bush showed no inclination for medical studies.

7. Today most fellowship training programs in pulmonary medicine include critical care medicine as well. In the late 1970s the specialties of anesthesiology, internal medicine, pediatrics and surgery included critical medicine within their curriculums. But it wasn't until 1985 that the American Board of Medical Specialties formally certified critical care medicine. In 1993 the American Thoracic Society changed the name of its journal to *American Journal of Respiratory and Critical Care Medicine*.

8. When one Kaiser Foundation Health Plan member was hospitalized in The Dalles, a city 60 miles east of Portland, for respiratory distress, a respiratory technician who had previously worked at BK called Vervloet to ask his advice about the appropriateness of bronchoscopy and tracheostomy. The Dalles hospital had no fiberoptic bronchoscope, so Vervloet, a licensed pilot, flew with McFarlane, a nurse, and a bronchoscope to The Dalles. On arrival, they performed the bronchoscopy and then coordinated the patient's return to Portland by ambulance.

9. Chong Lee, board-certified in allergy and immunology, provided services to the Allergy Department. He served as Area Medical Director for KSMC from 1992 to 1997, and was appointed to increasingly responsible administrative positions thereafter.

10. In the summer of 1992, The Scripps Clinic in La Jolla, California initiated what it called the Consolidated Medical Management Team, wherein an internist dedicated to hospitalized patients rotated weekly, directing a team that included a physician assistant and a case-management nurse. The following year the Mid-Atlantic CIGNA Health Care at Baltimore's St. Joseph and Good Samaritan hospitals rolled out a similar program with two full-time internists acting as "designated admitting physicians." In 1994, Park Nicollet Clinic in Minneapolis initiated its hospitalist program with a hybrid system comprising two full-time hospitalists, two rotating internists, and a rotating family practitioner. The hospitalist program for TPMG started at one facility in 1995; by 1999, 16 of the Region's Medical Centers had incorporated hospitalists.

11. McKinsey and Company, with 90 offices in 51 countries, offers consulting services to business and industry.

CHAPTER 14: SPECIALTIES OLD AND NEW

1. Mohs micrographic procedure, developed by Federic Mohs, MD, in the 1930s, treats basal cell and squamous cell cancers of the skin. It involves color coding excised specimens and mapping the area to identify the location of remaining cancer cells. Excised tissue is frozen with a cryostat at the time of surgery and specimens are examined for cancer cells at the edges and under the surface. Any residual cancer cells found using the Mohs map requires removal of additional tissue. The procedure is repeated as necessary.

2. Disciplines included orthopedists Donald Tilson and Robert Corrigan; general surgeon Arthur Denker; emergency physicians Ezra Rabie, Dean Barnhouse, and John A. McDonald; general and family practitioners Alex Carty, Derrick Yoshinaga, Jean Chapman, Timothy Craven, Janet Neuburg, Jock Pribnow, Willis Peacock, Victor Breen; urgency care physicians Curtis Thiessen and Craig Dougan.

3. Certified managed-care organizations (CMOs) are required to provide (1) a panel of providers of sufficient size and diversity to ensure workers' choice of appropriate provider and access; (2) a quality assurance program; (3) a peer-review program; (4) a dispute-resolution program to resolve complaints of workers, employers, medical providers, and insurers; (5) a program to provide early return to work; and (6) a workplace safety and health consultation program. By 2007 only four CMOs, including KP, remained; 13 others had become inactive or been decertified.

4. A graduate of the University of Manitoba Medical School, Thiessen took a job as physician in Heppner, a small town of 1,300 in Eastern Oregon. The following year he joined Portland Providence and the Department of Urgency Care. He joined NWP and its Urgency Care Department in 1988, and transferred to the Occupational Medicine Department in 1997.

5. A subsequent 2001 study published in the *New England Journal of Medicine* did not support Spiegel's earlier finding. It did, however, report quality-of-life benefits, including reduced pain and improved psychological symptoms. Still another study by Spiegel begun in 1991 and reported in 2007, did not duplicate his original findings to show a correlation between counseling and survival. But a subgroup of those patients with an estrogen receptor negative aggressive type of cancer showed a 21-month longer survival when combined with support and education.

6. Izetta Smith, former Program Director at the Dougy Center for Grieving Children and Families, is the author of *A Tiny Boat at Sea: How to Help Children Who Have a Parent Diagnosed with Cancer.*

CHAPTER 15: PSYCHIATRY AND PHYSIATRY:
HEALING THE MIND AND THE BODY

1. Nordstrom received the 1968 "Outstanding Young Men of America" award from the National Junior Chamber of Commerce. The following year he received the "Community Leader of America" award from the National News Publishing Service, Inc.

2. Levine received both a BA and MA in psychology, the BA at NYU and the MA at Columbia University. As well, he held a PhD in clinical psychology and an MA in public health administration and health education, both from the University of California, Berkeley.

3. Biskar, Fuller, and Nordstrom all received their PsyDs from the University of Southern California.

4. After his departure from KP in 1974, Abrams went into private practice as a polygrapher, testifying in more than 400 civil and criminal trials. Among these was the sensational 1976 trial of Patty Hearst, kidnapped heiress-turned-bank robber. Hearst's grandfather was publisher William Randolph Hearst, whose publishing empire was once the largest in the world. In the course of his career, Abrams established a polygraphic school in Oregon, served as President of the Northwest Polygraphic Association and as board member of the American Polygraphic Association. In 1990 he received that association's John E. Reid Award for excellence in teaching, research, and writing.

5. Other departments also provided telephone consultations: orthopedics with the "Bone Phone"; urology with the "Urophone."

6. KP's Center for Health Research began in 1964 as the Medical Care Research Unit of the Kaiser Foundation Hospitals. In 1968 it underwent a name change to Health Services Research Center and, in 1984, it assumed its present name: Center for Health Research.

7. After leaving his administrative position, Noel continued to practice both family and addiction medicine at the KP Longview-Kelso Medical Office in Washington. His decision in 1985 to accept a full-time position in addiction medicine seems ironic, given his earlier decision to devote more time to family practice. His new position was as Medical Director of a state-of-the-art alcohol and drug treatment center at Pomona Valley Community Hospital. With its two physicians and 12 nurses, the facility could treat over 40 inpatients; under Noel's direction the program reached a peak income of four million dollars a year. In 1990, Noel returned to NWP, resuming his former dual roles in both family and addiction medicine.

8. In 1945, the second son of Henry Kaiser developed multiple sclerosis. Kaiser learned about a treatment developed by neurologist Herman Kabat using prostigmine and a program of passive and active exercises. The son responded to the treatment and Kaiser, a devotee of Kabat and his methods, in 1946 established the Kabat-Kaiser Institute in Washington DC. In 1948 the institute relocated to Vallejo, California as a nonprofit charitable institute funded by The Permanente Foundation. The Kabat-Kaiser Institute evolved to become the comprehensive Kaiser Foundation Rehabilitation Center that treated multiple sclerosis, post-traumatic neurological problems, polio, and other neuromuscular disease.

9. Jawurek was a surgeon in Czechoslovakia when Hitler overran that country. Pressed into the Luftwaffe as a physician and glider trainer, he found himself without citizenship after the war and bicycled through Switzerland accepting locums tenens work in small towns. He managed to emigrate to the U.S. in 1972. He joined Permanente one year after Gerhardt at the BK emergency room.

10. Prolotherapy is a method of pain relief in which a hypertonic solution is injected at the site of a ligament sprain or tendon strain. Advocates believe that a "wound-healing cascade" occurs with deposition of new collagen that tightens the ligament, relieving pain.

PART V: ADDITIONAL PERMANENTE PERSUASIONS
CHAPTER 16: SOCIAL CONSCIENCE
OF PERMANENTE HEALTH CARE

1. Cotton Mather (1663-1728), a Puritan minister, was a prolific author and pamphleteer and one of the most influential religious leaders in the colonies. His *Magnalia Christi Americana* included Angelic Conjunction of Skill and the Study of Divinity.

2. Marci Clark's connection with KP predates her career at NWP. Her mother, Vivian Gammon Keppro, worked at the Swan Island Shipyard as a welder during the last year of the war. She recalled with fondness that unusual time, young women working together for a common cause. And she expressed her admiration for the progressive thinking of Henry and Edgar Kaiser, who provided child care for the children of working mothers, including Marci's toddler brother. The "Kaiser bus" picked up mother and son in their St. Johns neighborhood and dropped the little boy at the day care center before transporting Vivian to her nearby worksite.

3. The Employee Retirement Security Act of 1974 established minimum standards for pension plans in private industry, including rules regarding income

tax effects on employee benefits, as well as disclosure of financial information. The Act addressed the need to reform poorly funded pension plans.

PART VI: AFTER THE SIXTIES
CHAPTER 17: THE SEVENTIES

1. Paul Lairson was appointed Associate Medical Director of The Permanente Clinic under Lewis Hughes. In 1975 he accepted the position of Medical Director of the Georgetown University Community Health Plan. In 1978 he helped organize the Kaiser Foundation Health Plan and The Permanente Medical Association of Texas, becoming Medical Director of that program. In yet another move, this time to San Francisco, he was Director of the Permanente Medical Group Interregional Service, acting as liaison between Medical Directors of the various Permanente Medical Groups and the Kaiser Foundation Health Plan. During the course of a distinguished career, he served on numerous state and national committees including the Governor's Task Force on AIDS, the Group Health Association of America Board of Directors, the Board of Medical Examiners for physicians assistants, and Chair of the Board of Directors of On Lok (an organization within San Francisco's Chinese community to care for the frail and elderly).

2. Scott Fleming's career with KP spanned 35 years. In 1951 he joined the Legal Department of Henry J. Kaiser Company and, in 1955, became the company's first full-time attorney. In 1959 he played a major role in convincing the Eisenhower administration that the Federal Employee Health Program should provide choices in plans and should include KP among those choices. In 1970 his work with national health expert Paul Elwood, MD, and others, resulted in the 1973 passage of the HMO Act. In 1971 he joined HEW Secretary Elliot Richardson in Washington, DC for two years as Deputy Assistant Secretary for Health Policy Development. In 1998 he received the Distinguished Service Award from Group Health Association of America for his contribution to the HMO industry.

3. Other members of the task force included F.Y. Peterson; Barbara Robertson, RN, PhD; and Vivian Terral, RN.

4. Falstaff was an annual Permanente scientific meeting and social gathering, usually at the Sunriver Resort near Bend, Oregon or the Inn at Otter Crest on the Oregon Coast.

5. Miles Edwards, MD, head of the division of pulmonology and critical medicine at the University of Oregon Medical School (later Oregon Health Sciences University) from 1963 to 1983, helped establish the Center for Ethics in Health Care in 1989. Great grandson of the founder of the town of Newberg

and of George Fox University, and son of Lowell Edwards, the co-inventor of the Starr-Edwards heart valve, Edwards died in 2006. In 2006 OHSU established the Miles Edwards Chair in Professional and Comfort Care. Retired Permanente pulmonologist Robert Richardson, founder of the inpatient palliative care program at KPNW, was recruited to help develop the new OHSU program.

6. To maintain its tax-free status, KP Hospitals designated 5% of gross income to research, charity, and education. Each Region determined how these community service funds were to be allocated.

7. At KP in Northern California, it was the physicians who resisted incorporating. In 1976 Executive Director Bruce Sams tried to sell the idea of incorporating to the physicians, and a corporation committee met frequently from 1977 to 1979. But in a partnership vote in 1980 only 55% voted in favor, indicating the tepid support by the Medical Group. A second vote in May 1981 garnered 64% approval, and in January 1982 TPMG finally incorporated.

CHAPTER 18: THE EIGHTIES: NEW DIRECTIONS

1. An IPA is an association made up of solo or small-group practitioners who, in addition to maintaining a fee-for-service practice, provide services to an HMO.

2. PPOs are loose-knit organizations in which insurers contract with a limited number of physicians and hospitals who agree to care for patients, usually on a discounted fee-for-service basis.

3. Group Health Cooperative is a consumer-controlled organization governed by a Board of Trustees initially elected by the co-op members. Eventually non co-op members were allowed to vote for trustees, but they still are prohibited from serving on the Board or from voting for changes in the by-laws.

4. Experience rating looks at past utilization of specific groups rather than utilization of an entire community over time. In this way it differs from community rating, which is consistent with philosophies of both KP and Group Health. Market competition has since forced both health care programs to adopt experience rating.

5. Davis had held several positions on the Board of Trustees: Vice President, 1951 and 1952; President, 1953; Trustee, 1954 to 1962; and President, 1962 to 1964.

6. Haugen's son Cameron joined NWP in 1997. He is an obstetrician at the Salmon Creek Medical Office. In 2009 he received NWP's Distinguished Physician Award.

7. Chang came to Portland because of a magazine article that touted Portland, Oregon as the most livable large city in the U.S. Thinking he knew no one in

the Portland area, he was surprised to learn that surgeon George Chang (no relation to Kuo) a fellow student at national Taiwan College of Medicine was a Permanente staff physician. Because George was a more senior student during medical school days, Kuo sometimes referred to George as "uncle."

8. In 1983, a group of Multnomah County Medical Society physicians formed BestCare as a way to avoid losing control to hospitals and insurance companies. In 1986, BestCare affiliated with Healthlink to obtain needed capital; then in 1989 responding to overwhelming financial problems, it consolidated with HMO Blue Cross Blue Shield. In 1985 the Sisters of Providence purchased the first PPO, Vantage, and in 1988, Healthlinks' Caremark Services merged with Good Samaritan's NW Health Inc. to compete with Sisters of Providence's Good Health Plan.

9. Before taking over at PACC, Filosa had headed Good Samaritan's Health Incorporated, Health Affairs-Franciscan Sisters in Chicago, and Physicians Health Plan of Arizona. Among his credentials he had a PhD in Anthropology and was addressed as Dr. Filosa, although he was the first non-MD CEO.

10. At Permanente, Klevit practiced a subspecialty of endocrinology, was Chief of Pediatrics at KSMC, and Assistant Regional Medical Director. During his Permanente career he served on and chaired numerous committees instrumental in defining policies for the Medical Group.

11. The KP Community Fund provides grants to promote health and to improve health care access to the vulnerable, especially to those at risk because of race, gender, and social class.

CHAPTER 19: THE NINETIES

1. KP won the suit.

2. KP members in North Portland never gravitated to KP's presence at Legacy Emanuel in the numbers that were anticipated. After five years, KP quietly closed its little-used obstetrics presence at Emanuel. Not a single voice from community residents rose in opposition to the withdrawal.

AFTERWORD:
WHAT HAPPENED TO THE PIONEERS?

1. In 1949 Garfield hired Weinerman, an internist in the Department of Medicine at Yale and an enthusiast of group medical practice, as Medical Director for the Permanente Foundation Health Plan. He never became a partner in TPMG, however, and he resigned in 1951. In the 1950s McCarthyism cast a pall over political freedoms and fostered fear and suspicion about those who might be suspected of socialist or communist leanings. Some physicians

suspected that Henry Kaiser engineered Weinerman's ouster because of his suspected association with communist organizations. Partners in the Medical Group balked at Kaiser's interference in their affairs, and the event marked the beginning of contentious relations between the Medical Group and Health Plan.

2. Walter Wenkert, hired in 1951 to strengthen the health planning staff for Rochester social agencies, was to play a significant role over the years in the Rochester Health System.

3. Gustav Leinhard enjoyed a distinguished career with Johnson & Johnson, where, starting as an accountant, he rose to become President. The Robert Wood Johnson Foundation gives an annual Gustav O. Leinhard award of $25,000 to recognize outstanding achievement for improving health care in the U.S.

4. Evans Carlson gained fame in World War II as the organizer of an all-volunteer U.S. Marine battalion called Carlson's Raiders, also known as the Gung Ho battalion (Gung Ho is a Chinese term meaning work together). His work as a friend to China had its beginnings in 1937 when, as an intelligence officer in Shanghai, he traveled for two years with the Chinese communist Eighth Route Army to observe their tactics against the Japanese invaders. His battalion used the guerilla methods he had observed. After his retirement from the Marines, Carlson resided in Brightwood, Oregon. His former intelligence role imposed a prohibition against ever discussing his years in China. Charles Grossman provided Carlson's medical care until his death in 1947 at age 51.

5. During the 1854 cholera epidemic in London that killed 500 in the neighborhood of Broad Street Golden Square, physician John Snow visited the neighborhood where he discovered that almost all the deaths had occurred a short distance from the Broad Street water pump. Concluding that the pump was the source of the deadly outbreak, he advised removal of the pump handle and the outbreak subsided. Professors throughout the world tell this story to showcase the power of epidemiological techniques.

APPENDICIES

APPENDIX 1: ORIGINAL PARTNERSHIP MEMBERS, 1949

Ernest Saward

Roger George

Norman Frink

Barney Malbin

Morris Malbin

Frederick Waknitz

Charles Grossman

Harold Cohen

Lucius Button

Egon Ullman

Norbert Fell

Frank Mossman

APPENDIX 2: NORTHERN PERMANENTE MEDICAL STAFF, 1952

According to length of Service

Full Time
Norbert Fell
Ernest Saward
Harold Cohen
Egon Ullman
Norman Frink
Roger George
Frank Mossman
Virginia Gilliland
John Harrah
Robert Reubendale
Henry Kavitt
Edwin Quinn
Amelia Lipton
Theodore Dillman
Frank Sainburg
John Goldsborough

Part Time
Robert Buckinger
Bruce Best
James Causey
Douglas Davidson
R. Kay Hoover
Haynes Sheppard
Lowell Keizur
John D Hough
Curtis MacFarlane
Robert Honodel
Benjamin Herndon
David Hinshaw
Geral Huestis
Cleon Hubbard
George Asbury
Neil Alden

Residents
Claude Gennilard
Augusto Proano

Optometry
Jack Hilbourne

APPENDIX 3:
SPEECH TO THE MEDICAL
SOCIETY OF METROPOLITAN
PORTLAND, 1996

—⚏—

Ernie Aebi, MD, on Induction as President
April 18, 1996

I stand before you tonight as perhaps the only person who has read both of these volumes from cover to cover. (*The History of the Northwest Permanente Group* and the *History of the MCMS*). What that says about me, I'll let you decide. What I saw was two groups of physicians, linked briefly years ago, and only now coming together again with common interests and goals.

In the late 30s and early 40s, a group of physicians got together to figure out how to deliver health care to construction workers and their families at the site of Henry Kaiser's huge construction projects, including the aqueduct from the Colorado River to Los Angeles, the Grand Coulee dam and, during the war, the shipyards in Vancouver and Alameda.

They had none of the society's normal infrastructure for providing care at that time: no wealthy patients to pay for their own hospitalizations, no third party payers, no rich subsidizing the poor and not even county hospitals within access. They conceived of what became known as a health maintenance organization.

A little over 51 years ago—April 4, 1945—Dr. Sidney Garfield, the founder of the California Permanente groups, and Henry Kaiser's brother-in-law spoke to the Multnomah County Medical Association of Portland and outlined the principles of the Permanente groups—these were referred to by Dr. Ernie Saward, the Northwest Region's founder as the "genetic code."

These were:

Prepayment: This was felt to bring the patient to the physician more frequently and earlier in the illness and permit the practice of true preventive medicine. In the early years of the shipyards, a team of doctors and nurses would actually go down to the docks to do multiphasic health examination on the longshoremen.

Group Practice: Garfield believed that medicine was, by nature, a cooperative enterprise and likened it to the medicine that was taught and practiced in the university setting.

Adequate Facilities: Bringing all the facilities under one ownership and one roof allowed the physicians to practice more efficiently.

New Economy of Medicine: This was a reversal of the FFS system. Instead of only the sick paying for themselves, the healthy paid to maintain their own health, and capital coalesced with which to care for the sick.

Dual Choice: They felt that enrollment in the plan should be voluntary, and that an employer should always offer an alternative, or indemnity plan.

Physician Responsibility in Management: The group believed in physician responsibility in management as well as in medical matters. Of course that all had to be worked out with Henry Kaiser!

It still sounds amazingly current, and given how medicine was practiced at the time, I guess you could call it revolutionary.

They applied these principles to their practice and initiated such things as well baby clinics and work site safety inspections.

During the war they pulled in a number of good doctors from the west coast. After the war, most of them left. The Permanente group in Vancouver was down to seven MDs. They began to face the scrutiny and disapproval of the Washington State Medical Association—and not all of it was unearned. Dr. Ernie Saward was hired away from the Hanford Nuclear Reservation where he had set up a medical program for Hanford workers and their families. He found the group in poor shape—with few doctors remaining and a health plan with almost no members. Some of the seven physicians remaining had quality problems, and a few were self-declared Communists who had joined for philosophical reason. The latter won the group support of the Reed College faculty, but did not endear them to mainstream medicine.

They later found that, while they supported the concept of prepaid medicine, the remainder of their ideals were not closely aligned with Henry Kaiser's. Ernie Saward set about dealing with the quality problems and rebuilding the group.

The Washington State Medical Association charged them with the unethical practice of medicine on the basis of practicing medicine for a salary. Dr. Saward was asked to appear before the judicial council of the AMA where the charges were dropped.

Kaiser Permanente's growth didn't really take off until they opened Bess Kaiser Hospital in 1959. Previously they were tied to a small hospital in Vancouver and all the growth was on the Portland side of the river (times change!).

For years the program revolved around its medical centers—first Bess Kaiser, and later the addition of Kaiser Sunnyside. For decades the relationship with the medical association never improved much. In the early 60's, the MCMS rejected en masse, all twenty-two of Permanente's applicants. Though they were eventually accepted, after discussions by the lawyers, hard feelings remained.

Well I am here to say that things change. This was brought home to our group by the pending closure of Bess Kaiser Hospital—our flagship institution has become an aging, expensive building in a world of medicine that is becoming less tied to the inpatient care setting.

Over the years our similarities to our colleagues in the medical community have grown more rapidly than our differences. All of us, by necessity, have learned the economics of health care, and all of us bear the responsibility of delivering the most efficacious care to our patients. And there is no one that I trust more to do so than my fellow physicians do. Ethical controversy will always exist as long as we provide medical services for compensation, but I don't believe, as some do, that physicians will make decisions that will adversely affect their patients because of prepayment, capitation, or any other compensation incentive.

APPENDIX 4:
REFLECTIONS OF
A LAME DUCK, 1975

Lewis E. Hughes, MD

(Presented at Falstaff, September 1975)

For several years this Program has been headed for trouble, and I think most of us now recognize that. It is becoming difficult to live within a marketable dues structure and at the same time membership dissatisfaction is at an all time high. To the extent that the causes of that trouble are within the Program, they are, I submit, to a very substantial degree due to actions of this Medical Group. There has been a "let George do it" attitude in the Group as a whole, abdication of the responsibility to make hard judgments by the Executive Committee, and I must admit, a lack of firm direction, plain talk, and timely decisions by the Medical Director. We have pursued some sort of idyllic utopia where work schedules are relaxed, hours of work are short, vacations are long, all the while expecting that Health Plan will find the wherewithal to provide the help and facilities to rival the big name centers around the country; and by the exercise of "good management" keep it all within a cost range which our blue collar/white collar membership can afford.

Five years ago, the old tyrant went East, and many cheered his going. He was ruthless they said, had little regard for the opinions of his colleagues, cared more for cost control than for quality, put the interest of the Health Plan ahead of the physicians he was supposed to represent. Good riddance.

Welcome to the new leader, one who would listen, who would be fair, who some were kind enough to say had integrity, who would be a friend to all and hurt nobody. Right away, he helped arrange a tidy increase in most drawing accounts, coupled with the guarantee that the substantial additional earnings level we had come to enjoy would be maintained regardless of the Program's results. He tried to accommodate everyone, submitted controversial decisions to the Executive Committee, pretty much went along with its verdicts, whether his own best judgment agreed or not.

The Executive Committee enthusiastically set about making things right for the doctors, in fact spent most of its time making things right for the doctors. Vacations were lengthened, compensatory time was liberalized, release outpatient time was granted for numerous non-outpatient department activities, moonlighters were hired to relieve us of onerous night call duties. The Medical Director did question the wisdom of some of these moves, but not very loudly, and the goodies continued to flow.

Democracy ruled supreme, everyone could have his say, and almost everyone could have his way. When something didn't work out right, and work out right now, that was said to be the fault of the Health Plan - too many members enrolled, vital facts hidden, mismanagement. When the Medical Director's objections were heard, it was easy for some to see that he was becoming a puppet of the Health Plan and was now mainly interested in advancing Health Plan schemes, often to the detriment of his colleagues' interests.

Meanwhile, for some reason, Health Plan's cash position was deteriorating, slowly at first and nothing to be alarmed about. Our spectacular history of success assured us that we were good, that Health Plan could always find enough to pay us whatever we decided they should pay, as they had for as long as most of us could remember.

When the word was spread, a year-and-a-half ago, that Health Plan's preliminary forecast showed an alarming slippage in earnings potential for the Program, the concern rally wasn't for the Program's health, but that Health Plan would want us to help to do something about it. The picture improved for a time, giving rise to comments about manipulation of figures to give an illusion of a problem, and thus manipulate us. Then came the rapid deterioration of a year ago. By now, it was pretty clear that there was really a problem. The response of many seemed to be, "So what, it's Health Plan's problem. After all, that sort of thing has to be due to mismanagement. There must be a lot of fat at Crown Plaza to get six million dollars in the red, so they should tighten up over there."

No doubt, Health Plan agreed that they should tighten up at Crown Plaza, but that was hardly going to take care of the whole problem, since the entire budget for Crown Plaza wasn't equal to half the deficit. They did strive mightily, laying off some, reducing salaries of others, reducing the hours of still others, but in no way could that six percent of the organization make a very big dent in the shortage. So it turns out that if you need to find a lot of money, you need to look where the money is, and in this program, the money is in Hospital operations and medical services.

There wasn't much fat in the hospital. Many of you already felt that Peter August's efficiency experts had stretched Bess Kaiser too thin. What with trying to hang on until Sunnyside opened, she really had no slack. There just wasn't any way that medical services and clinic operations could be spared if any kind of a solution was going to happen.

I am sure that some still doubt that what was done to the physicians and the clinic personnel had to be done, still questioning the ability of the Medical Group to do much about the financial results, feeling that we physicians take care of the patients, the administrators take care of the money, so it's up to them to take care of the money problems.

Well I beg to differ, and I propose to tell you why.

I'm going to talk about several of the items in the expense section of the monthly financial report from the standpoint of how physicians influence costs, whether they realize it or not. With the exception of Crown Plaza, Dentistry, and our Community Service Program, this physician's group, individually or collectively, or both, has a profound impact on all of those expenses.

The first item is Hospital Operations Costs, and that means both the cost of running our own hospital and the costs of services necessarily referred elsewhere. It's the administrator's job to run the hospital efficiently, but he's not always in a position to do it strictly on a cost effectiveness basis. His decisions have a way of being affected by the want lists of the Medical Staff. In addition, he is quite unable to control the utilization of the hospital. In this regard, I can only say that I wish we did half as well in our control of other cost centers as we do in hospital utilization. Utilization control has long been magnificent, thanks to a dedicated Utilization Committee, and the cooperation of the staff. And that's exactly the point; physicians do have a profound influence on the costs of the hospital. The costs of the hospital represent a quarter of our entire operational costs.

Moving on, the next line says Medical Services. That's us, and it represents almost another quarter of Program expenses in physician income and retirement costs. Not much doubt about whose responsibility that is.

Next, we have Clinic Operations; in other words, the non-physician costs of staffing and running our outpatient clinics. In this area Health Plan helps with things like hiring and firing and getting the toilets scrubbed, but the decisions that cause them to spend more money or less money are almost all made by physicians. If Medical Group says, "get another nurse," they get another nurse. Lab, Pharmacy, x-ray are obviously there because doctors are going to decide that this patient needs that service. It's also up to us to decide how many physicians' assistants and nurse practitioners and other allied health types will be used. All that accounts for yet another quarter of the expense, and it's almost entirely ours to control, even though we don't pay the bill.

It turns out then that we either spend or direct the spending of half of the operation's expense money, Health Plan spends about 15 percent, and the responsibility for the other 35 percent is about evenly split between us; or to summarize it, the Medical Group controls the spending of two-thirds, administration one-third.

I know that it's kind of obscene to bring money into patient care decisions, but I suggest that it's equally obscene to have folks forced to drop the Health Plan because they just can't afford it anymore, and that obviously will happen if expenses, and therefore dues, get too high. I think we can accomplish a lot of economy without depriving them of essential ingredients of care.

I don't think there's much question that high dues are the surest way to drive away many members and potential members, but bad service is a good way too, particularly if dues aren't much cheaper than the competition. We've had service problems for a long time. We couldn't be proud of it, but as long as our dues were a lot cheaper, we could get away with it. Those days are past, or passing. Pride and concern for our reputation should be reason enough for sprucing up our services, but health and survival of the Program make a pretty good additional reason.

We used to say that our service problem was short staffing, pure and simple. After all, we had 1 physician for 1300 or 1400 members; other similar programs had about 1 to 1000. So we increased our staff by 30 percent, and that alone probably increased the members' dues by at least 3 million dollars per year. And what did they get for that money? Apparently nothing. They keep saying that something is wrong when they still wait 6 weeks or more for an appointment unless they get pushy. They are filing complaints at 3 times the rate they did 3 years ago. Maybe you think they're just making more visits now, thus using up all those new doctors. Not so. Only 1 of the years since 1969 had less visits per member than has 1975. So they're using no more services, we're using a third more doctors, and they wait as long as ever and are certainly more dissatisfied.

We hear quite a number of excuses for this. I've even heard that some think it might be due to a decrease in physician productivity. More comfortable, however, seem to be the theories related to increased administrative time, greater time necessary for special procedures and subspecialty consultations; in other words, an increase in technology. I checked into this a bit. Percentage wise, administrative time never did amount to much, and percentage wise it hasn't changed much, even though our friendly legislators have given us all sorts of added chores, such as P.S.R.O. Increase in O.R. time is less than the staff increase. All the time set aside from clinic for special procedures and consultations takes the equivalent of 1 or 2 physicians. So all of those things required 4 to 6 physicians, but just to change the ratio we added over 40. Maybe today's disease or today's technology needs more time, but my hunch is that most of your time is still spent with the same old trivia that filled our days 10 or 20 years ago and needs about the same amount of your attention. What I'm saying is, the explanation for this apparent decrease in productivity is probably a decrease in productivity.

Looking back to the days when we had staffing ratios of 1:1600 or 1:1300, it did make sense to increase the staffing, but increasing by 30 percent and improving the service not at all is a disgrace. I've heard from physicians a lot of comments, complaints, accusations relating to this state of affairs in the Oregon Region, most of them blaming the Health Plan, Hospital Administration, and Clinic Administration. Those can certainly be assigned a share. It is, however, time for the Medical Group to realize that some of the responsibility, and indeed a hell of a lot of that responsibility, belongs to us. If the physicians of this Group, either collectively or individually, control two-thirds of the spending, and almost totally direct the delivery of ambulatory services, it seems quite clear that there is no way the financial problems and the service problems we now face will ever be solved by our partners in administration unless we too, and each of us, take a very active part.

Every department that is not grossly understaffed, and I recognize only one or two in that category now, needs to figure out a way to get things cleaned up and keep them that way. The patient who thinks he's sick shouldn't have to worry about it for 5 or 6 weeks, whether he feels all that bad or not. You've probably heard the term "worried well," and some of these patients will, in fact, be well, but they've paid their money and they deserve to be reassured. I am sure many expect more well care than they need, but the media pushed it and we promised it, so we'd better deliver or find a way to educate them away from it; otherwise, our name is mud. Six weeks is too long to wait, even for physicals or pap smears.

Quite a few of the members are also turned off considerably by what happens after they finally get in. Most of them don't presume to judge the quality of their medical care, but they do presume to judge whether an encounter with the system was a satisfying encounter or not. Both as patients and as members, they deserve to be satisfied if they're not totally unreasonable. Most of them are not totally unreasonable, and most of their complaints of lack of satisfaction with their visit have some reasonable basis. It is reasonable for patients to expect that they will not have to sit in the waiting room for long periods of time on most of their visits. They will understand if occasionally things are delayed; they will not understand if it happens more or less routinely. It is reasonable for the patients to expect courteous attention, whether it is by the receptionist, or by the nurse, or by the doctor. It is reasonable for patients to expect that personnel show interest. They kind of think that the purpose of those personnel is to take care of them. It is reasonable for patients to expect that they will receive an explanation of the results of their visits, and candid answers to their questions. There may be some who wish to be told nothing, but a frequent complaint from patients is that they want to be told something and are told nothing. Granted, some of those were told and paid no attention, but I'm sure there are also some who weren't told. No doubt, in our business, we have exceptions to the old businessman's rule, "The customer is always right," but if we expect to retain their loyalty and their enthusiasm for this Program, we had jolly well better find ways to make our members more satisfied than they are now, and keep them that way.

Okay, so what now? Can I expect that now that I have scolded you, you will all return to your respective offices with high purpose and firm resolve to set everything right and forthwith do so? Obviously, it takes more than a scolding. It also takes more management and better management, and I mean Medical Group management. A carrot here, a stick there, a set of guidelines laid down so that you understand what specifically is expected of you and firm managerial direction to obtain compliance.

I fully realize that there have been numerous deficiencies in the Medical Group management during my administration. I understood from the beginning that you can't please everybody, but then set out to find a way to please everybody. I understood the principle that getting decisions made in a timely manner, even if the decision is sometimes wrong, is better than no decision while agonizing over the proper course, but I still agonized and delayed, trying to be sure. As the pressures built, it should have been obvious that some delegation was necessary, but I put that off too. As a result, things that needed to be done were either delayed or didn't get done at all. Running a successful business requires discipline, hard-nosed cost consciousness and a willingness at times to subordinate the desires and perhaps even the needs of individuals to the hard realities of making the business run in a competitive world.

I have no idea how long it will be until a new Medical Director is chosen. The duties of the office cannot be put in limbo until that time, however, particularly under the present circumstances. Having recognized the needs as discussed above, it is incumbent upon me to make some changes in that interim. Provision for the delegation of some duties has already been made. Dr. Nomura has been appointed Associate Medical Director At Large, working on a number of needed Medical Group projects. Doctors Senft and Hurtado have been appointed as Associate Medical Directors to be in charge of the two Medical Centers and provide a much-needed liaison with Administration and direction of the operations within those Centers.

As for myself, the greatest need is probably a change of style, and I intend to effect that. If I succeed, you probably won't like it. Decisions will be made more quickly and no doubt more arbitrarily. Special privileges, such as vacations on short notice, may well be challenged. Proposals will be made which will mean more work, less goodies. I intend to advocate that outstanding performance be rewarded and substandard performance penalized. That sort of thing will produce some anguish, since its administration will necessarily be arbitrary. Most successful businesses, however, do make provision for recognition of merit. It may be impossible to administer it with total fairness, but it is far more unfair to simply ignore exceptional performance. I will expect to exert the administrative prerogatives of the office of the Medical Director as long as I hold that office and will ask the Executive Committee and the Partnership to respect those prerogatives. As the policy-making body of The Permanente Clinic, I will expect the Executive Committee to direct its attentions first towards those decisions which build strength in the Program and second to the personal amenities for the members of the Group.

Much has been said about achieving better communications. You will see more of me in the clinics, and you will hear more of me through the mail. Communication, however, is a two way process and quite frankly, your communications to me have been just as lousy as mine to you. I'm perfectly willing to talk with anyone, and you don't have to wait for me to come around, although I hope those occasions will evoke useful conversations. I am, however, also available by telephone or interoffice mail. Since I can't please everyone, I'm not suggesting that I necessarily will go along with your pet schemes or peeves, but I'd still like to hear about them.

Some of the above make it sound that I intend to be less democratic than in the past. I do. I'm afraid I have lost faith in democracy as a means of governance of what is essentially a business organization. A successful large business operation is almost invariably an autocracy, although hopefully having enough built-in checks to prevent it from becoming a tyranny. Certainly equity, fairness and precision are necessary goals, but the interminable delays in decision making should not be regularly accepted as a price for achieving such goals.

This change in style will not be easy for me, and I suspect it will not be easy for many of you. I am absolutely convinced that this kind of change is necessary, whether it is accomplished by me or by my successor, and that it will be just as painful if it waits for him.

Despite the problems we all recognize, I think our Program has done quite well. Despite our imperfections, I think we have made available to our members better health care by far than most of them would otherwise have been able to obtain. There are plenty of barriers and frustrations in the fee-for-service world, too. Unfortunately, for our image, the patient tends to see the fee barrier as his own problem, but to see an appointment barrier as a problem of the Program. Certainly the challenges are greater than 15 years ago. Competition is sharper, particularly in the area of hospital utilization, expanding technology threatens to overwhelm our ability to maintain acceptable cost levels while continuing to provide comprehensive care, our very size obscures our own incentives and make it difficult for us to view clearly the relationship between productivity and reward. I think these problems are manageable, and I think we can do better.

There are a lot of things going for us. There has, as all of you are aware, been a great public recognition of the benefits of a prepaid group practice type of program. Almost all of the national health insurance programs, which have been proposed in the Congress, recognize and make provision for this alternative method of delivery of care. It is now recognized in the Medicare legislation, and the Health Maintenance Act of 1973 was a specific effort of Congress to stimulate the growth of the prepaid group practice type of programs.

Programs such as ours have the capacity not only to improve the health care of the population but also to provide a satisfactory professional/personal life for the provider. They are not utopia and won't provide all things for all people. They can organize a better way to do the work, but the work still has to be done. They can hope to reduce costs, but whatever services are delivered will cost, then these costs must be borne. As the

Program component most responsible for decisions affecting cost and services, physicians are the key to the whole operation. Lay administration can expedite, but unless the physicians, and each of them, are willing to accept responsibility for taking positive action to make the Program work, it will not function well and could eventually fail. That would be a tragedy, not only for ourselves but also for the community. If we utilize appropriately and fully our talent and energy, we can achieve precisely the opposite: a Program which is widely regarded as a model of quality care at a reasonable cost.

APPENDIX 5:
NORTHWEST PERMANENTE
EXECUTIVE MEDICAL
DIRECTORS

J. Wallace Neighbor, MD
1943-1948

Ernest Saward, MD
1948-1969

Lewis Hughes, MD
1969-1976

Marvin Goldberg, MD
1976-1985

Fred Nomura, MD
1985-1992

Allan Weiland, MD
1993-2004

Andrew Lum, MD
2005-2007

Sharon Higgins, MD
2007-

APPENDIX 6:
NORTHWEST PERMANENTE
DISTINGUISHED PHYSICIANS

1979

John A. Grover, MD
Ronald Jones, MD
William R. Knox, MD
Albert C. Martin, MD
Clarence L. Morgan, MD
Charles J. Zerzan, MD

1980

H. Raymond Blair, MD
Robert H. Blomquist, MD
John C. Bondurant, MD
Richard C. Cohen, MD
Robert L. Miller, MD
Richard A. Romaine, MD

1981

Stephen Adelman, MD
Susan E. Cox, MD
Virginia M. Feldman, MD
Thomas Morris, MD
Martin L. Schwartz, MD

1982

Norman I. Birndorf, MD
Harold R. Cohen, MD
Arthur D. Hayward, MD
Sharon M. Higgins, MD
James N. Powell, MD

1983

David D. Long, MD
John A. Pearson, MD
Henrik P. Porter, MD
Jerry M. Slepack, MD
Ekhard K. Ursin, MD

1984

Eric E. Brody, MD
Lenora B. Dantas, MD
J. Thomas Leimert, MD
Stephen F. Lieberman, MD
Gunnar A. Waage, MD
Roger A. Wicklund, MD

1985

Charles W. Emerick, MD
Joseph A. Kane, MD
Robert Lawrence, MD
Ian C. MacMillan, MD
David L. Moiel, MD
Bhawar Singh, MD
David L. Tilford, MD

1986

Nathan K. Blank, MD
Thomas C. Carey, MD
Paul C. Droukas, MD
Luis E. Halpert, MD
Michael Lewis, MD
Leslie R. Naman, MD
Jacob A. Reiss, MD
Perry R. Sloop, MD

1987

Ferenc F. Gabor, MD
Jerry E. King, MD
Stuart L. Oken, MD
Robert H. Richardson, MD
Edward H. Stark, MD

1988

William K. Harris, MD
Jeffrey M. Israel, MD
John H. Nelson, MD
John J. Thompson, MD
Maximo C. Yao, MD

1989

Kuo C. Chang, MD
George W. Feldman, MD
Harvey D. Klevit, MD
Karen Leider, MD
James R. Loch, MD
Thomas R. Syltebo, MD

1990

David D. Clarke, MD
Harry S. Glauber, MD
Michael A. Krall, MD
Alan Rosenfeld, MD
David R. Scott, MD
Mark L. Tochen, MD

1991

Michael R. Blahnik, MD
Andrew G. Glass, MD
Joseph W. Kaempf, MD
Kadavil R. Satyanarayan, MD
Matthew H. Zukowski, MD

1992

Eldon D. Andersen, MD
Alvin R. Graham, MD
Manuel D. Karlin, MD
William R. Nelson, MD
David S. Weil, MD

1993

Maurice J. Comeau, MD
Richard E. Grazer, MD
Calvin Y. Leong, MD
Barbara Manildi, MD
Ronald S. Sklar, MD

1994

Richard W. Bills, MD
Scott I. Feuer, MD
David W. Hill, MD
Kathleen P. Holahan, MD
Robert A. McFarlane, MD

1995

Thomas A. Hickey, MD
Fred M. Nomura, MD
Jayant M. Patel, MD
Mary A. Shepard, MD
Mian M. Tahir, MD

1996

Kathryn S. Evers, MD

Christopher P. Nelson, MD

Maty T. Rhatsad, MD

Angelito C. Saqueton, MD

Terry R. Williams, MD

1997

Michael J. Barrett, MD

Robert W. House, MD

Jeffrey S. Liebo, MD

Gregory L. Swift, MD

David Zeps, MD

1998

Lawrence A. Dworkin, MD

Susan M. Kauffman, MD

James D. Norris, MD

Mary Lynn O'Brien, MD

Richard W. Steinberg, MD

Maureen A. Wright, MD

1999

Stephen R. Bachhuber, MD

Marianne Dwyer, MD

Diana Habrich, MD

Paul O. Jacobs, MD

Sean E. Jones, MD

Jeremy K. Ota, MD

Robert J. Shneidman, MD

Donna D. Strain, MD

2000

Kendall H. Barker, MD

Martha L. Brooks, MD

Larry P. Cooper, MD

Alida N. Rol, MD

Margaret S. Vandenbark, MD

R. Edwin Wright, MD

2001

Mark A. Kleinman, MD

Susan C. Laing, MD

Thomas A. Lorence, MD

George R. Oh, MD

Daniel M. Rappaport, MD

Betty E. Reiss, MD

Robert T. Speirs, MD

2002

Beryl M. Burns, MD

Edwin K. Chinn, MD

Keith H. Griffin, MD

Thomas D. Harburg, MD

Keith B. Riley, MD

Scott A. Weaver, MD

2003

Homer L. Chin, MD

Mary Jo Clarke, MD

Wayne F. Gilbert, MD

Michael K. Herson, MD

Linda Lorenz, MD

Melanie M. Plaut, MD

Bradley J. Roemeling, MD

Steven M. Sandor, MD

2004

Aaron L. Angel, MD

Edward A. Chasteney, MD

Colleen S.Y. Chun, MD

Antonio A. Daniels, MD

Marcia J. Dunham, MD

Byron W. Hanson, MD

Mark R. Hurt, MD

Neil R. Olson, MD

2005

Mary L. Knox, MD
Rasjad K. Lints, MD
Brian J. Markey, MD
Michael P. McNamara, MD
Stephen E. Renwick, MD
Alden W. Roberts, MD
David M. Schmidt, MD
David W. Westrup, MD
Richard W. Wise, MD
John T. Woo, MD

2006

Wiley V. Chan, MD
Elizabeth A. Frederick-Ragsdale, MD
Leila M. Hotaki, MD
Anthony I. Kostiner, MD
Steven E. Laxson, DPM
Janet M. Leigh, MD
Scott H. Mandel, MD
David P. Parsons, MD
Deborah A. Sailler, MD
Richard Strauss, MD
William A. Ward, MD
James B. Wentzien, MD

2007

Christine Choo, MD
Dieter F. Hoffmann, MD
Peter M. Krook, MD
Joyce C. Liu, MD
Luanne B. Nilsen, MD
Cara N. Steinkeler, MD
Robert S. Unitan, MD
Masatoshi Yamanaka, MD

2008

Richard R. Beam, MD
David L. Boardman, MD
Stella M. Dantas, MD
Ronald D. Jaecks, MD
Daniel A. Ladizinsky, MD
Albert Luh, MD
Michelle L. Ritter, MD
John R. Steeh, DO

2009

Diana Antoniskis, MD
Jennifer Bard, MD
Marcia Bechtold, MD
Bill Borok, MD
Cameron Haugen, MD
Cynthia McPhee, MD
Atanu Prasad, MD
Andrew Zigman, MD

APPENDIX 7:
NORTHWEST PERMANENTE
MEDICAL FAMILIES

George Barton, MD, and son Lane Barton, MD

Raymond Blair, MD, and son Neil Blair, MD

Mark Butzer MD, and daughter Michele Ruby, MD

Husband and wife Robert Buys, MD, and Susan Buys, MD

Harold Cohen, MD,* and daughter Vicki Cohen, CNM

Changshee "George" Chang, MD, and son Naun Chang, MD

Lenora Dantas, MD, and daughter Stella Dantas, MD

Husband and wife Terry Morrow, MD, and Peggy Eurman, MD

Husband and wife George Feldman, MD, and Virginia Feldman, MD

Husband and wife Peter Feldman, MD, and Donna Strain, MD

Husband and wife Steven Forrest, MD, and Laurie Forrest, MD

Arnold Hurtado, MD, and daughter Laurie Hurtado, MD

Anthony Kostiner, MD, and daughter Dana Kostiner, MD

Noah Krall, MD,* and son Michael Krall, MD

Husband and wife William Wojeski, MD, and Karen Leider, MD

Husband and wife John Linman, MD, and Sally Linman, MD

Ian MacMillan, MD, wife Shirley MacMillan, RN, NP, and son Brian MacMillan, OD

Charles Pinney, MD,* and Tanner Pinney, MD

James Powell, MD, and daughter Lisa Powell-Els, MD

Husband and wife Jacob Reiss, MD, and Betty Reiss, MD

Angelito Saqueton, MD, and daughter Cecilia Saqueton, OD

Husband and wife Richard Strauss, MD, and Karen Franz, RN, NP

Husband and wife John Thompson, MD, and Catherine Thompson, MD

*deceased

SOURCES

INTRODUCTION

PART I: A LENGTHY PROLOGUE

CHAPTER 1: THE ROOTS

Smillie, John G. The story of the Permanente Medical Group. Oakland, CA: The Permanente Federation; 1996.

Gilford, Steve. On This Date in KP History #133: Return to Desert Center.

Gilford, Steve. On This Date in KP History #265: Garfield as a Surgeon.

Gilford, Steve. On This Date in KP History #304, #305 Young Sidney Garfield: Part 4.

Lewis Weeks interview with Sidney Garfield. Hospital Administration Oral History Collection: Lewis E Weeks Series. American Hospital Association; 1986.

Gilford, Steve. On This Date in KP History #342: Garfield Centennial Year: First he was a Surgeon.

Inside KP Northwest: Quints birth forges lifelong link with delivering doctor. Portland, OR: NW History; 2003.

Gilford, Steve. Blasts From the Past 1996;I(7).

Gilford, Steve. The road from Desert Center Video; KP Audiovisual Center Steve Gilford.

Communication from Steve Gilford, April 2002.

Stewart, Walter. The life and political times of Tommy Douglas. Toronto, Canada: McArthur and Co; 2003.

Starr, Paul. The social transformation of American medicine. New York: Basic Books; 1982.

75th Finnish Hall Anniversary Program, April 1985.

Author interview with Merle Reinikka, President United Finnish Kaleva Brothers and Sisters Lodge #23, 2004 June.

Heltzel EE. Finn Hall's history often turbulent. The Oregonian 1979 April 28; p B1.

History of Portland UFKB and S Lodge #23: translation from Finnish; Grand Lodge History Committee.

Town Hall—Then and Now. The Pulse 1979 Oct;8(10).

Press release: Finnish group return to historic Portland landmark. Portland: OR, Kaiser Permanente Northwest Department of Public Affairs; 1991 Apr 3.

Cutting, Cecil. An oral history of KP medical program Vol. IV. Berkeley, CA: Bancroft Library; 1986.

Author interview with Cecil Cutting, June 2003.

Spitzer, Paul C. Grand Coulee: harnessing a dream. Pullman, WA: WSU Press; 1994.

Foster Mark S. Henry J Kaiser: builder in the modern American West. Austin, TX: University of Texas Press; 1989.

Interview with Wallace Neighbor, Sept 20, 1974. TPMG Archives.

Hendricks, Rickey. A model for national health care: The history of KP. New Brunswick, NJ: Rutgers University Press; 1993.

Author interview with Becky Kaiser, August 2005

Gilford, Steve. Inside KP: KP days of yesterday in the wild west.

Robins George M. History of the Multnomah County Medical Society: 1884-1954.

The Oregonian. September 19 1935.

Cleland John GP. Essentials of an industrial health program. NW Medicine 1956 Sep;44:973-4.

The Oregonian. July 19, 1935.

Cleland John GP. The history of medical care in Clackamas County. 1976 May.

Author interview with Janet Hochstatter, June 2006.

Author interview with John Cleland, July 2006.

Author interview with Paul Brown, July 2006.

The Scribe. March 1988.

The Scribe. Vol. XII # 6 1995.

The Scribe. June and Nov 1997.

The Scribe. Mar, Aug 1998.

The Oregonian. April 15, 1993.

Noehren W. A proposal concerning prepayment medical care. J Pediatr 1947 Dec;31(6):704-9.

What is the Clackamas County plan? The Bulletin: MCMS 1962;SVII(4).

Resolution 16, House of Delegates. Chicago, IL: American Medical Association; 1961.

Correspondence: Clackamas County Plan. N Engl J Med 1961 Nov 23.

The Oregonian. June 25, 1962.

Noehren WA. Briefs Plan. The Sandy Post 1962 May 10. p 3.

Noehren Walter, Hegrenes Jack Jr. Medical care of everyman. Report to the American Medical Association. 1962 May 15.

PACC Report to the State of Oregon Consumers and Business Services. 1995 Sep 28.

Crowley Walt. To serve the greatest number. Seattle, WA: University of Washington Press; 1996.

Glickstein D. Group Health Cooperative of Puget Sound—A short history. Perm J 1998 Spring;2(2):60-1.

39 Wh2d586 GHC appellant vs King County Medical Society Medical Society, et al. November 15, 1951.

Rhodes, Richard. The making of the atomic bomb. New York: Simon and Schuster; 1986.

Wells, H.G. The world set free. London: MacMillan & Co; 1914.

Libby, Marshal. The uranium people. New York: Charles Scribner and Sons; 1979.

Author interview with Lady Elizabeth Saward, April 2003.

Author conversations with Ernest Saward, 1962.

MacKenzie GM. Experiment in collective medical service; JAMA 1932 July 9;99.

Noehren, Walter A. Psychiatry I Hanford. Am J Psychiatry 1946 Sept.

Smillie interview with Ernest Saward, June 2, 1982.

Hawn, Clinton VanZandt. History of Mary Imogene Bassett Hospital [monograph on the Internet]; excerpted from The Mary Imogene Bassett Hospital. Cooperstown, NY: Bassett Healthcare Network; 2010 Mar 17 [cited 2010 Mar 17]. Available from: www.bassett.org/history.cfm.

Lewis Weeks interview with Sidney Garfield. Hospital Administration Oral History Collection: Lewis E Weeks Series. American Hospital Association; 1987.

Saward interview. University of Rochester Medical School; August 7, 1985.

Sanger, SL. Working on the bomb: an oral history of WW II: Hanford. Portland, OR: Continuing Education Press, Portland State University; 1995.

Stannard, J Newell, editor. Radiology and health, a history. Interview with Stafford Warren. Springfield, VA: Office of Scientific and Technical Information; 1988.

Merceau, Thomas E. Historic Overview: History of the plutonium production facilities at the Hanford site. Washington, DC: U.S. Dept of Energy; 2002 June.

Freer Brian. Worker health and safety: History of the plutonium production facilities at the Hanford site. Washington, DC: U.S. Dept of Energy; 2002 June.

Richlander Villager. April 12, 1945.

Gerber, Michele. On the Home Front. Lincoln, NE and London: University of Nebraska Press; 1992.

Hevly, Bruce and Finley, John M, editors. The atomic west. Seattle, WA: University of Washington Press; 1998.

Groves, General Leslie. Now it can be told. New York: DaCapo Press; 1962.

Diary of Col. Frank T. Mathias. 1942 Nov -1945 Aug.

Hanford Engineer Works monthly reports May June July Oct Nov 1944.

Correspondence with W.K. MacCready, Richland resident, January 24, 2004.

Correspondence with Hope S. Amacker, Richland resident, January 20, 2004.

Author interview with Roger Rohrbacher, engineer retired from Hanford Works.

Greenlick M, Garber Seth. History of the NW Region: Dr Ernest Saward story [video]. Portland, OR: Kaiser Permanente Northwest Department of Public Affairs; 1990.

Mull, Robert W. Something to win the war: The Hanford diary [video]; 1991.

PART II: THE EARLY DECADES
CHAPTER 2: WARTIMES 1941-1945

Bunker, John Gorley. Liberty ships: the ugly ducklings. Annapolis, MD: Naval Institute Press; 1972.

Foster, Mark S. Henry J Kaiser: builder in the modern American West. Austin, TX: University of Texas Press; 1989.

Author interview with Hank Harrison, WWII Merchant Seaman, 2006.

Benedetto, William R. Sailing into the abyss. New York: Citadel Press; 2007.

Smillie, John G. The story of the Permanente Medical Group. Oakland, CA: The Permanente Federation; 1996.

Heines, Albert P. Henry J. Kaiser: American empire builder. New York: Peter Lang; 1953.

Maben, Manley. Vanport. Portland, OR: Oregon Historical Society Press; 1987.

Jallotta, Pat. Downtown Vancouver. Chicago, IL: Arcadia Press; 2004.

Housing in war and peace. Vancouver, WA: City of Vancouver Housing Authority; 1972.

Imagining home: Stories of Columbia Villa [video]. Portland, OR: Hare in the Gate Productions; 2005.

Stories told at shipyard workers reunion at Dept of Defense End of WW II 60 Year Commemoration. Vancouver, WA; 2005.

Portland Observer. March 16, 1966.

The Oregonian. July 14, 1966.

Gilford, Steve. On This Day In KP History #255: HJK's creative shipbuilding: the USS Alazon Bay.

Kaiser Company Group Sickness and Accident Insurance Plan brochure, 1942.

Author interview with Morris Collen, April 2003.

Author conversations with Sowles, Dick, Freitag, and Sims;Vanport residents, 2004.

The Oregonian. May 24 1998.

Perkins J. Jane Powell. Life Magazine 1946 Sep 9-Oct 12:p98.

Goodwin, Doris Kearns. No ordinary time: Franklin and Eleanor Roosevelt. New York: Simon and Schuster; 1994.

Author interview with James DeLong, June 2002.

Gersbach interview with James DeLong. KPNW Archives; 1985.

The Columbian. August 11, 2003.

Author interview with Clementine Thomas, Edgar Kaiser wartime secretary; May 2004.

Daily Shipping News. September 4, 1992.

A forgotten revolution in child care. Oregon Times Magazine 1976 Feb-Mar.

Zinsser, Caroline. The best day care there ever was. Working Mother 1984 Oct.

O'Brien EG. Pepper hearings on medical manpower. J Am Med Assoc 1942;120(17:1414.

Vancouver health care expands. Bo's'n's Whistle 1943 June 17.

Author conversation with Vivian Terral RN, 2003.

Gersbach interview with Vivian Terral, RN, April 9, 1993. KPNW Archives.

Author interview with Leora Baldwin Roche, April 2003.

Author interview with Jaimie Noehren, December 2004.

Author interview with Charles Grossman, July 2002.

Grossman CM. The first use of penicillin in the United States. Ann Intern Med 2008 Jun 14;149(2):135-6.

Tager M. John F Fulton, coccidioidomycosis, and penicillin. Yale J Biol Med 1976 Sep;49(4):391-8.

Neighbor recruitment letter to Charles Grossman, August 7, 1944.

The Oregonian. February 11, 1944.

Janisse T. A voice of Permanente. Perm J 1997 Summer;1(1):2.

Brinkley, Douglas. Wheels for the world. New York: Penguin Books; 2003.

Author communications with Charles Grossman, 2003.

CHAPTER 3: HARD TIMES 1945-1950

Minutes of The Permanente Clinic partnership meetings, 1949-1950.

Memo to author from Norman Frink, 1986.

Smillie interview with Ernest Saward, June 1982.

Ernest Saward: An oral history of KP medical care. Vol. XV. Berkeley, CA: Bancroft Library; 1986.

Author conversation with Ernest Saward, 1962.

Lewis Weeks interview with Sidney Garfield. Hospital Administration Oral History Collection: Lewis E Weeks Series. American Hospital Association; 1986.

Annual report of The Northern Permanente Foundation, December 12, 1947.

Letter from Bernice Oswald to Charles Grossman, March 7, 1949.

Letter from Ernest Saward to Charles Grossman, April 14, 1949.

Letter from Charles Grossman to Ernest Saward, Sept 16, 1949.

Legal opinion re Grossman status, Thelan, Martin, Johnson and Bridges, May 24, 1948.

Articles of Partnership of The Doctors Clinic, January 14, 1949.

Balance sheet, The Doctors Clinic, September 30, 1950.

Author interview with Virginia Malbin, January 2005.

Author interview with Charlotte Cohen, August 2002.

Author interview with Frank Mossman, June 2003.

Maben, Manley. Vanport. Portland, OR: Oregon History Society Press; 1987.

Flood of change: The 1948 Vanport flood. The Sunday Oregonian 1998 May 24; Special section.

Author interview with Norman Malbin, June 2006.

Telegram from Edgar Kaiser to Rex Hamby, May 27 1950.

Garfield note to Charles Grossman, July 1950.

CHAPTER 4: THE FIFTIES: FIRM FOUNDATION

Smillie, John G. The story of the Permanente Medical Group. Oakland, CA: The Permanente Federation; 1996.

Garfield, SR. A report on Permanente's first ten years. Permanente Foundation Medical Bulletin 1952;X(1-4):1.

The Permanente Plan's First Ten Years. N Engl J Med 1952 Oct 30;247(18):692-3 .

Starr, Paul. The social transformation of American medicine. New York: Basic Books; 1982.

Gross Mark L. The doctors. New York: Random House; 1966.

deKruif, Paul. Kaiser wakes the doctors. London: Jonathan Cape; 1946.

Supermarket medicine. The Saturday Evening Post 1953 Jun 20:22-3,46-8.

The Larson report. JAMA Special Edition 1959 January 17.

Prepaid medical care: nation's biggest private plan. Time Magazine 1962 Sept 14:60-1.

Communication from Morris Collen, September 2, 2005.

Solemn rites dedicate Bess Kaiser Hospital. The Oregonian, July 8, 1959.

Author interview with Laurence Duckler, March 2004.

Happy Birthday Bess Kaiser Medical Center. The Pulse 1979 Jul;8(7).

Author interview with Noah Krall, March 2004.

CHAPTER 5: VIENNA, VLADIVOSTOK AND VANCOUVER: THE NORBERT FELL STORY

Gersbach interview with Norbert Fell, September 1990. KPNW Archives.

Communication with Ekhard Ursin, re: experience with the Duke of Hohenberg in the spring of 1958, October 12, 1996.

Communication with Ekhard Ursin, re: tribute to a beloved physician: Norbert Fell, 2003.

Ursin interviews with Connie Saunders, RN, and Margaret Frederickson, RN, September 1990.

Palmer, Alan. Twilight of the Hapsburgs. New York: Atlantic Monthly Press; 1994.

Gunther, John. Inside Europe. New York: Harper and Bros; 1936.

Bukey, Evan Burr. Hitler's Austria. Chapel Hill, NC: University of North Carolina Press; 2000.

Author interview with Alyce Fell Rene, February 2006.

CHAPTER 6: PARIAHS AND PRESIDENTS

Starr, Paul. The social transformation of American medicine. New York: Basic Books; 1982.

Gross, Mark L. The doctors. New York: Random House; 1966.

Gilford, Steve. Time line of KP history; 2002.

deKruif, Paul. Kaiser wakes the doctors. London: Jonathan Cape; 1946.

Through the eye of a man who has been here twenty years: Paul Trautman, 1980. KPNW Archives.

Author interview with Paul Trautman, November 2005.

Author interview with Ernest Aebi, November 2005.

Author interview with Maurice Comeau, October 2005.

Author interview with Colin Cave, April 2006.

Author interview with David Watt, June 2006.

CHAPTER 7: ISLAND PARADISE

Smillie, John G. The story of the Permanente Medical Group. Oakland, CA: The Permanente Federation; 1996.

Friedman, Emily. The aloha way: health care structure and finance in Hawaii. Hawaii Medical Service Foundation; 1993.

John Smillie interview with Ernest Saward, June 1982.

Author interview with James DeLong, June 2002.

Author interview with T. K. Lin, May 2006.

Author interview with Norah Walker, Executive Secretary to Regional Manager, June 2006.

Author interview with Sumie Kroyden, RN, June 2006.

Author interview with Noah Krall, March 2004.

Author interview with Arnold Hurtado, June 2004.

Author interview with Ekhard Ursin, January 2004.

Hawaii Permanente Medical Group: In the beginning 1957-1963 [video]. Mike Bacon Productions.

Kaiser Kommentary Hawaii Region Medical Staff 1971;4(1).

Series. Honolulu Star-Bulletin 1958 May 22, Sept 25, Oct 13, Oct 24; 1960 Aug 22 - 1960 Sept 1.

Series: Pacific Medical Associates conflict with Henry J. Kaiser. Honolulu Star Bulletin 1966 Dec15; 1967 May 23.

Series: Pacific Medical Associates conflict with Henry J. Kaiser. Honolulu Advertiser 1967 Sept 20; 1968 April 15, Dec 15.

PART IV: SPECIALTIES
CHAPTER 8: THE ER AND THE OR

Your first aid. The Pulse 1943 Dec 1;2(1). Portland, OR: The Northern Permanente Foundation.

Heads lab. The Pulse 1944 Mar 14;2(7). Portland, OR: The Northern Permanente Foundation.

One cast deluxe. The Pulse 1944 Jun 1;2(11). Portland, OR: The Northern Permanente Foundation.

EKG studies as diagnostic procedure. The Pulse 1944 Oct 1;6. Portland, OR: The Northern Permanente Foundation.

Smillie, John G. The story of the Permanente Medical Group. Oakland, CA: The Permanente Federation; 1996.

Flint, Thomas. Emergency treatment and management. Philadelphia, PA: Saunders & Co; 1965.

Albert Martin interview with Lawrence Duckler, March 2004.

Albert Martin interview with Ekhard Ursin, April 2003.

Albert Martin interview with Paul Trautman, April 2003.

Albert Martin interview with Dean Barnhouse, July 2003.

Albert Martin interview with Sigrid Chambers, RN, March 2004.

Albert Martin interview with Peg Pemberton, ERT, March 2004.

Meet an employee. The Pulse 1977 Nov;6(3).

Albert Martin interview with Michael Hoevet, September 2003.

Albert Martin interview with Ronald Potts, August 2003.

Albert Martin interview with Josephine Colbach, July 2003.

Author interview with David Hale, August 2003.

Author interview with Dean Barnhouse, November 2003.

Author interview with Tom Ruedd.

Hamacinski J. Emergency room violence growing concern. Massachusetts Nurse 2005 April.

Postgraduate Medicine 1994 June; 105.

Author interview with Norman Frink Jr, April 2005.

Author interview with Robert McFarlane, November 2006.

Author interview with George Chang, January 2007.

Author interview with Edward Stark, May 2006.

Author interview with David Long, July 2006.

Author interview with George Adlhoch, December 2005.

www.carrietingleyhospitalfoundation.org [Web page on the Internet]. Albuquerque, NM: Carrie Tingley Hospital Foundation; [cited 2010 Mar 10]. Available from: http://www.carrietingleyhospitalfoundation.org/.

Hunsberger B. Community activist Josiah Hill dies at age 61. The Oregonian 2000 Oct 17;C14.

Author interview with Joseph Neary, DPM, October 2007.

Author interview with Mian Tahir, September 2006.

Author interview with Jane Stradley Jones, RN, NP.

Author interview with Herohisho Ono, October 2006.

Author interview with Harold Paxton, December 2006.

Communication with Michael Weinstein, November 2006.

Nesbitt RM. A history of prostate transurethral resection. Rev Mex Urol 1975;35:349-62.

Author interview with Luis Halpert, December 2003.

Author interview with Thomas Carrie, June 2006.

Author interview with Stephen Lieberman, August 2006.

Author interview with Matti Totonchy, August 2006.

Author interview with Ferenc Gabor, September 2006.

Huggins C, Hodges CV. Studies on prostate cancer I. Cancer Res 1941;1:293-7.

Author interview with Lee Baldwin Roche, April 2003.

Klein, Roger; Kendrick, Angela. The history of anesthesia in Oregon. Portland, OR: Oregon Trail Publishing Co; 2004.

Author interview with Rex Underwood, May 2004.

Nuland, Sherwin B. Doctors: The biography of medicine. New York: Vintage Books; 1995.

CHAPTER 9: PEDIATRICIANS, OBSTETRICIANS AND QUINTS

Van Leeuwen, K. The Permanente health plan. J Pediatr 1946 Nov;29(5):667-3.

"Mac" heights keeps busy. The Pulse 1943 Dec 3;11(1).

Author interview with Charles Grossman, July 2002.

Jean Bradley interview with Lannie Hurst, October 2003

Oshinsky, David M. Polio: An American story. New York: Oxford University Press; 2005.

Mikelova LK, Halperin SA, Scheifele D, Smith B, Ford-Jones E, Vaudry W, Jadavji T, Law B, Moore D; Members of the Immunization Monitoring Program, Active (IMPACT). Predictors of death in infants hospitalized with pertussis: a case-control study of 16 pertussis deaths in Canada. J Pediatr 2003 Nov;143(5):576-81.

Author interview with Fred Colwell, June 2004.

Jean Bradley interview with Jacqueline Varga, September 2003.

Pediatric history communication to Helena Purcell from Virginia Feldman, November 4, 1990.

Inside KPNW August 2003; December 2003.

Bo's'N's Whistle, June 17, 1943.

We like kids too. The Pulse 1944 Jan 1;2(4).

Penny saved is earned. The Pulse 1944 Sep 1;2(15).

Author interview with Fred Colwell, September 2004.

Author interview with Mark Butzer, October 2006.

Author interview with Raymond Blair, November 2006.

Author interview with Jody Klevit.

Author interview with Dallas Hovig.

Author interview with Gunnar Waage, May 2006.

Author interview with Philip Brenes, August 2006.

The Oregonian. September 28, 1973.

Author interview with Virginia Feldman, June 2008.

Author interview with Charlotte Cohen.

The Oregonian. July 14, 1977.

Gersbach interview with Harold Cohen. KPNW Archives.

Babies, laser and Liberty Ships. The Pulse 1990 May-June.

Harold Cohen retires. The Pulse 1993 Jan-Feb.

Author interview with Shelley Spielman.

Harold Cohen Memorial service comments, December 2004.

Northwest Permanente Executive Committee minutes, 1970-1979.

Author communication with Carolyn Stadter, CNM.

Author interview with Albert Vervloet.

Anderson, Karen; Robinson, Jo. Full House. New York: Little Brown and Co.; 1986.

CHAPTER 10: OPHTHALMOTO-RHINOLARYNGOLOGY

Socialist rule in Vienna said to hurt professions. The Oregonian April 10 1927.

Gersbach interview with Jack Hilbourne, OD, [video], 2003. KPNW Department of Public Affairs.

Author interview with Jack Hilbourne, OD, December 2006.

Author interview with Frank Mossman, March 2004.

Author interview with Charles Emerick, February 2005.

Author interview with William Harris, December 2006.

Author interview with Ernest Aebi, November 2005.

Albert Martin interview with Byron Fortsch, December 2004.

Author interview with Byron Fortsch, December 2006.

Author interview with Steve Van Hee, OD, December 2006.

Author interview with Leslie Chan, OD, July 2004.

Author interview David Campagna, OD, January 2007.

Green D. When optometrists strike. Optometric Management 1975 Sep.

Exhibit # 7 Northwest Permanente Board of Directors meeting January 21, 1978.

CHAPTER 11: PATHOLOGICAL NEEDS

Heads lab. The Pulse 1944 March 15;2(8).

Author interview with Charles Grossman.

Lehman letters to Ernest Saward, September 18, 1969; December 10, 1969.

The Oregonian. July 1, 1991.

Lab reports. The Pulse 1970 Feb;2(2).

Medical staff additions. The Pulse 1970 July;2(5).

Medical staff additions. The Pulse 1983 Dec.

Medical staff additions. The Pulse 1985 Feb.

Medical staff additions. The Pulse 1992 July.

Medical staff additions. The Pulse 1988 Dec.

Author interview with Gene Bogaty, January 2007.

Author interview with Dan Baer, January 2007.

Author interview with David Scott, March 2007.

Author interview with Katherine Holihan, January 2007.

Author interview with Neil Olson, January 2007.

Author interview with John Thompson, February 2007.

Author interview with Ronald Jones, January 2007.

Author interview with Lawrence Dworkin, February 2007.

Author interview with Jacob Reiss, February 2007.

Regional lab tackles array of testing jobs. The Pulse 1988 Nov-Dec.

The Pulse 1992 July-Aug.

CHAPTER 12: RADIOLOGY

Stevens R. The Pulse 1944 March 15;2(8).

CHAPTER 13: INTERNISTS AND THE EARLY MEDICAL SUBSPECIALISTS

Stevens R. Issues for American internal medicine through the last century. Ann Intern Med 1986 Oct;105(4):592-602.

Lemley BR. The American College of Physicians: the first 75 years. Ann Intern Med 1990 Jun 1;112(11):872-8.

EKG studies as diagnostic procedure. The Pulse 1944 Oct;2(16).

Author interview with John Wild, October 2004.

Author interview with John Grover, February 2005.

Coronary care unit. The Pulse 1969 Feb;2(1).

Communication with Phillip Au, November 2007.

Author interview with Arnold Hurtado, November 2004.

Author interview with Norman Birndorf, April 2006.

Author interview with Eric Liberman, November 2005.

Author interview with Harold Nevis, March 2006.

Author interview with Harry Glauber, March 2007.

Author interview with Claudio Lima, PA, April 2007.

Communication with Roderick Hooker, PhD, PA, March 2008.

Author interview with Vincent Chiu, February 2006.

Author interview with Henrik Porter, July 2006.

Medical staff additions. The Pulse 1970 July;2(5).

Author interview with Charles Zerzan, November 2007.

Author interview with Eberhard Gloekler, February 2007.

Foa R. Back from Cape Cod: reflections on choosing to return to practice. Neurology Today 2004 Jul;4(7):4,7.

Author interview with Jerry Slepack, May 2006.

Author interview with Jan Collins, April 2007.

Author interview with Marvin Harner, November 2006.

Planning For Health 1984;2.

Author interview with John Solters, June 2007.

Author interview with Susan Kauffman, August 2007.

Tobin MJ. Pulmonary and critical care medicine a peculiar American hybrid. Thorax 1999 Apr;54(4):286-7. Erratum in: Thorax 1999 Jun;54(6):564.

Author interview with Robert Richardson, June 2007.

Author interview with Albert Vervloet, March 2006.

Author interview with Manny Karlin, December 2007.

Author interview with Tom Lorence, November 2007.

Wachter RM, Goldman L. The emerging role of "hospitalists" in the American health care system. N Engl J Med 1996 Aug 15;335(7):514-7.

Brandner J. Will hospital rounds go the way of the house call? Manag Care 1995 Jul;4(7):19-21;25-8.

Caplan WM. The hospital-based specialist program. Perm J 1997 Fall;1(2):37-40.

Freese RB. The Park Nicollet experience in establishing a hospitalist system. Ann Intern Med 1999 Feb 16;130(4 Pt 2):350-4.

Craig DE, Hartka L, Likosky WH, Caplan WM, Litsky P, Smithey J. Implementation of a hospitalist system in a large health maintenance organization: the Kaiser Permanente experience. Ann Intern Med 1999 Feb 16;130(4 Pt 2):355-9.

Some internists bid farewell to rounds. Internal Medicine News 1995 Mar 1.

Moore JD Jr. The inpatient's best friend. 'Hospitalists' specialize in managing care of the very ill. Mod Healthc 1997 Feb 3;27(5):54-6,58-62.

CHAPTER 14: SPECIALTIES OLD AND NEW

Author conversations with Charles Grossman, 2008.

Author interview with Paul Contorer, November 2006.

Author interview with Richard Romaine, January 2007.

Author interview with Angelito Saqueton, March 2007.

Author interview with Clark Sisk, July 2007.

Author interview with Marge Patera, June 2007.

Author interview with Mary Lyons, January 2008.

Author interview with Laurence Duckler.

Industrial medicine market perspective report to Northwest Permanente Board, November 11, 1986.

Industrial medicine report to Northwest Permanente Board, February 19,1987.

Industrial medicine proposal to Northwest Permanente Board, April, 1989.

Industrial Medicine Task Force report to Northwest Permanente Board, February 21, 1991.

Author interview with David Nelson.

Author interview with Ezra Rabie.

Author interview with Donald Tilson.

Author interview with Adrianne Feldstein.

Author interview with Curtis Thiessen.

Author interview with Mary Wilson Rock.

Communication from Joseph Davis, May 20, 2007.

Communication from Allan Weiland, August 22, 2007.

Oregon Workers Compensation Division M.C.O. list August 3, 2007.

Feldstein, A. Kaiser Works, Inc.: a new way to transfer best practices in occupational health. Perm J 1998 Fall;2(4):76-9.

Author interview with Andrew Glass, October 2007.

Author interview with David Tilford, November 2007.

Author interview with Marge Patera, October 2007.

Communication from Thomas Leimert, November 2007.

Author interview with Ruth Bach, December 2007.

KPNW Cancer Education Center Bulletin 1977 March 10.

Henderson, J. Counseling helps breast cancer patients regain control. Prowoman Magazine 1990 Oct-Nov:36-8.

Spiegel D, Bloom JR, Kraemer HC, Gottheil E. Effect of psychosocial treatment on survival of patients with metastatic breast cancer. Lancet 1989 Oct 14;2(8668):888-91.

Goodwin PJ, Leszcz M, Ennis M, et al. The effect of group psychosocial support on survival in metastatic breast cancer. N Engl J Med 2001 Dec 13;345(24):1719-26.

CHAPTER 15: PSYCHIATRY AND PHYSIATRY: HEALING THE MIND AND THE BODY

Starr, Paul. The social transformation of American medicine. New York: Basic Books; 1982.

LeFannu, James. The rise and fall of modern medicine. Hoboken, NJ: Carroll & Graf Publishers; 1999.

Kay, Raymond. Historical review of the Southern California Permanente Medical Group; 1979.

Shorter, Edward. A history of psychiatry: from asylum to prozac. New York: John Wiley and Sons; 1997.

Hurtado A, Greenlick M, Saward E. Health Services Monogram series: Home care and extended care in a comprehensive prepayment plan. Chicago, IL: Hospital Research and Educational Trust; 1972.

Author interview with Eugene Nordstrum, PhD, May 2006.

Author interview with Jean Monahan, MC, May 2006.

Author interview with Allan Fuller, PhD, May 2006.

Author interview with Dennis Florendo, MSW, May 2006.

Author interview with Herb Biskar, PhD, June 2006.

Author interview with Robert Senft, July 2006.

Author interview with Donald Lange, PhD, July 2006.

Author interview with Stanley Abrams, PhD, August 2006.

Author interview with Judi Brenes, RN, MS, September 2006.

Author interview with Ona Allan, RN, September 2006.

Author interview with Ray Noel, October 2006.

Author interview with Kitty Evers, December 2006.

Author interview with Stuart Oken, December 2006.

Author interview with Lauretta Young, January 2007.

Robert Senft memo to Robert Miller, January 7, 1991.

Glenda Hall memo to Robert Miller, December 19, 1990.

Medical staff additions. The Pulse 1971;3(7).

Making the rounds. The Pulse 1944 April 1;2(9).

Smillie, John G. The story of the Permanente Medical Group. Oakland, CA: The Permanente Federation; 1996.

Gilford, Steve. On This Day in KP History #206.

The history of physiatry [monograph on the Internet]. Hawaii: Physiatry and Rehabilitations Services, LLP; 1999 [cited 2010 Mar 10]. Available from: www.rehabmedicine. org/FAQs/History/history.html.

Author interview with John Gerhardt, August 2006.

Author interview with Kadavil Satyanarayan, September 2006.

Author interview with Paul Jacobs, October 2006.

PART V: ADDITIONAL PERMANENTE PERSUASIONS
CHAPTER 16: SOCIAL CONSCIENCE OF PERMANENTE HEALTH CARE
by Kitty Evers, MD

Smillie, John G. The story of the Permanente Medical Group. Oakland, CA: The Permanente Federation; 1996.

Foster Mark S. Henry J. Kaiser: builder in the modern American West. Austin, TX: University of Texas Press; 1989.

Interview with Becky Kaiser, July 2005

Jobs for disabled. The Call Bulletin, An Independent Newspaper. San Francisco, CA 1944 Jun 1;p1.

Stories told at the U.S. Department of Defense WW II 60th Commemoration Anniversary, August 27, 2005; Vancouver, Washington.

Kesselman, Amy. Fleeting opportunities: women shipyard workers in Portland and Vancouver during World War II and reconversion. Albany, NY: State Univeristy of Albany; 1990.

Burrow GN, Burgess NL. The evolution of women as physicians and surgeons. Ann Thorac Surg 2001 Feb;71(2 Suppl):S27-9.

Evers interview with Sharon Higgins, August 2008.

Group Profile report to Northwest Permanente Board of Directors meeting March 20, 2008.

Saward, Ernest. An oral history of Kaiser Permanente medical care, Vol. XV. Berkeley, CA: Bancroft Library; 1985.

Author interview with Merwyn Greenlick, May 12, 2004.

Weeks interview with Merwyn Greenlick, June 1988.

Oregon Labor Press. August 9, 1968.

Suffian, Sandy. Doctorate Thesis: The historical emergence of social mission in nonprofit HMO's. 2006.

Greenlick, Merwin R; Freeborn, Donald K; Pope, Clyde R, editors. Health care research in an HMO: two decades of discovery. Baltimore, MD: Johns Hopkins University Press; 1988.

Evers interview with Carol Polanski, August 2008.

Evers interview with Marci Clark, September 2008.

Evers interview with Jerry Slepack, September 2008.

Keaveney B. Healthcare's quiet tragedy. Physician Practice 2008 July/Aug.

Senft RA, Evers K, Savery RJ. Outreach to physicians with problems: a four-year experience. Perm J 1999 Winter;3(1):39-43.

Gilford S. The rediscovery of Contractors General Hospital—birthplace of Kaiser Permanente. Perm J 2006;10(2):57-60.

PART VI: AFTER THE SIXTIES
CHAPTER 17:
THE SEVENTIES

Smillie interview with Ernest Saward, 1982.

Department of Surgery letter to the Executive Committee of The Permanente Clinic, April 12, 1973.

Department of Obstetrics business meeting minutes, August 28, 1974.

KPNW Cost Effectiveness Task Force report, March 20, 1975.

Spectrum. Fall 1989.

Kay, Raymond M. Historical review of the SCPMG. Los Angeles, CA: Southern California Permanente Medical Group; 1979.

Fleming, Scott. Evaluation of the KP medical care program: historical perspective. May 15, 1985.

Smillie, John G. The story of the Permanente Medical Group. Oakland, CA: The Permanente Federation; 1996.

The Permanente Clinic Executive Committee minutes, 1970-1978.

Author interview with Albert Vervloet, July 2006.

Author interview with Fred Nomura, November 2007.

Correspondence re: Professional Corporation Miles Ormseth of Davis, Biggs, Strayer, Stoel, and Boley, September 11, 1970.

Nomura, Fred. Report on pros and cons of incorporation versus remaining a partnership. 1975 July 20.

Correspondence re: incorporation Douglas Thompson of Souther, Spaulding, Kinsey, Williamson, and Schwabe, 1977.

Hudson, Leonard; Spence, William. Report on Pulmonary Function Laboratory. 1975 Feb 21.

Author interview with Ken Myers,
January 2007.

Portland Physician May 197

Kaiser proposes hospital. The Oregon Journal
1970 Feb 28.

Medical center need outlined at hearing.
The Oregon Journal 1972 April 12.

Proposed Kaiser hospital: evaluation due
in July. Enterprise Courier 1972 June
8;106(113).

Review petition filed on hospital proposal.
The Oregonian 1972 Oct 4.

Decision on hospital postponed.
The Oregonian 1972 Nov 18.

Hayward interview with Marvin Goldberg,
Oct 2003.

Author conversation with Marvin Goldberg,
May 1976.

Author communication with Marvin
Goldberg, August 10, 2005.

Region news: Packwood. The Pulse; 1987
Nov-Dec.

Allen, Terry Ann. Southern California Permanente Medical Group: The first 50 years.

Author interview with Gregory Swift,
February 2007.

Group Health, Seattle Family Practice on-site
visit Ekhard Ursin, January 29, 1970.

Family Practice Program report; John Emery,
March 19, 1974.

Family Practice Committee report; John
Emery, November 3, 1975.

The Permanente Clinic Executive Committee
minutes, April 1, 1977.

Bess Kaiser Area Statement on Family
Practice; Perry Sloop, May 4, 1977.

Northwest Permanente Board of Directors
meeting minutes, May 16,1980.

The changing PA. The Pulse1986;1:10.

Hooker, Roderick S; Cawley, James F.
Physician assistants in American medicine.
St. Louis, MO: Churchill Livingstone; 2003.

PAs at KP: 20 years. The Pulse 1990
Nov-Dec.

Report to the NWP Board of Directors on
Allied Health Issues; Fred Nomura, January
24, 1989; February 25, 1989.

Healthgram Kaiser Foundation Health Plan,
1976 Spring.

Healthgram Kaiser Foundation Health Plan,
1976 Winter.

CHAPTER 18:
THE EIGHTIES:
NEW DIRECTIONS

Author interview with Gregory Swift,
February 2007.

Author communication with Gregory Swift,
March 22, 2007.

Author interview with Carlos Giralt, PA,
June 2007.

Author interview with David Moiel,
July 2007.

Author interview with Edward Arinello,
August 2007.

Author interview with William De'ak,
September 2007.

Author communication with William De'ak,
October 10, 2007.

Longview Daily News, 1984 June 26.

Author interview with Raymond Dockery,
December 2007.

Author interview with William Nelson, December 2006.

Author communication with Joseph Davis, May 21, 2007.

Author interview with Thomas Syltebo, February 2007.

Author interview with Scott Feuer, February 2007.

Author interview with Nicholas DeMorgan, January 2007.

Author interview with Jon Blackman, June 2007.

Author interview with William Nyone, February 2008.

Glickstein D. Group Health Cooperative of Puget Sound—A short history. Perm J 1998 Spring;2(2):60-1.

Crowley Walt. To serve the greatest number. Seattle, WA: University of Washington Press; 1996.

Inside dope on x-rays. The Pulse 1944 April;2(10).

Author interview with Henry Kavitt. April 2002.

Gorsbach film with Henry Kavitt [video], 2002. KPNW Public Affairs Department.

O'Boyle, Bobby. From x-ray to imaging services. Portland, OR: KPNW Printing and Graphics; 1999.

Author interview with Ben Brown, February 2007.

Author interview with Darlene Fortuny, RN, March 2007.

Author interview with Robert Lawrence, March 2007.

Author interview with Michael Noonan, April 2007.

Author interview with Chuo Chang, April 2007.

Author interview with Keith Riley, April 2007.

www.finegold.org [home page on the Internet]. Rocky Pointe, NY: Finegold Association of the United States; updated 1/20/10 [cited 2010 Mar 10]. Available from: www.finegold.org.

Kaiser Permanente Planning For Health. 1988 Spring.

Regionalization of Ob/Neonatal Services: an outline of issues. Exhibit #3. Northwest Permanente Board of Directors meeting January 15 1987.

Hayward interview with David Lawrence, November 2003.

Northwest Permanente Board of Directors meeting minutes, April 19,1985.

Blomquist letter to Maurice Comeau, Chairman of Compensation Committee, April 23, 1985.

Northwest Permanente Compensation Committee meeting minutes, May 6, 1985.

Northwest Permanente Board of Directors meeting minutes, May 14, 1985.

Author interview with Fred Nomura, October 2007.

Author interview with Ronald Potts, October 2007.

The Columbian. July 7, 1988.

The Columbian. July 8, 1988.

Weiland, Allan. The nurse strike of 1988. 2007.

Summer strike, record growth headline: 1988 events. The Pulse 1989 Spring [Special edition].

Nomura memo to NWP Board March 11, 1989

Schecter P. History of the Oregon Nurses Association: The labor of caring. Oregon Historical Quarterly 2007 Spring;14,16,18-19,24-29.

Robins, George. History of the Multnomah County Medical Society: 1884-1954. Portland, OR: Multnomah County Medical Society;1990.

Cleland, John GP. The history of medical care in Clackamas County. Oregon City, OR: Clackamas County Medical Society; 1976.

Cleland John GP. Essentials of an industrial health program. NW Medicine 1956 Sep;44:973-4.

Author interview with Janet Hochstatter, June 2006.

Author interview with John Cleland, July 2006.

Author interview with Paul Bowen, August 2006.

Collins C. Good Sam, HealthLink consider merger. Portland Physician Scribe 1988 Mar 7;4(5).

Davis B. PACC taps Klevit to head medical affairs. Portland Physician Scribe 1995 Mar 17;7(6).

PACC physician members OK sale to FHS: merge with Qual Med. Portland Physician Scribe 1997 Jun;15(11).

Collins C. Shake up at Qual Med. Portland Physician Scribe 1998 Aug 21;16(16).

CHAPTER 19: THE NINETIES
by Allan J. Weiland, MD

AFTERWORD: WHAT HAPPENED TO THE PIONEERS?

Author interview with Elizabeth Gallagher Saward, April 2003.

Smillie, John G. The story of the Permanente Medical Group. Oakland, CA: The Permanente Federation; 1996.

Kneeland, Donald. An oral history: Interview with David W. Stewart. Rochester, NY: Blue Cross/Blue Shield of the Rochester Area; 1987.

Comments from Joseph Dolittle, Rochester health care executive, July 2008.

Telegram to Ernest Saward (invitation to attend signing of Medicare Bill) from Laurence O'Brien, Assistant to the President, July 29,1965.

Saward, Ernest. Statement of Kaiser Medical Care Program before the Senate Committee on Government Operations, July 11, 1968.

Saward E. Health Care Crisis, The University and Society Rochester Medical Review 1970 Fall;3(2).

Saward E. Physician Education in the Peoples Republic of China. Connecticut Medicine 1976 Jan;39(1).

National health insurance and the internist (comments from Ernest Saward). The Internist 1975 Jun:10-11.

Saward Ernest; Axelrod, Solomon; Sigmond, Robert. Report of the Health Education and Welfare Task Force on Appalachian Regional Hospitals to Joseph Califano, Jr. September 15, 1977.

Letter to Ernest Saward from Edward M Kennedy, Chairman, Senate Subcommittee On Health and Scientific Research, May 14, 1979.

PERMANENTE IN THE NORTHWEST

Saward EW, Gallagher EK. Reflections on change in medical practice. The current trend to large-scale medical organizations. JAMA 1983 Nov 25;250(20):2829-5.

Maritato, Anna Maria. Saward Eulogy, Interfaith Chapel, University of Rochester. September 7, 1989.

Author interview with Jaimie Noehren, April 2005.

Author conversations with Charles Grossman, 2006.

Grossman Charles M, editor. Evans Carlson's legacy of friendship: 30 years of the Evans F Carlson Friends of the People's Republic of China. Portland, OR: Evans F. Carlson Friends of the People's Republic of China; 2005.

Author correspondence from Norman Frink, Sr, 1984-1987.

Northwest Permanente Retirement seminar, 1982.

Communication with Norman Frink, Jr, November 23, 2004.

The Oregonian. April 21, 1991.

Author interview with Alyce Fell Rene, February 2006.

Author interview with Norman Malbin, June 2006.

Conversation with Charlotte Cohen, May 25, 2007.

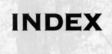

INDEX

INDEX